'This thought-provoking and rich edited volume explores the concepts of violence, care and cure as part of the growing interdisciplinary scholarship on the medical encounter. Contributions by leading and emerging scholars from an impressive range of disciplines engage the reader in historical, practical, philosophical and creative reflections that open up new dimensions of research across the fields of medicine and humanities. An eye-opening read for scholars and professionals interested in new and self-reflective approaches to the study and practice of medicine through the humanities and *vice versa*'.

**Heike Bartel**, *Professor of German Studies and Health Humanities, The University of Nottingham, UK*

'In healthcare and medicine, efforts to care and cure are entangled with violence in complex ways. The contributions in this book highlight the potential of medical humanities to uncover systemic biases and broaden our understanding of medical encounters. The volume is an essential contribution to scholarship, opening new avenues for research and reflection'.

**Anna Ovaska**, *Research Fellow in Narrative Studies, Tampere University, Finland*

# Violence, Care, Cure

This book explores the notions of violence, care, and cure within the medical encounter and seeks to foreground the ways in which, whether individually or as a triad, they are prone to ambiguous interpretations. The chapters of this book attend to the complex interlacing of these three key terms and what to make of their entanglement by offering historical, practical, philosophical, personal, and aesthetic analyses of different medical scenes, objects, and concepts.

Besides the three main concepts that give the collection its title, the volume deals with bodily experience, medical neglect or scepticism, pain and suffering, diagnosis and recovery, and epistemic injustice, through the lens of, among others, biopolitics, ethics, gender medicine, and critical medical humanities. Altogether, the chapters pay particular attention to the role of images and other narratives, including social media platforms. The case studies in this collection invite the reader to observe medical encounters that take place in and are shaped by a variety of both material and 'immaterial' spaces, from the consulting room to the antechamber of medical bureaucracy, and from artistic venues to biopolitical discourses. Taken together, this book argues that a hermeneutic of violence, care, and cure is inseparable from individual and collective perceptions of the medical encounter; that is, it is inextricable from an understanding of the tensions and consensus that surge among perceptions orchestrated by both internal (subjective) and external (social, cultural, political) 'gazes'. Moreover, the volume aims to provide, both directly and indirectly, a meta-reflection on the disciplines that fall under the umbrella of 'medical and health humanities', interrogating the field's potential to unearth systemic bias, to open different possibilities of existence, and to make visible the complexity of its research objects, as well as to caution against their possible pitfalls.

By bringing together different methodological approaches, this volume provides its readers with conceptual resources for thinking about the intersections of violence, care, and cure. By providing a space where the voices of both emerging and established scholars mingle and respond to one another, this book will be essential reading for anyone across the social sciences and humanities interested in the sociology of health and medicine, the medical humanities, and gender studies.

**Marta-Laura Cenedese** is UKRI (MSCA Horizon Guarantee) Postdoctoral Fellow at the Institute for Medical Humanities at Durham University. Marta is a literary scholar specialising in postcolonial literatures, memory studies, critical medical humanities, queer death studies, and decolonial feminism. She is the author of *Irène Némirovsky's Russian Influences: Tolstoy, Dostoevsky and Chekhov* (2021) and editor of *Written on the Body: Narrative (Re)constructions of Violence(s)* (2023). Her research has been published in *Comparative Literature, Storyworlds, Journal of Medical Humanities, Modern and Contemporary France*, and elsewhere. Marta was an associated researcher at the Centre Marc Bloch Berlin (2020–2024) and has been a visiting fellow at the Dahlem Humanities Center, Humboldt University Berlin (2020) and at the Centre d'Histoire, Sciences-Po Paris (2023).

**Clio Nicastro** is a researcher in Philosophy, Cultural Studies, and Film Studies affiliated with Bard College Berlin. She studied philosophy at the University of Palermo, where she completed her PhD in Aesthetics and Theory of Arts. She was DAAD postdoctoral fellow as well as fellow at the ICI Berlin Institute for Cultural Inquiry, where she held an additional one-year postdoctoral position research thanks to a VolkswagenStiftung grant. She is the author of *La Dialettica del Denkraum in Aby Warburg* (2022) as well as the co-editor with Cristina Baldacci and Arianna Sforzini of the volume *Over and Over and Over again. Reenactment Strategies in Contemporary Arts and Theory* (2022). She is a member of the board of directors of the Harun Farocki Institut.

## Routledge Research in Gender and Society

**Masculinity in Lesbian "Pulp" Fiction**
Disappearing Heteronormativity?
*Paul Thompson*

**Exploring Autistic Sexualities, Relationality, and Genders**
Living Under a Double Rainbow
*Edited by Hanna Bertilsdotter Rosqvist, Anna Day, and Meaghan Krazinski*

**Gender Fields**
The Social Organisation of Gender Identity
*Sofia Aboim and Pedro Vasconcelos*

**Overcoming Objectification**
A Carnal Ethics
*Ann J. Cahill*

**Mapping Queerness in Times of Uncertainty**
Stories of Struggle, Invisibility and Space
*Arnaud Kurze, Sarah Sturken and Steve The*

**Intimate Partner Femicide**
Contesting the Legal Story
*Bethany Wilkinson with Susan Goodwin*

**Violence, Care, Cure**
Self/perceptions within the Medical Encounter
*Edited by Marta-Laura Cenedese and Clio Nicastro*

For more information about this series, please visit: https://www.routledge.com/Routledge-Research-in-Gender-and-Society/book-series/SE0271

# Violence, Care, Cure

## Self/perceptions within the Medical Encounter

**Edited by**
**Marta-Laura Cenedese and Clio Nicastro**

Routledge
Taylor & Francis Group
LONDON AND NEW YORK

First published 2025
by Routledge
4 Park Square, Milton Park, Abingdon, Oxon OX14 4RN

and by Routledge
605 Third Avenue, New York, NY 10158

*Routledge is an imprint of the Taylor & Francis Group, an informa business*



*British Library Cataloguing-in-Publication Data*
A catalogue record for this book is available from the British Library

ISBN: 9781032660141 (hbk)
ISBN: 9781032660158 (pbk)
ISBN: 9781032660165 (ebk)

DOI: 10.4324/9781032660165

Typeset in Times New Roman
by codeMantra

# Contents

*List of figures* *xiii*
*List of contributors* *xv*
*Acknowledgements* *xix*

**Introduction: Violence, care, cure: (Self-)perceptions within the medical encounter** 1
MARTA-LAURA CENEDESE AND CLIO NICASTRO

**Musing 1: Narrative medicine, racial justice, and the Black maternal mortality crisis** 17
MITA BANERJEE

**PART 1**
**Medical histories and biopolitics** 25

1 **Touching matters of care: A visual approach to care and violence in Dr Marie Stopes' birth control campaign** 27
NORA HEIDORN

2 **Politics in the time of cholera: COVID, table manners, and bio-politics** 47
FEDERICO DAL BO

3 **Bio-story: Michel Foucault and the history of social medicine** 61
XENIA CHIARAMONTE

**Musing 2: Counteracting psychiatric violence through critical heritage studies and cooperation** 74
ELISABETH PUNZI, HELEN JOHANSSON AND ANNICA ENGSTRÖM

PART 2
Unsettling and working through practices and languages of cure 79

4 The 'interpretation workshop' as artistic research: A methodological approach to original biographical national socialist writings 81
LENA DITTE NISSEN

5 'The way out is via the door': R.D. Laing and the cure from the family 97
JANINA KLEMENT

6 'Io sono matta': Psychiatric violence, militant madness, and sexual difference in Alberto Grifi's 'anthropology of disobedience' 113
SOPHIA ROHWETTER

7 The denied poetics of global psychiatry and Frantz Fanon's poetisation of science 132
LISA SCHMIDT-HERZOG

Musing 3: Fanon, epistemic injustice, and the colonial medical encounter 144
DANIELE LORENZINI

PART 3
Agency in illness and ethics of suffering 149

8 Narrative autonomy to the test of illness 151
SILVIA PIEROSARA

9 Plumbing the perpetual loss of paradise: Susan Taubes and sacred suffering 163
RACHEL PAFE

10 Almodóvar's anatomies 175
HANNAH PARLETT

Musing 4: On care and violence in medical humanities research collaborations 190
ANGELA WOODS

**PART 4**
**Anatomy of a transformation** 195

**11 T for trans: An outraged investigation of non-binary medical transition in Germany** 197
CLAUDE KEMPEN

**12 I am not my MRI** 210
MARIA MORATA

**13 Surprised by the night: On the traversal of a dysphoric phantasy** 218
MYRIAM SAUER

**14 Afterword: Moral value in medicine: Violence, cure, and care** 230
SANDER L. GILMAN

*Index* *247*

# Figures


| | | |
|---|---|---|
| 0.1 | Poster of the conference *Violence, Care, Cure*. Image credit © Claudia Peppel, 'Who's afraid of…?', paper collage, 2013 (detail), poster design: Studio BENS | 2 |
| 1.1 | 'Prorace' and 'Racial' brand cervical caps and condoms associated with Marie Stopes' Society for Constructive Birth Control (CBC) on display in the Medicine Galleries, Science Museum, London. Photograph by the author. | 28 |
| 1.2 | Nora Heidorn, research-collage, 2021 | 37 |
| 1.3 | Scan this QR code to enter *Touching Matters of Care ('Prorace' cervical cap, 1915–20)*, interactive digital object, 2022. It may take a few seconds to load | 39 |
| 1.4 | Still from Nora Heidorn, *Touching Matters of Care ('Prorace' cervical cap, 1915–20)*, digital object, 2022. Courtesy of Birth Rites Collection | 40 |
| 1.5 | Still from Nora Heidorn, *Touching Matters of Care ('Prorace' cervical cap, 1915–20)*, digital object, 2022. Courtesy of Birth Rites Collection | 41 |
| 1.6 | Latest price list of approved contraceptive appliances. Lamberts Prorace LTD, 1946. Accessed at Wellcome Library, London. Photograph by the author | 41 |
| 4.1 | First page of the memoir by Camilla Nissen. Image by the author | 84 |
| 4.2 | Circle of chairs for Interpretation Workshops at Künstlerhaus Büchsenhausen, 2020. Image by the author | 85 |
| 4.3 | Performance TAKE IT AS IT IS at Standortfriedhof Lilienthalstraße, Berlin, September 2020. Image by the author | 93 |
| 6.1 | Still from Alberto Grifi and Massimo Sarchielli, *Anna*, 1975. Courtesy Associazione culturale Alberto Grifi | 117 |
| 6.2 | Still from Alberto Grifi, *Lia*, 1977. Courtesy Associazione culturale Alberto Grifi, 00:16:01 | 120 |
| 6.3 | Still from Alberto Grifi, *Lia*, 1977. Courtesy Associazione culturale Alberto Grifi, 00:08:36 | 121 |

6.4 A close-up of the packaging of Normalina, the pharmaceutical product used by the psychiatric video-police to normalize deviant citizens. From Alberto Grifi, *Dinni e la Normalina, ovvero la videopolizia psichiatrica contro i sedicenti nuclei di follia militante*, 1978. Courtesy Associazione culturale Alberto Grifi 123
6.5 Still from Alberto Grifi, Dinni e la Normalina, ovvero la videopolizia psichiatrica contro i sedicenti nuclei di follia militante, 1978. Courtesy Associazione culturale Alberto Grifi 123
10.1 A still from *The Skin I Live In* (*La piel que habito*, dir. Pedro Almodóvar), Pathé 2011 179
10.2 'Anatomía': A still from *Pain and Glory* (*Dolor y gloria*, dir. Pedro Almodóvar), Sony Pictures 2019 185
12.1 Exhausting, still picture from video. Image credit © Daniele Lucchini 210
12.2 Three, still picture from video. Image credit © Daniele Lucchini 211
12.3 Beating, still picture from video. Image credit © Daniele Lucchini 212
12.4 Fearful, still picture from video. Image credit © Daniele Lucchini 213
12.5 Seventeen, still picture from video. Image credit © Daniele Lucchini 214
12.6 Terrifying, still picture from video. Image credit © Daniele Lucchini 214
12.7 Sickening, still picture from video. Image credit © Daniele Lucchini 215
12.8 Radiating, still picture from video. Image credit © Daniele Lucchini 216

# Contributors

**Mita Banerjee** is a Professor of nineteenth- and twentieth-century American literature and culture, with a particular focus on Ethnic and Indigenous Studies, at Johannes Gutenberg Universität Mainz. Her publications explore the intersection between literary studies and other fields, especially medicine, law, and economics. She has looked at the ways in which literary and cultural narratives contribute to processes of nation-building and decolonization and, most recently, the ways in which medical categories can inform cultural identities and in which medicine, in turn, is narratively constructed.

**Marta-Laura Cenedese** is UKRI (MSCA Horizon Guarantee) Postdoctoral Fellow at the Institute for Medical Humanities at Durham University. She is the author of *Irène Némirovsky's Russian Influences: Tolstoy, Dostoevsky and Chekhov* (2021) and editor of *Written on the Body: Narrative (Re)constructions of Violence(s)* (2023). Marta was an associated researcher at the Centre Marc Bloch Berlin (2020–2024) and has been visiting fellow at the Dahlem Humanities Center, Humboldt University Berlin (2020) and at the Centre d'Histoire, Sciences-Po Paris (2023).

**Xenia Chiaramonte** is an Associate Professor at Ca' Foscari University of Venice. She is the author of *Governare il conflitto. La criminalizzazione del movimento No Tav* (2019) and has contributed to numerous publications on law and social struggles, political trials, instituting practices, and social transformations. She specialises in critical theories of punishment and co-animates the blog for the Italian Critical Criminological journal: *Studi sulla Questione Criminale*. Currently, she is completing a monograph on law and ecology.

**Federico Dal Bo** (b. 1973) (PhD, University of Bologna, 2005) (PhD, Free University of Berlin, 2009) is a senior lecturer in Jewish Studies at the University of Modena and Reggio Emilia, Italy. He has published monographs and many articles on Judaism and Philosophy, including *Deconstructing the Talmud, The Absolute Book* (Routledge, 2019), *Judaism, Philosophy, and Psychoanalysis in Heidegger's Ontology: Harrowing the Heath* (Palgrave Macmillan, 2023), *Jesus in the Latin Talmud. Judaism and Christianity during the Disputation of Paris in 1240 and Other Transcultural Issues* (2024), and *Print, Power, and Cultural Hegemony. A Material History of Early Hebrew Prints* (2024).

**Annica Engström** is an artist, master of fine arts, and graphic designer. She works as a project manager, counsellor, and curator of artistic projects, books, and exhibitions, often in cooperation with people who experience mental distress. She is also a producer at the Museum of Medical History in Gothenburg.

**Sander L. Gilman** is a Distinguished Professor Emeritus of the Liberal Arts and Sciences as well as Emeritus Professor of Psychiatry at Emory University. A cultural and literary historian, he is the author or editor of over 100 books. His *"Gebannt in diesem magischen Judenkreis": Essays* appeared with Wallstein Verlag (Göttingen) in 2022; his most recent co-edited volume is *Readers for Life: How Reading and Listening in Childhood Shape Us* (London, 2024). He is the author of the basic study of the visual stereotyping of the mentally ill, *Seeing the Insane*, published in 1982 (reprinted: 1996 and 2014) as well as the standard study of *Jewish Self-Hatred*, the title of his monograph of 1986, which is still in print. He has held positions at Cornell University, the University of Chicago, and the University of Illinois at Chicago and has been a visiting professor at numerous universities in North America, South Africa, The United Kingdom, Germany, Israel, China, and New Zealand.

**Nora Heidorn** is an interdisciplinary researcher, curator, and writer with a background in contemporary art. She investigates the complex politics of health, sexual reproduction, and care through an intersectional feminist lens using curatorial and artistic methods. Her practice-led PhD at the Royal College of Art in London (2025) was funded by the Arts and Humanities Research Council.

**Helen Johansson** has studied classical archaeology, ancient history, and religion, and is also a poet. She has worked as a peer supporter within psychiatry, mainly with people diagnosed with psychosis and has also worked with user-led audits of psychiatric health care units. She is currently tutoring and educating peer support workers.

**Claude Kempen** is a white and trans nonbinary writer from Berlin, currently pursuing a PhD at the Universities of Melbourne and Potsdam. Their research focuses on contemporary nonbinary memoirs, with the aim of developing a nonbinary theory. Their previous work has examined Islamophobia in pornography (ZMO Working Papers, 2020), queer activism in Jordan (de Gruyter 2021) and Nonbinary Theory (Continuum Journal, 2026). Claude's other non-fiction writing has addressed grief and transgender spirituality (AnthroDesires, 2021) as well as the trauma of surviving coercive and corrective surgery during childhood (Archer Magazine, 2024).

**Janina Klement** studied history, sociology, and political and cultural theory at the University of Bonn, UCL, and Yale. She is currently completing her PhD on global histories of avant-garde psychiatry, antipsychiatry, and critiques of psychoanalysis from the 1950s to the late 1970s at UCL's Centre for Multidisciplinary and Intercultural Inquiry.

**Daniele Lorenzini** is an Associate Professor of Philosophy at the University of Pennsylvania. He is the author, most recently, of *The Force of Truth: Critique, Genealogy, and Truth-Telling in Michel Foucault* (2023).

**Maria Morata** is an independent curator, researcher, artist, and PhD candidate at the Universidad Complutense in Madrid (Spain). She explores the encounters of sick bodies with technical medical dispositives from a queer and *crip* perspective. She is a member of the *Sickness Affinity Group* and founder of the art collective *cripxcess*. Currently, she works on her long-term project 'SOMA ARCHIVES' with artistic and activist groups.

**Clio Nicastro** is a researcher in Philosophy, Cultural Studies, and Film Studies affiliated with Bard College Berlin. She studied philosophy at the University of Palermo, where she completed her PhD in Aesthetics and Theory of Arts. She was DAAD postdoctoral fellow as well as fellow at the ICI Berlin Institute for Cultural Inquiry, where she held an additional one-year postdoctoral research thanks to a VolkswagenStiftung grant. She is the author of *La Dialettica del Denkraum in Aby Warburg* (2022) as well as the co-editor with Cristina Baldacci and Arianna Sforzini of the volume *Over and Over and Over again. Reenactment Strategies in Contemporary Arts and Theory* (2022). She is a member of the board of directors of the Harun Farocki Institut.

**Lena Ditte Nissen** works as artistic researcher and filmmaker at the intersection of documentary and performative practice with reference to classical experimental film and ethnographic research strategies. Her films, performances, and installations have been shown in international institutions and film festivals. Her PhD is funded by the Austrian Academy of Sciences.

**Rachel Pafe** is a writer and researcher based in Berlin. Her PhD project (Goethe University of Frankfurt/ University of Lille) deals with Gillian Rose, a sociologist and philosopher who had a fraught relationship with mysticism, religion, and political action, bouncing between the Frankfurt School and modern Jewish and Christian thought. She explores this by charting Rose's real and imagined conversations with Susan Taubes, Theodor Adorno, Emmanuel Levinas, Simone Weil, Walter Benjamin, and Daniel Bensaïd.

**Hannah Parlett** recently completed her PhD at the Centre of Film & Screen, University of Cambridge. Her doctoral thesis explored maternal transgression in contemporary cinema, focusing on the work of Claire Denis, Andrea Arnold, Lynne Ramsay, and Sean Baker. Her other publications include a chapter on gesture and affect in feminist installation art and a forthcoming article on rage and suicide in Francophone cinema from the 1960s.

**Silvia Pierosara** (PhD in Philosophy and Theory of Human Sciences) is an Associate Professor of Moral Philosophy at the University of Macerata, Italy. Her research interests include theories of recognition, foundations and applications of narrative ethics, universalism and contextualism, transcendentality and historicity, critical theories of justice, moral autonomy, relational autonomy, narrative autonomy, history of ethics and moral philosophy, and critical philosophies of history including progress, memory, and nostalgia. She is the author of several monographs and articles.

**Elisabeth Punzi** (PhD) is a clinical psychologist, Associate Professor, and lecturer in social work at Gothenburg University. Her research concerns mental health, disability, and substance use. She has a specific interest in creative expressions and their importance for recovery and wellbeing, as well as in the meaning of heritage and culture.

**Myriam Sauer** is a writer based in Berlin. Her most recent publication is her novel, *Eine Passage durch den reißenden Strom* (A Torrential Passage), which came out in 2023 with Querverlag. Her academic interests include the history and theory of psychoanalysis, sociology, and literature.

**Lisa Schmidt-Herzog** is a PhD student of Philosophy at the Freie Universität Berlin and Institut für Medizingeschichte und Wissenschaftsforschung Lübeck. After working on Merleau-Ponty's phenomenology of perception, she has been engaged with questions of madness, alterity, and scientific positivism. Her doctoral project is a critical theory of the normal and the normative within the transcultural psy-disciplines.

**Sophia Rohwetter** is a writer, researcher and art critic interested in the history and philosophy of modern and contemporary art, the visual culture of anti-psychiatry, psychoanalysis, and Marxist aesthetics. Currently, she is a University Assistant and PhD candidate at the Department of Art History at the University of Vienna.

**Angela Woods** is a Professor of Medical Humanities at Durham University, UK. From 2012 to 2022, she was co-director of Hearing the Voice, a large interdisciplinary project investigating the experience of hearing voices. She is now the Director of the Institute for Medical Humanities and the Discovery Research Platform for Medical Humanities.

# Acknowledgements

Marta-Laura Cenedese and Clio Nicastro are grateful to ICI Berlin Institute for Cultural Inquiry, the Nordic Summer University, the VolkswagenStiftung, and the Centre Marc Bloch for generously funding the original conference – *Violence, Care, Cure: (Self-)perceptions within the Medical Encounter* (ICI Berlin, 3–4 February 2022). Thanks to Koneensäätio and the project INTERACT: Intersectional Reading, Social Justice, and Literary Activism (PI Kaisa Ilmonen) for generously funding the language revision and proofreading of the volume. Many thanks to Albion M. Butters for his careful work in that regard.

Thanks to ICI's directors Christoph Holzhey and Manuele Gragnolati, and to Claudia Peppel, for making the conference possible. We also want to thank Claudia for allowing us to use her artwork for the visual image of the conference.

We are indebted to Rosa Barotsi, Heike Bartel, Anna Ovaska, and Hannah Wallenfeld for their support and friendship.

We wish to gratefully acknowledge the permission from publishers to draw on the following earlier publications, which appear in this book: Chapter 3 is a revised version of Xenia Chiaramonte's 'Notes on Bio-history: Michel Foucault and the political economy of health', published in *Acta Universitatis. Lodziensis. Folia Iuridica*, 96 (2021), 111–23;[1] Chapter 8 is a translated and revised version of Silvia Pierosara's chapter 'L'autonomia narrativa alla prova della malattia', published in *Per un'autonomia narrativa. Etica, storia, educazione* (2022, 55–74).[2]

1 https://doi.org/10.18778/0208-6069.96.09.

2 https://www.edizionistudium.it/libri/unautonomia-narrativa.

# Introduction

## Violence, care, cure: (Self-)perceptions within the medical encounter

*Marta-Laura Cenedese and Clio Nicastro*

In the desktop documentary 'Watching *The Pain of Others*' (2018), French researcher and filmmaker Chloé Galibert-Laîné tries to make sense of their uncomfortable experience watching Penny Lane's *The Pain of Others* (2018), a documentary film that assembles footage about Morgellons disease. The latter is a 'perplexing' and 'poorly understood' skin condition involving the spontaneous appearance of 'ulcerative skin lesions that contain unusual filaments lying under, embedded in, or projecting from the skin' (Middelveen et al. 2018, 71). In the film, Lane makes use of fragments from videos by three famous YouTubers with Morgellons, to which she interposes excerpts with medical experts. As Galibert-Laîné remarks, the film seems to be built around two parallel narrative arcs: the first one is that of the three YouTubers – Carrie, Tasha, and Marcia – whose stories, initially believable, become more and more improbable as the film advances and the camera obsessively moves closer and closer to the skin's pores; conversely, the second narrative includes excerpts in which doctors' statements lead the viewer from doubting the reality of the illness towards starting to take the patients seriously. The ambivalence of the disease is further increased by the nature of its peculiar alleged means of contagion, since the women purportedly developed their symptoms when exposed to images of the skin lesions on social media. Galibert-Laîné themselves, at the end of the video essay, suspiciously looks at a little wound on their leg, critically interrogating the power of empathy, which is far from neutral. Reflecting on their own experience as a viewer, Galibert-Laîné posits that Lane's film invites spectators to 'formulate their own diagnostic' and to either believe 'the disembodied voice of Science' or the intimate evidence provided by the women, whose only expertise is their bodily experience and self-observation. As the video essay progresses, and with it also Galibert-Laîné's meta-reflexive investigation, viewers are compelled to ponder the legitimacy of lived experience, the supposed objectivity of medicine as well as its gender bias, the scrutiny to which we subject our bodies as 'other' from us, the limits of empathy, and the exhibitionist, voyeuristic drive that morphs illness into a social encounter(/experience).

'Watching *The Pain of Others*' was of great inspiration when we started conceiving the conference 'Violence, Care, Cure: (Self-)perceptions within the medical encounter' (ICI Berlin 2022), which is at the basis of this collected volume (Figure 0.1). As we were reasoning on the ambivalence between violence and care,

DOI: 10.4324/9781032660165-1

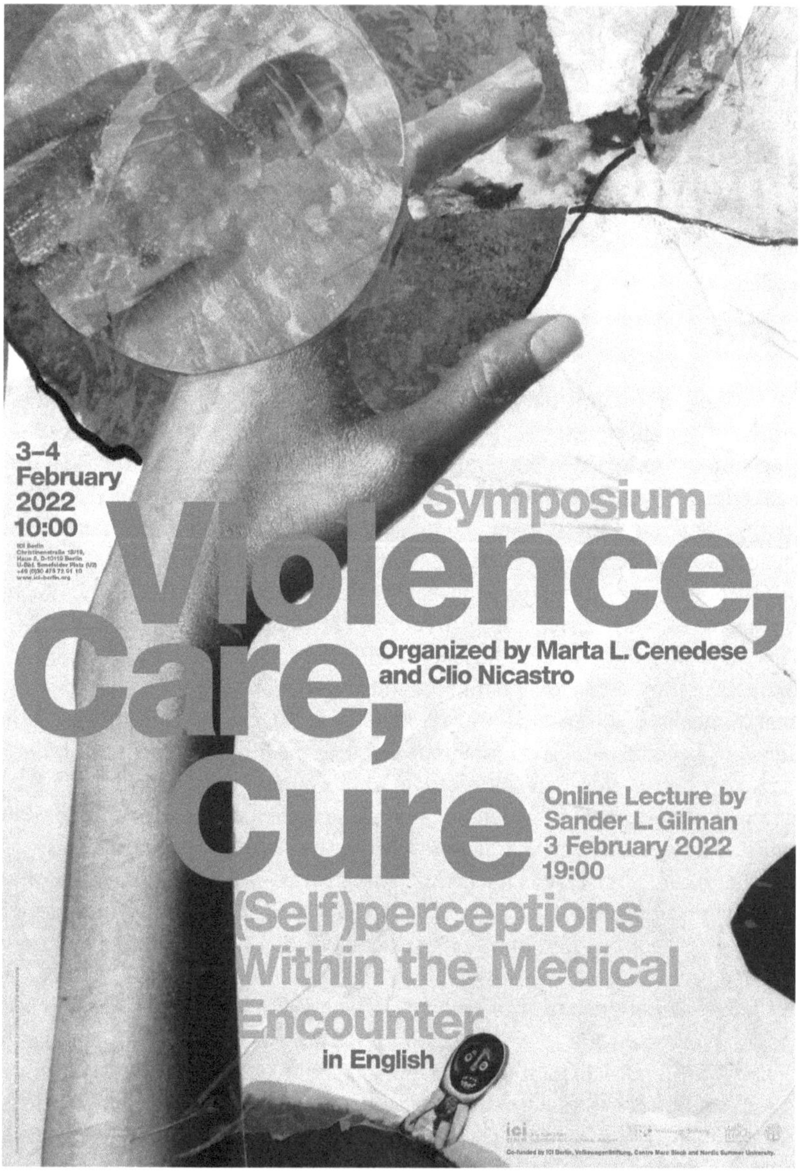
3–4
February
2022
10:00
Symposium
Violence,
Care,
Cure
Organized by Marta L. Cenedese
and Clio Nicastro
Online Lecture by
Sander L. Gilman
3 February 2022
19:00
(Self)perceptions
Within the Medical
Encounter
in English

*Figure 0.1* Poster of the conference *Violence, Care, Cure*. Image credit © Claudia Peppel, 'Who's afraid of…?', paper collage, 2013 (detail), poster design: Studio BENS.

and care and cure, in stories of illness and medicine *tout court*, Galibert-Laîné's video essay helped us to reflect in more complex ways and consider possible ramifications outside of our own disciplinary fields (philosophy and literary/cultural studies). It also provided us with an anchor to the most immediate socio-political event of the early 2020s, the COVID-19 pandemic, which inevitably influenced our need to confront the polarising climate, between conspiracy and security, and life and death, that we were living through. Aside from one contribution, however, we have chosen to let the pandemic take a backseat in the volume, in order to privilege other *cases* that illuminate the intersections between violence, care, and cure. Here, we borrow Lauren Berlant's (2007, 633) description of 'a case', which is not necessarily and not merely an illustrative example of an already existing more general issue but 'a problem-event that has animated some kind of judgement'.[1] Indeed, Berlant (2007, 633) makes a long and heterogeneous list of cases – from symptoms to crimes – that recognise as their common denominator 'an irritating obstacle to clarity'. The variety of fields and approaches included in this volume mirrors Berlant's idea of 'a case' in exploring the several forms and situations in which violence, care, and cure can intersect within the medical realm. In this respect, Galibert-Laîné's 'Watching *The Pain of Others*' encapsulates several of the themes that are discussed in this book: besides the three main concepts that give the collection its title, it deals with bodily experience, medical neglect or scepticism, biopolitics, ethics, pain and suffering, diagnosis and recovery, gender medicine, epistemic injustice, and the role of images and other narratives, including social media platforms.

## Where the three concepts meet: A glossary

**Violence:** Lacking a preconceived definition in order to remain receptive and open to complexity, the volume suggests a conceptualisation of violence that is necessarily broad and that, significantly, views violence as an instrument of power (see, e.g., Bourdieu 1977, 2001; Foucault 1982; Žižek 2008; Dorlin 2019; Vergès 2020). In this volume, violence stands not only as the act of inflicting harm or injury on an individual or a group (physical and psychological violence), but also as a mode of constructing individuals, communities, and the world (symbolic and systemic violence). We do not posit that violence is inherent to science and/or to the medical encounter but rather that it emerges from the intersection of the social relations, performative activities, and structures of power (both symbolic and material) that permeate such institutions. While we acknowledge arguments about the inherent potential of violence within language, narratives, and sense-making practices (e.g., Bourdieu 1991; Levinas 1987; Derrida 1997), we contend that to name, to tell, and to make visible are essential for 'finding nonviolent ways of understanding subject formation and embodied life' (Fareld 2022, 189). The potential violence of language and scientific discourse is at the centre of Lisa Schmidt-Herzog's contribution (Chapter 7), in which she questions the neglect of Frantz Fanon's work in the medical and psy disciplines. According to Schmidt-Herzog, this effacement is due to the rigid relation between language and epistemic structures, which Fanon's work – uniting the poetic, the scientific, and the political – subverts and dismantles. The recent heated debate surrounding Giorgio Agamben's (2020) position against the restrictive measures adopted during the COVID-19 pandemic – especially in Italy where the philosopher lives – has reignited scrutiny of the role of 'biopolitics'. Foucauldian scholar Daniele Lorenzini (2021a, 2021b) argues that 'biopolitics' primarily functions as a descriptive tool for grasping the present and does not inherently imply an obscure or necessarily dangerous form of power. What is especially relevant for this volume is what Lorenzini (2021b, 42) terms the '(bio)politics of differential vulnerability', which highlights how the unprecedented exacerbation of social inequalities intensified by the pandemic is much more urgent to observe and to fight than a health dictatorship. In this sense, the health crisis has produced a range of new vulnerabilities and new social inequalities as a way of governing people; according to Lorenzini, this phenomenon is not limited to instances where the statistical impact of the coronavirus (and associated deaths) correlates with variables such as social class, salary, and race but extends globally, with the distribution of vaccinations following geopolitical logics. Xenia Chiaramonte (Chapter 3) shares the same concern in wanting to retrace the original meaning of biopolitics as used by Foucault to find a valuable analytical framework for a cogent approach to the relationship between medicine and power dynamics.

The above considerations shed light upon the different scales that appear when mapping the points of juncture between violence, care, and cure. In a volume concerned with 'medical encounters', it comes as no surprise that the micro dimension[2] coincides with the *body* as, to use a contentious metaphor, the 'battlefield' where wounding and caring occur:

> The body implies mortality, vulnerability, agency: the skin and the flesh expose us to the gaze of others, but also to touch, and to violence, and bodies put us at risk of becoming the agency and instrument of all these as well.
> (Butler 2004, 26)

In his seminal work on migraines, Oliver Sacks navigates the different explanations and remedies for one of the most mysterious yet common disorders of the nervous system – one that afflicts millions of people.[3] After a thorough examination of the main types of migraines and the prevalent treatments against them, Sacks (1995, 234) concludes that there is only one cardinal rule to deal with the diagnostic challenges of migraines: 'one must always listen to the patient'. At least at the time Sacks completed his research, migraine patients had a frequent second complaint beside their pain, namely, that of not being listened to by physicians: 'Looked at, investigated, drugged, charged: but not listened to' (Sacks 1995, 234). Novalis has famously and poignantly considered disease as a musical problem, whose cure is a musical solution,[4] which definitely offers a generative metaphor to move away from the visual fields of the medical gaze. Since the 1970s, when Sacks published his above-mentioned book, significant changes have undeniably occurred in the interaction between doctors and patients. These have undoubtedly been aided by the work of authors such as French-Canadian doctor Martin Winckler (1989, 1998, 2004, 2009, 2016, 2019) as well as by over two decades of research and dissemination of narrative medicine (Charon 2006; Charon et al. 2017), the recent yet long history of which is the focus of Sander L. Gilman's afterword to this volume. Nonetheless, in many countries, the recent implementation of healthcare cuts (as well as inflation) has impeded the practical application of awareness regarding the importance of listening: despite the 'lessons' of the COVID-19 pandemic, in the public sector healthcare workers are poorly paid, overworked, and understaffed.[5] We, of course, do not want to oversimplify or idealise the dialogical dimension of the medical encounter; instead, we have sought to compile various instances that consider intentional, unintentional, systemic, and/or individual forms of misunderstanding. The latter plays a crucial role in a study by German medical historian and scholar of Gender Studies, Barbara Duden, which productively resonates with Galibert-Laîné's video essay. Another medium, another land, another time in history—yet the question remains similar: what does it mean within the medical encounter to take someone at their word? This is a question that is also behind Maria Morata's 'performative text' (Chapter 12), where she confronts the absence of visual indicators for pain – especially chronic pain – and the power structures behind vision machines used by medical imaging technology.

By delving into the records of eighteenth-century German gynaecologist Johann Storch, who carefully transcribed how his female patients described their symptoms, Duden (1991) aims to understand how women from another time perceived their bodies and talked about their different bodily manifestations before anatomy reconfigured and remapped sensations, as Foucault notably discusses in *The Birth of the Clinic* (1963). Duden praises women's organic metaphors for allowing access to a richer and painful intertwining between bodily symptoms, feelings, and (often abusive) relationships with men. Defining herself as the first 'historian of the body' in the early 1990s, Duden wished to overcome the opposition between the body as a series of natural, biological, stable, and unchanging phenomena, and the socio-historical dimensions of ever-changing life. An example of this would be the fear of solidification of blood, the movement and flow of which comprise a central element in women's complaints and therefore became a key concept for Duden's study. The fixation on expulsion to cure a disease reflected the theory that emotions can get trapped inside the organs; for instance, a heavy stomach was considered to be the consequence of anger, which could be released and cleansed by rhubarb. Duden is here fascinated by the connection between the mental and the physical, which together constituted the fabric of experiences and sensations, and by the role of Storch's patients in apprehending the origin of the interpretative power of the natural sciences and medicine (Duden and Schminke 2019). Hannah Parlett's addition to this volume (Chapter 10) is, in this respect, a fascinating travel into the director Pedro Almodóvar's obsession of the body, showing anatomy as both a medical practice and a fantasy about the inner lives of organs and tissues. Parlett analyses salient scenes of Almodóvar's films that depict the encounter between patient and physician, while at the same time revealing the historical interconnection between the cinematic and medical gaze.

**Care:** We understand *care* as a concept that holds ethico-political import – both as tangible labour and as a political and cultural construction. We are aware that over the last years the term 'care' has been widely circulating in academia and in the art field, almost becoming a buzzword that can easily fit the neoliberal discourse. Yet, not only do we want to follow German filmmaker Harun Farocki's suggestion that one should not hand a notion over to the enemy but rather reclaim it (Farocki 2008, 21–22), we also wish to add a new perspective on care by reading it in constellation with violence and cure. In doing so, we want to call into question the neutrality of caring. Therefore, we hold simultaneously broad definitions, such as 'a species activity that includes everything that we do to maintain, continue, and repair our "world" so that we can live in it as well as possible' (Tronto and Fisher, in Tronto 1993, 103) and 'a critical theory that denounces and exposes the processes through which caring for the most vulnerable has become marginalized, and through which the recognition of care-related practices, people, and institutions has been undermined' (Brugère 2019, 59). As a notion and a praxis, care precedes Western academic interest; however, theories of care originate within the North American feminist, civil rights, and liberation movements of the 1960s and 1970s (Fine and Tronto 2020, 302). Foundational in the field are Carol Gilligan's *In a* Different Voice (1982) and Joan Tronto's *Moral Boundaries: A Political Argument for an Ethic of* Care (1993), which brought subaltern voices to matter for moral and political theory, and thus turned *care* into a critical political concept (Laugier 2011, 185). In *Moral Boundaries*, Tronto (1993, 136) argues that care has a role in our everyday life as a *practice*; in this regard, she identifies four phases, each of which defines a particular quality of what caring entails: 'attentiveness, responsibility, competence, and responsiveness'. To these qualities of an ethics of care, in *Who Cares? How to Reshape a Democratic Politics*, Tronto (2015, 14) subsequently adds a fifth element, 'caring with', which she sees as essential for building a caring democracy that 'imagines the entire polity of citizens engaged in a lifetime of commitment to and benefiting from these principles'. The ethical tension between the personal and political dimensions of care are thematised in this volume by Rachel Pafe (Chapter 9), who looks at how Hungarian-American writer and thinker Susan Taubes engages with Simone Weil, whose critique of modern violence she appreciates while at the same time still challenging the idea of a total solution to suffering. This chapter contends that the unresolved tension between Taubes and Weil raises crucial questions about the communal dimensions of an ethics to address suffering within the realm of political life. Taking a cue from Tronto's encompassing understanding of care as 'not restricted to human interactions' (see Tronto 1993, 103 ff.), María Puig de la Bellacasa (2017, 1) has more recently explored the relevance of care 'for thinking and living in more than human worlds'. In this volume, Nora Heidorn's thinking with and about historical objects (Chapter 1) is framed in terms of Puig de la Bellacasa's ethics of care. As Heidorn (35) writes, 'all kinds of objects and artefacts – "things" – could become Matters of Care through caring and critical attention to what they represent and what they do in the world'. Puig de la Bellacasa's (2017, 5–12) conception of care retains the tension between its ontological dimensions (affective, practical, ethico-political) in order to stay with its potential to disrupt and displace.

As these feminist thinkers, among many others, show, an ethics of care stresses relationality, vulnerability, and interdependence, and therefore is 'always about power' (Tronto 2020, 185), yet it is also about imagination (Fleury 2019, 11). Imagination is at the core of Myriam Sauer's contribution (Chapter 13), where, by blending fiction and theory, she emphasises the fantasies (in their psychoanalytical sense) produced by gender dysphoria, a wound that can never be completely sutured. Within a medical context, Cynthia Fleury observes, 'Care is a shared function, arising from the dialectical, creative alliance of caregivers and care-receivers, who, together, open up to a unique dynamic that is woven thanks to the specificity of their own subjectivity'.[6] And Annemarie Mol (2008, 6) reminds that care is 'not opposed to, but includes, technology'.

**Cure:** As we have seen above, the concepts of both violence and care have been amply discussed from a variety of disciplinary fields, and several prominent scholars have written about them. Yet, what motivates this volume is the lack of scholarship engaging with both at the same time – that is, with the ambiguities of care and its overlaps with different forms of violence. Even more profoundly, these works overlook a space that, we believe, marks a primary stage for their conflicting intersections: the medical setting and encounter. By these terms, we do not mean solely the doctor–patient encounter at the hospital/clinical space; instead, we refer to a variety of spatio-temporal contact zones that, beyond the consulting room, also include bureaucratic systems, artistic venues, and the discursive space or the digital sphere – as well as all the in/corporeal agents involved. In this respect, we follow Anne Whitehead and Angela Woods (2016, 2), who call to expand and 're-envisage' the 'primal scene' of the medical humanities to include the exploration of 'new scenes and sites' outside of medical institutions – those that are potentially 'occluded from view' and that may prompt 'more critical questions'.

Two important notions that emerge within this encounter, and that underscore the mismatch that often arises between the medical gaze (Foucault 1963) and the individual's gaze in the face of the same event, are those of 'disease' and 'illness'. Once established, the distinction between the two shifted the focus from the official descriptions and definitions of syndromes (their scientific/medical classification) to the individual's experiences and articulations of them (see, e.g., Kleinman 1988; Toombs 1992; Frank 1995). Particularly salient for this volume is Sander L. Gilman's (1995) work, whereby he distinguishes between 'illness' as the subjective experience of a condition that affects (to a greater or lesser extent) the physical and mental health of an individual, and 'disease' as a medical category that emerges within a given historical and cultural context and offers a model for understanding and treating a certain constellation of symptoms. The latter, therefore, corresponds to a social construction and not to a mere label, thus suggesting an approach that seeks to take distance from both dogmatic scientism and relativism. The perception of a symptom is not necessarily 'truer' than its scientific description because symptoms are, most often, an expression of the psychosomatic relationship between the physical and the psychic. Aware of the inevitable interaction between the two dimensions of illness, as an experience ('illness') and as a category ('disease'), Gilman is particularly interested in their distinction when he investigates the relationship between images and medical science, which, in his opinion, the history of medicine has long underestimated and not fully understood in all its complexity. For Gilman, the presence of such images throughout history suggests a tension between the real and the imagined, and therefore tells us about the social construction of diseases, especially chronic and contagious ones (1988). As shown above in our discussion of Duden's work, the ways diseases have been portrayed with words and images have also affected the (self-)perception of the body through history.

At the same time, however, the distinction between 'illness' and 'disease' has also highlighted the gulf (and incommunicability) between the patient's experience and the physician's understanding of it (see Toombs 1992, 11). This aspect, in particular, is concerned with the flawed equivalence between cure and care (see Mol 2008, 1–2), and especially cracks open the prescriptive and linear assumption that after 'diagnosis', a cure will channel a 'recovery' towards 'health'. Phenomenologist S. Kay Toombs (1992, 112) explains, 'If the end of the medical encounter is defined solely in terms of diagnosis and cure of the "disease," the suffering of those with chronic illness seems intractable. The focus on "cure" suggests that the physician has little to offer the person who is incurably ill'. Toombs (1992, 114) goes on to add that

> If "cure" is perceived to be the goal, disease is the enemy and the patient's body the battlefield. The emphasis is on winning the war, whatever the cost. The "disease" is confronted as an abstract entity residing in, but in some way separate from the one who is ill.

The 'curing function' of medicine is thus opposed to its 'healing function'. Here, cure implies a normative expectation of recovery as returning to the original healthy body (i.e., prior the disease derailed its normative functioning); on the contrary, healing encompasses an understanding of the body as lived. The former, normative conception of 'cure' has also been challenged by disability studies scholars: Alison Kafer (2013, 27–28), for instance, speaks of 'curative time' and 'curative imaginary' to designate a temporal framing that, by normalising 'the dominant narrative of progress', casts disabled people aside, leaves out addictions and chronic diseases, eliminates any form of impairment, and assumes the imperative of treatment. Instead, recovery is not a linear return to a pre-fixed state of absolute and universal health (i.e., identical to a 'before' comparable for everybody and which, according to Kafer (2013, 27), is concerned with 'compulsory able-bodiedness/able-mindedness') and health is commensurate to one's temporally fluctuating abilities (Woods et al. 2022; Cheston et al. 2025). Healing implies the 'mourning' of recovery identified as a return to a prior state (Canguilhem 1966) and the shift towards a perspective of continuum between living with and without illness (Fleury 2019, 29, 31). As Xenia Chiaramonte writes in this volume, 'illness is not measured as a deviation from pre-established norms; it is a change in the quality of life' (69).

**Individuals and communities:** The privileged perspective of the patient's experience has contributed to the rise of prominence of scholarship on stories of illness, which the 'narrative turn' of the 1990s certainly nurtured. Anne Hunsaker Hawkins (1999), for instance, coined the term *pathographies* to address discrete illness narratives. Narratives, broadly construed, allow the ill person to reconfigure and reorganise their experience at a time of, as Silvia Pierosara writes in this volume, 'loss of personal and moral autonomy' (152). Such loss, Pierosara notes in her contribution (Chapter 8), can become an incentive to reconstruct meaning and, therefore, it calls for a different kind of autonomy – *narrative autonomy* – through a process of mutual reliance between the patient and care network which demands acting with 'narrative humility' (DasGupta 2008). In this volume, we continue to foster the production of individual stories of 'medical encounters'; however, their forms challenge canonical tropes of linearity and coherence and instead offer new, performative, episodic narrations interlaced with rigorous critical, theoretical, and reflective examination. For instance, in this book – besides Sauer's previously mentioned exploration of the lived experience of gender dysphoria through an exchange between poetic and theoretic modes of expression and Maria Morata's attempt to represent on the written page her performative account of her life with chronic pain – we find Claude Kempen's praxiographic autoethnography, which, drawing on their personal experience of transitioning in Germany as a non-binary person and making use of their own insurance-purposed medical records, theorises 'trans as gap' and revels in its vastness and multiplicity (Chapter 11).

Nonetheless, we are also cognisant of the criticism towards an emphasis on the individual, which oftentimes is not fully integrated into the larger structures and contexts that accompany illness and medical practice in general (see, e.g., Woods 2011; Wasson 2018). In her book *The Logic of Care. Health and the Problem of Patient Choice*, Annemarie Mol (2008) explores how the 'individual' and the 'collective' are related in the context of healthcare, and suggests that a logic of care starts with collectives. Individuals do not aggregate into a collective based on already present, fixed categories; rather, they first belong to collectives that, within a 'logic of care' (as opposed to a 'logic of choice'), are horizontally categorised and differentiated (Mol 2008, 66–83). And indeed, the above-mentioned chapters are not mere individual accounts but rather stories entangled with social phenomena and structures. They are 'collective narratives' in a double sense: they are inextricable from their context, made up of more than the simple individual, embedded in institutional and social interdependence, as well as aided and upheld by different groups and communities (see, e.g., Kempen; Morata); they are shared here as part of a communal practice of making visible. This attention – turned towards the peripheral to spotlight who and what the institutions discard and communities marginalise, and the loss entailed by this exclusionary logic – is present in Janina Klement's (Chapter 5) and Sophia Rohwetter's (Chapter 6) contributions, which aim to broaden the frame of anti-psychiatry. Whereas Klement thoroughly digs into R.D. Laing's practice as a psychiatrist who created new therapeutic strategies and considered schizophrenia a social event, Rohwetter's chapter delves into the Italian radical psychiatry movement of the late 1970s, revealing how, in its encounter with proletarian struggles, feminist politics of sexual difference, and avant-garde counterculture, the psychiatric scene underwent a transformation, becoming a contested social site that was amplified and mediated by audio-visual media.

Invoking shared experiences, however, does not imply the existence of a universal 'we' that, similarly to Mol's (2008) 'logic of choice', entails 'inclusion in some already constituted thing or entity' (Mbembe 2019, 40). Whereas 'universal' stands in as a vague synonym for a (Eurocentric) exclusionary system that, de facto, ideologically serves the superior position of the enlightened Western world (Suaudeau and Niang 2022), here we privilege a 'we' that fosters what is 'in-common', which, according to Achille Mbembe (2019, 40), 'presupposes a relation of co-belonging and sharing'. At the opening of her video essay 'Watching *The Pain of Others*' (2018), Chloé Galibert-Laîné includes a quotation from Susan Sontag's *Regarding the Pain of Others* (2003, 7): 'No "we" should be taken for granted when the subject is looking at other people's pain'. Similarly, and without denying its own subjectivity and positionality, 'we' in this book is not taken for granted but seen as fluid and flawed, relational and variegated, always in-the-making, and subject to question. Still, we are witness to how collective positionings are easily taken up in public discourse in order to separate between 'us' and 'them' in simplistic, essentialist, preconceived ways.

These issues have gained momentum with the outbreak of the COVID-19 pandemic. Yet, although the pandemic itself is referred to by only one of the volume's contributors (Dal Bo), the peculiar and often extreme ways in which it has been approached, and in which it has propelled categorical debates about violence, care, and cure, linger over the volume. Such a black-and-white opposition between internal/external, care/neglect, and cure/violence may seem reductionist; however, to engage with these seemingly contrasting attitudes reveals the genesis and features of a number of scientific dogmatic drifts, social and racial inequalities within healthcare systems, and idiosyncratic projections of individual and collective fears that often lead to stigmatising certain collectivities for the origin or transmission of a contagious disease. For instance, in this volume, Federico Dal Bo (Chapter 2) proposes a rich biopolitical analysis of a racist comment that a right-wing Italian politician made just before the pandemic hit Italy and Europe. In his chapter's incipit, Dal Bo refers to Sander L. Gilman's (2021) recent work about the COVID-19 pandemic and the resurgence of historical and sociological stereotypes in the naming and blaming of specific groups for the origin and transmission of infectious diseases. Looking at case studies of Ultra-Orthodox Jewish (Haredi) communities and the Chinese in the Popular Republic of China, Zhou Xun and Gilman (2021) explore the symbolic value of health and illness defined by the community and in defining the boundaries of communities, which are both impermeable and flexible. Public health measures, they write, may be necessary, but they also reinforce existing boundaries that provoke placing the blame on others: 'They may indeed save lives, but what kind of life? and whose life?' (Xun and Gilman 2021, 43).

**Critical:** Diving deep into a variety of case studies – such as the Black maternal mortality crisis (Banerjee), the blaming of a racialised group (Dal Bo), the anti-psychiatry movement (Klement and Rohwetter), gender dysphoria (Sauer), chronic pain (Morata), the collaboration between researchers and patients/health practitioners (Punzi et al., Woods), etc. – in this volume we address continuities among episodes of violence that highlight the structural rather than the exceptional, which confute claims of stability in favour of a long global history that reaches back to the early twentieth century. Thus, this volume is also a critical response to the COVID/post-COVID peak in violence – including within the medical setting.

Our wish is that, after reading the different contributions, readers will have better critical tools to understand the nuances at stake in the medical encounter, and be less inclined to take polarised positions – something that often happens when this topic is discussed in the public arena.

Finally, by examining the state of the art and testing its methodological boundaries, the volume also aims to provide, both directly and indirectly, a meta-reflection on the disciplines that fall under the umbrella of 'medical and health humanities'. Although not all contributors recognise their work as belonging to this field, several chapters (e.g. Banerjee, Heidorn, Punzi et al., Pierosara, Woods) directly interrogate certain approaches (whether established or emerging) at the core of the medical humanities – such as narrative medicine, visual medical humanities, engaged research, and collaborative research with non-academic partners – for their potentiality to unearth systemic bias, to open different possibilities of existence, and to make visible the complexity of objects and artefacts, as well as to caution against their possible pitfalls. In his afterword to the volume (Chapter 14), Sander L. Gilman offers an overview of the status of moral education and the role of the humanities in fulfilling this mission. As he argues, as the fortunes of the humanities slowly dwindled and collapsed, and skill-based education (i.e., STEM) took over, the medical humanities came to fill the moral gap of professional education. Gilman criticises the early naiveté of a field, especially in its declination as 'narrative medicine' (Charon 2001), for claiming that 'literature can teach empathy and that empathy is what was lacking in the training of physicians' (234). Similarly to Gilman's critique, the claim today that the humanities shape better people and thus better professionals would be disputed by many medical humanities scholars, including proponents of narrative medicine, whose development includes a heightened attention to the issue of social justice and, indeed, to forms of violence within the discipline (see, e.g., DasGupta 2017). For Gilman, the humanities act 'as a sort of contra-factual universe, the "as if" world' (241) that better serves as a means of orienting ourselves within the reality we inhabit, to test (and perhaps reinforce) 'our own blind spot and presupposition' (241):

> The humanities can add another dimension to the study and practice of medicine and vice versa. No stronger sense of moral virtue is implied unless we embed this moral goal in one or the other ways of imagining and shaping the world.
>
> (243)

All in all, we wish to offer a 'critical' lens on the discipline (as is the case for the *critical* medical humanities) to account for a field that is inherently fluid, mobile, ever-developing, and, in our opinion, critically attuned to fostering new avenues for research – whether thematic, theoretical, or methodological – that do not fear to reflect on and challenge its own forms and practices. In this regard, by including novel and provocative ideas and objects of analysis as well as forms of expression, the volume's chapters contribute to the growing scholarship concerned with a variety of non/narrative and non/linguistic forms that interrogate and convey the embodied experience of medical matters but also different methods, geographies, and territories of knowledge.

## Coda

Overall, this edited volume addresses the notions of 'violence', 'care', and 'cure' within the medical encounter and seeks to foreground how, as a triad as well as individually, they are prone to ambiguous interpretations. Altogether, the book's chapters – which are organised around four sections – attend to the complex interlacing of these three key terms and what to make of their entanglement by offering historical, practical, philosophical, personal, and aesthetic analyses of different medical scenes, objects, and concepts. As the book's title infers, we argue that a hermeneutic of violence, care, and cure is inseparable from individual and collective perceptions of the medical encounter; that is, it is inextricable from an understanding of the tensions and consensus that surge among perceptions orchestrated by both internal (subjective) and external (social, cultural, political) 'gazes'. In this book, we invite the reader to observe medical encounters that take place in and are shaped by a variety of both material and 'immaterial' spaces, from the consulting room to the antechamber of medical bureaucracy, and from artistic venues to biopolitical discourses. We engage here not only with the most apparent forms of medical violence but also with those hidden forms of aggression that circulate in everyday medical/health/care practices and settings, and which affect predominantly marginalised and minority groups. What individuals experience, at either end of the consultation room, is a complex intertwinement of personal vicissitudes, global structures, and community practices, a prismatic network in which 'care' and 'violence' are reflected and refracted in a variety of often overlapping and divergent interpretative modes. The interlacing of personal experience and critical reflection that the book engages with eschews the confessional mode and instead creates a productive distance that turns even more personal experiences into something worth sharing, and thus it allows readers to apprehend their own bodily and medical experiences in a new light.

As mentioned, the book is divided into four sections punctuated by four 'musings'. These are short, thought-provoking pieces by established scholars in the field, which encapsulate the main ideas and questions this volume wishes to tackle – namely, the ambiguous, thorny, productive intertwinement of violence, care, and cure.[7] After this introduction, Mita Banerjee's musing on colour-blindness in healthcare, and specifically within childbirth, leads us to the first part of the book, where Heidorn's, Dal Bo's, and Chiaramonte's contributions engage with 'Medical histories and biopolitics'. The following section, 'Unsettling and working through practices and languages of cure', brings together four contributions by Lena Ditte Nissen, Janina Klement, Sophia Rohwetter, and Lisa Schmidt-Herzog, which address different forms of therapeutic encounters for coping with social, historical, or psychological forms of violence. This part is introduced by Elisabeth Punzi, Helen Johansson, and Annica Engström, who reflect on how critical heritage studies and cooperation can serve as important means to counteract psychiatric violence. Drawing from Frantz Fanon's critique of objectification within the medical encounter in the colonial context, Daniele Lorenzini's musing builds a generative bridge from the second to the third section, 'Agency in illness and ethics of suffering', where Silvia Pierosara, Rachel Pafe, and Hannah Parlett inquire into how one can actively make sense of and react to conditions that generate overwhelming (physical and psychological) pain and loss of meaning. This part is concluded by Angela Woods' musing on her experience in co-directing the project 'Hearing the Voice' (University of Durham), where care emerges in terms of attention, investment, and ethical practice. To encourage a transformative approach to the issues we have tackled in this volume, we dedicate the last section, 'Anatomy of a transformation', to three contributions – by Claude Kempen, Maria Morata, and Myriam Sauer – that use imagination and performative practises of (self-)expression to overcome narrative and material gaps in the medical sphere. The book concludes with Sander L. Gilman's afterword where, as previously detailed, he takes a broader view to interrogate the role of the humanities within professional education, particularly when it pertains to physicians and healthcare workers.[8]

Overall, we hope that, in bringing together different methodological approaches, this volume will provide its readers with conceptual resources for thinking about the intersections of violence, care, and cure. By providing a space where the voices of both emerging and established scholars mingle and respond to one another, we hope to also encourage future scholars – highlighting novel areas of investigation; nurturing interdisciplinary thinking on the intersections between medicine and critical thinking; developing a medical understanding of the human at both individual and collective levels; and showcasing marginal creative and intellectual practices.

## Notes

Open Access of this chapter is kindly supported by the UKRI Horizon Europe Guarantee, Grant Reference EP/Y014057/1

1 Clio Nicastro is grateful to Tom Holert for bringing to her attention Berlant's concept in the context of the project *Terms and Conditions* (Harun Farocki Institut Berlin 2024–2025).
2 Here we refer to Asia Bazdyrieva's (2023) poignant reflection on scales of violence, divided into the macro, the meso, and the micro.
3 See https://www.who.int/news-room/fact-sheets/detail/headache-disorders.
4 Novalis, *Das allgemeine Brouillon*, entry 386, HKA 3, 310 (2007, 58).
5 See, e.g., https://www.lastampa.it/cronaca/2023/10/10/news/tagli_sanita_inflazione-13774265/; https://www.linkiesta.it/2023/08/sanita-italia-tagli-investimenti/ in the case of Italy. For the UK, see, for example, https://nhscuts.org.uk/about/; https://www.theguardian.com/society/article/2024/jul/23/nhs-finances-so-dire-that-whole-service-may-collapse-says-spending-watchdog.
6 'Le soin est une fonction en partage, relevant de l'alliance dialectique, créative, des soignants et soignés, qui, ensemble, font éclore une dynamique singulière, notamment tissée grâce à la spécificité des sujets qu'ils sont' (2019, 20). Translation from the French by Marta-Laura Cenedese.
7 At the conference held at ICI Berlin in February 2022, the authors of the four musings took part in a roundtable discussion that was conceived as a collective moment

to reflect on the main themes of the conference, as seen from the different disciplinary perspectives and experiences of the panelists.

8 At the conference, Sander L. Gilman gave the keynote lecture 'Let's Talk about Vaccination' (3 February 2022). A recording is available on the ICI Berlin website: https://www.ici-berlin.org/events/lets-talk-about-vaccination/.

## References

Agamben, Giorgio. 2020. *A che punto siamo? L'epidemia come politica*. Roma: Quodlibet.

Bazdyrieva, Asia. 2023. "Micro, Meso, Macro." *Transmediale Journal* 5. https://transmediale.de/en/journal/micro-meso-macro.

Berlant, Lauren. 2007. "On the Case." *Critical Inquiry* 33(4): 663–672.

Bourdieu, Pierre. 1977. *Outline of a Theory of Practice*. Cambridge: Cambridge University Press.

Bourdieu, Pierre. 1991. *Language and Symbolic Power*. Cambridge: Polity Press.

Bourdieu, Pierre. 2001. *Masculine Domination*. Stanford, CA: Stanford University Press.

Brugère, Fabienne. 2019. *Care Ethics: The Introduction of Care as a Political Category*. Translated by Armelle Chrétien, Olivia Cooper-Hadjian and Brian Heffernan. With a Preface by Joan Tronto. Leuven, Paris, Bristol, CT: Peeters.

Butler, Judith. 2004. *Precarious Life: The Powers of Mourning and Violence*. New York: Verso.

Canguilhem, Georges. 1991. *The Normal and the Pathological* (1966). Translated by Carolyn R. Fawcett in collaboration with Robert S. Cohen. New York: Zone Books.

Charon, Rita. 2001. "A Model for Empathy, Reflection, Profession, and Trust." *JAMA* 286(15): 1897–1902.

Charon, Rita. 2006. *Narrative Medicine: Honoring the Stories of Illness*. Oxford: Oxford University Press.

Charon, Rita, Sayantani DasGupta, Nellie Hermann, Craig Irvine, Eric R. Marcus, Edgar Rivera Colsn, Danielle Spencer, and Maura Spiegel (eds). 2017. *The Principles and Practice of Narrative Medicine*. Oxford: Oxford University Press.

Cheston, Katharine, Marta-Laura Cenedese, and Angela Woods. 2025. "The Long or the Post of It? Temporality, Suffering, and Uncertainty in Narratives Following COVID-19." *Journal of Medical Humanities* 46: 3–20. https://doi.org/10.1007/s10912-023-09824-y.

DasGupta, Sayantani. 2008. "Narrative Humility." *The Lancet* 371(9617): 980–981.

DasGupta, Sayantani. 2017. "The Politics of the Pedagogy: Cripping, Queering and Un-homing Health Humanities." In *The Principles and Practice of Narrative Medicine*, edited by R. Charon et al., 137–154. Oxford: Oxford University Press.

Derrida, Jacques. 1997. *Of Grammatology* (1967). Translated by Gayatri Chakravorty Spivak. Baltimore, MD: The Johns Hopkins University Press.

Dorlin, Elsa. 2019. *Se défendre. Une philosophie de la violence*. Paris: La Découverte.

Duden, Barbara. 1991. *The Woman Beneath the Skin: A Doctor's Patients in Eighteenth-Century Germany*. Translated by Thomas Dunlap. Cambridge, MA: Harvard University Press.

Duden, Barbara, and Schmicke, Imke. 2019. "Die Geschichtlichkeit der Körperwahrnehmung in der Tiefe ausbuchstabiert. Ein Interview mit Barbara Duden." *Body Politics* 7(11): 41–54.

Fareld, Victoria. 2022. "Vulnerability, Violence and Nonviolence." In *Interpreting Violence: Narrative, Ethics and Hermeneutics*, edited by Cassandra Falke, Victoria Fareld and Hanna Meretoja, 179–191. Milton: Routledge.

Farocki Harun. 2008. "Einfühlung." In *100 Jahre* Hebbel *Theater. Angewandtes Theaterlexikon nach Gustav Freytag*, edited by Hebbel am Ufer, 21–22. Berlin: Hebbel am Ufer.

Fine, Michael, and Tronto, Joan. 2020. "Care Goes Viral: Care Theory and Research Confront the Global COVID-19 Pandemic." *International Journal of Care and Caring* 4(3): 301–309.

Fleury, Cynthia. 2019. *Le soin est un humanisme*. Paris: Gallimard.
Foucault, Michel. 1982. "The Subject and Power." *Critical Inquiry* 8(4): 777–795.
Foucault, Michel. 2002. *The Birth of the Clinic* (1963). Translated by A. M. Sheridan. London: Routledge.
Frank, Arthur. 1995. *The Wounded Storyteller: Body, Illness, and Ethics*. Chicago, IL: Chicago University Press.
Galibert-Laîné, Chloé. 2018. "Watching *The Pain of Others*." https://www.chloegalibertlaine.com/watching-the-pain-of-others.
Gilligan, Carol. 1982. *In a Different Voice*. Cambridge, MA: Harvard University Press.
Gilman, Sander L. 1988. *Disease and Representation: Images of Illness from Madness to AIDS*. Ithaca, NY and London: Cornell University Press.
Gilman, Sander L. 1995. *Picturing Health and Illness: Images of Identity and Difference*. Baltimore, MD: Johns Hopkins University Press.
Gilman, Sander L. 2021. "Placing the Blame for Covid-19 in and on Ultra-Orthodox Communities." *Modern Judaism – A Journal of Jewish Ideas and Experience* 41(1): 1–30.
Hawkins, Anne Hunsaker. 1999. *Reconstructing Illness: Studies in Pathography*. West Lafayette, IN: Purdue University Press.
Kafer, Alison. 2013. *Feminist, Queer, Crip*. Bloomington, IN: Indiana University Press.
Kleinman, Arthur. 1988. *The Illness Narratives: Suffering, Healing, and the Human Condition*. New York: Basic.
Laugier, Sandra. 2011. "Le *care* comme critique et comme féminisme." *Travail, Genre et sociétés* 26: 183–188.
Levinas, Emmanuel. 1987. "Meaning and Sense." In *Collected Philosophical Papers*, 75–109. Translated by Alphono Lingis. Dordrecht: Springer.
Lorenzini, Daniele. 2021a. "Passe sanitaire, gestes barrières: avons-nous basculé dans le 'biopouvoir'?" *Marianne*, 11 August.
Lorenzini, Daniele. 2021b. "Biopolitics in the Time of Coronavirus." *Critical Inquiry* 47(2): 40–45.
Mbembe, Achille. 2019. *Necropolitics*. Translated by Steven Corcoran. Durham, NC: Duke University Press.
Middelveen, Marianne J., Melissa C. Fesler, and Raphael B. Stricker. 2018. "History of Morgellons Disease: From Delusion to Definition." *Clinical, Cosmetic and Investigational Dermatology* 11: 71–90. https://www.ncbi.nlm.nih.gov/pmc/articles/PMC5811176/.
Mol, Annemarie. 2008. *The Logic of Care. Health and the Problem of Patient Choice*. London and New York: Routledge.
Novalis. 2007. *Notes for a Romantic Encyclopaedia: Das Allgemeine Brouillon*. Translated by David W. Wood. Albany: State University of New York Press.
Puig de la Bellacasa, María. 2017. *Matters of Care. Speculative Ethics in More Than Human Worlds*. Minneapolis: Minnesota University Press.
Sacks, Oliver. 1995. *Migraine. Revised and Expanded*. London: Picador.
Suaudeau, Julien, and Mame-Fatou Niang. 2022. *Universalisme*. Paris: Anamosa.
Sontag, Susan. 2003. *Regarding the Pain of Others*. New York: Farrar, Straus and Giroux.
Toombs, S. Kay. 1992. *The Meaning of Illness: A Phenomenological Account of the Different Perspectives of Physician and Patient*. Dordrecht: Kluwer.
Tronto, Joan C. 1993. *Moral Boundaries: A Political Argument for an Ethic of Care*. New York and London: Routledge.
Tronto, Joan C. 2015. *Who Cares? How to Reshape a Democratic Politics*. Ithaca, NY: Cornell University Press.
Tronto, Joan C. 2020. "Caring Democracy: How should Concepts Travel?" In *Care Ethics, Democratic Citizenship and the State*, edited by Petr Urban and Lizzy Ward, 181–197. Basingstoke: Palgrave Macmillan.

Vergès, Françoise. 2020. *Une théorie féministe de la violence. Pour une politique antiraciste de la protection*. Paris: La fabrique éditions.
Wasson, Sara. 2018. "Before Narrative: Episodic Reading and Representations of Chronic Pain." *Medical Humanities,* 44: 106–112.
Whitehead, Anne, and Angela Woods. 2016. "Introduction." In *The Edinburgh Companion to the Critical Medical Humanities*, edited by Anne Whitehead and Angela Woods, 1–31. Edinburgh: Edinburgh University Press.
Winckler, Martin. 1989. *La Vacation*. Paris: P.O.L.
Winckler, Martin. 1998. *La Maladie de Sachs*. Paris: Gallimard.
Winckler, Martin. 2004. *Les trois médecins*. Paris: P.O.L.
Winckler, Martin. 2009. *Le Chœur des femmes*. Paris: Gallimard.
Winckler, Martin. 2016. *Les Brutes en blanc*. Paris: Flammarion.
Winckler, Martin. 2019. *L'école des soignantes*. Paris: P.O.L.
Woods, Angela. 2011. "Post-Narrative – An Appeal." *Narrative Inquiry* 21(2): 399–406.
Woods, Angela, Akiko Hart, and Helen Spandler. 2022. "The Recovery Narrative: Politics and Possibilities of a Genre." *Culture, Medicine and Psychiatry* 46(2): 221–247.
Xun, Zhou, and Sander L. Gilman. 2021. *'I Know Who Caused COVID-19': Pandemics and Xenophobia*. Chicago, IL: Chicago University Press.
Žižek, Slavoj. 2008. *Violence. Six Sideways Reflections*. New York: Picador.

# Musing 1

## Narrative medicine, racial justice, and the Black maternal mortality crisis

*Mita Banerjee*

The present volume addresses a question which is perhaps one of the most difficult questions to ask in the domain of medicine. Are there instances in which the cure – or the attempt to cure – can itself become a form of violence? Or, asked differently, can there be at least implicit violence in some conceptions of cure? In this contribution, I would like to address three interrelated questions. First, I would like to interrogate the notion of medicine as 'colour blind' (Cunningham and Scarlato 2018; Williams 1998). Second, I look at the current Black maternal mortality crisis as one instance in which this ideal of medical colour blindness may actually turn out to have devastating consequences. Third, I propose that the methodology of narrative medicine, with its 'importing' of the practice of close reading taken from literary studies, may be one way of addressing issues of social and racial justice in the contemporary practice of US American medicine.[1]

The notion of universality, it could be argued, is at the core of the practice of medicine. Medicine, like the law (Crenshaw et al. 1996), needs to be colour blind. In order to be medical *care*, medicine needs to be universal; it must strive to cure human beings, regardless of their gender, race, or social status. What I would like to ask in this chapter, on the other hand, is whether there may be in fact a degree of violence in this universalist notion of medicine. This critique is in line with increasing debates on the notion of 'universalism' outside medicine as well (see Niang and Suaudeau 2022; Messling 2019).

I would like to talk about the particular instances where the notion of universal – and hence 'colour-blind' – medical care turned out to be devastating. In 2016, Kira Johnson was pregnant with her second child. She and her husband Charles already had a son, Charles Jr., and they were very much looking forward to their second child. On all counts, they were well prepared: they were highly educated, could afford good medical care, had had all the check-ups and prenatal care, and had made plans for the hospital in which Kira would give birth. At first, everything seemed to go well: Kira gave birth to their second son, Langston, a healthy baby boy. It was after the delivery that things began to go awry. Kira's husband Charles sensed that things were not going well, and that after the C-section something seemed to be off with his wife. He alerted the doctors, but they assured him that things were fine. It was here that the script of race began to kick in. Charles Johnson has said in retrospect that he tried to restrain himself, because he did not

DOI: 10.4324/9781032660165-2

want to fit the script of the angry Black man. He says that ever since, he has been asking himself whether things might have turned out differently – if his wife would have lived – had he and Kira been white.

Studies have shown that doctors tend to prescribe less pain medication for Black patients. Interns have stated that they feel that Black bodies are less susceptible to pain than white ones.

> In 2016, a study by researchers at the University of Virginia examined why African-American patients receive inadequate treatment for pain not only compared with white patients but also relative to World Health Organization guidelines. The study found that white medical students and residents often believed incorrect and sometimes "fantastical" biological fallacies about racial differences in patients. For example, many thought, falsely, that Blacks have less-sensitive nerve endings than whites, that Black people's blood coagulates more quickly and that Black skin is thicker than white. For these assumptions, researchers blamed not individual prejudice but deeply ingrained unconscious stereotypes about people of color, as well as physicians' difficulty in empathizing with patients whose experiences differ from their own.
>
> (Villarosa 2018, n.p.)

It must be noted in this context that as a practice, medicine is not aloof from social conditioning; it, too, is shaped by the society in which it is practised. One question that needs to be asked in this context is how the legacy of slavery, where Black women had no reproductive rights and where Black people were seen as non-human, has also impacted conceptions of 'Black pain' even to the present day.

How do race and narrative intersect here? At the centre of Charles and Kira's plight, there is the concept of narrative and there is the story of race. Two aspects are significant in this context. First, the question is whether race can affect the way in which doctors listen to a Black woman's story. It is in this context that, as a methodology attuned to the way that patients' stories are being listened to, narrative medicine may be crucial as an intervention. According to Rita Charon (2017, 8), the founder of Narrative Medicine, '*close reading* [is a] form of reading in which every word counts, in which no textual feature is squandered for its contribution to the meaning of the words'. Thus, 'honoring the stories of illness' (Charon 2006) means being able to listen to all the nuances inherent in the patient's story.

What may be even more important in this context is the fact that one of the express aims of narrative medicine is to enhance the self-reflexivity of medical practitioners. In other words, it wants to train healthcare providers to look at the way in which they 'read' (or listen to) their patients' stories. Over the last years, practitioners of narrative medicine have extended this question to include questions of racial and social justice. Rita Charon has described this development as follows:

> Narrative medicine began as a rigorous intellectual and clinical discipline to fortify healthcare with the capacity to skillfully receive the accounts persons

> give of themselves – to recognize, absorb, interpret, and be moved to action by the stories of others. It emerged to challenge a reductionist, fragmented medicine that holds little regard for the singular aspects of a patient's life and to protest social injustices of a global healthcare system that countenances tremendous health disparities and discriminatory policies and practices.
>
> (Charon et al. 2017, 1)

It is in this context that narrative medicine, as a practice of what Charon (2017, 8) calls 'close listening',[2] is especially well suited to detect moments of implicit bias. For the practice of healthcare, critics have spoken of the relationship between implicit bias and what is termed the 'racial empathy gap'. As Jason Silverstein suggests,

> Let's do a quick experiment. You watch a needle pierce someone's skin. Do you feel this person's pain? Does it matter if the person's skin is white or Black? For many people, race does matter, even if they don't know it. They feel more empathy when they see white skin pierced than Black. This is known as the racial empathy gap. [...] In this experiment, when viewers saw white people receiving a painful stimulus, they responded more dramatically than they did for Black people.
>
> (Silverstein 2013, n.p.)

What is so significant about the notion of implicit bias, moreover, is that this bias has been imbibed by all members of a given society; if there is implicit bias in the act of listening, then this means that it affects all of us, regardless of our own ethnic background. What is at stake here, then, is not simply a question of being White; rather, it is that implicit assumptions about Whiteness and Blackness may affect the ways in which we act.

One of the questions that has been central to Charles Johnson's account of his wife's pregnancy and post-natal care concerns precisely the act of listening, or rather the act of being listened to. If both he and Kira had been White, Charles Johnson has asked time and again, would doctors have listened differently when he told them that he feared that his wife was not recovering from childbirth? From Charles Johnson's perspective, it was clear that he felt constrained by the script of race, and by his own perception of how he might be perceived by others. As a White man, he noted, he would have allowed himself to be angry; but as a Black man, he felt that he should keep his feelings in check. When he finally got doctors to check on his wife, it was already too late. When they wheeled her back into the operating room hours after Langston's birth, Kira's medical team found that she had developed complications from the C-section, and they were ultimately unable to save her life. Charles Johnson has since founded the organization '4 Kira 4 Moms' and has tried to battle the Black maternal mortality crisis with his own testimony. The point that he has made in his campaign for racial and social justice is that Kira's death is part of a larger crisis in US healthcare.

In this crisis situation, Black women have found that their stories were not being listened to, or they were being listened to differently. People monetarily perked up when Serena Williams said in interviews that she almost died giving birth to her daughter Olympia (Ledbetter 2018). It was then that people began to say that if this could happen to Serena Williams, who by her own account had some of the best healthcare in the world, something had to be wrong with the American healthcare system. What emerges from this is a fundamental question: what is the relationship between medical care and social care? In other words, where does the story of medicine begin? It is here, I would argue, that the intervention of narrative medicine is key; these are precisely the questions that literary studies would ask. For the ways in which we interpret a story, it is of key significance just where the story opens. The emplotment, in other words, is not incidental but decisive to the meaning of the entire story. There may be one problem inherent in this 'literary' reading of the Black maternal mortality crisis, however. What I would like to suggest in bringing narrative medicine to an understanding of Black maternal mortality is by no means a flattening out of this major crisis in US healthcare today. Rather, following the tenets of narrative medicine, I am trying to ask how the questions asked by literary studies may be useful, in order to interrogate and enhance medical practice. That said, it is essential to acknowledge that the practice of medicine is infinitely more complex than reading a literary text, and the consequences of 'misreading' are incomparably graver.

These caveats notwithstanding, in trying to understand the Black maternal mortality crisis, it may be important to ask where the story begins. Studies have found that in a very specific sense, being Black in America already puts you at a higher health risk, since the effects of racism and the pressure of having constantly to perform are likely to raise your blood pressure, as are many other effects. As Joia Crear-Perry, an OB-GYN and founder of the National Birth Equity Collective, has noted in an interview,

> Part of the reason I'm doing this work, so I'm an OB-GYN by training, I also had a baby at 22 weeks when I was 25 years old, and my son, who is now 20, weighed 40–45 grams. So, part of this work and part of [...] what I understand now is that we cannot buy or educate our way out of having babies early as Black women, that our bodies are stressed. The stress of that while you are pregnant is compounded even more. We are built as a race to survive, to take care of yourself, so when you're pregnant and you have another body inside of you the stressors that come along with life build up on top of that and sometimes your body says, you are doing too much, Black woman, you need to relax, and so our body wants to live and we have our babies really early. That's a really simplified way of saying that the stress of being Black in America is one of the reasons why we have babies too early and they die too fast.
>
> (HealthIssues.org 2016, 00:03:02–00:04:00)[3]

What is at stake here is the notion of pre-existing conditions. This is what the nature of the twin pandemics of race and COVID-19 implies (Wegemer and von

Keyserlingk 2022). The COVID-19 pandemic has shown in blatant clarity that both pandemics are related: the pandemic of racism, given the pre-existing conditions it entails, put people at a higher risk of dying from COVID-19 (Bambra et al. 2020). The concept of the 'twin pandemics' may also be related to the Black maternal mortality crisis: here, too, pre-existing conditions may put Black women at a higher risk for pregnancy-related complications (Lister et al. 2019). What further exacerbates this situation is the question of economic disparity and uneven access to healthcare. The Black maternal mortality crisis is also made worse by the fact that, while Kira and Charles Johnson were able to choose and actually get to one of the best hospitals in the area, this may not be the case for the majority of Black women, or for other women of colour (Villarosa 2018).

How, then, may narrative medicine serve as an intervention here? The paradigm of narrative medicine would tell us that we need to 'honor the stories of illness', to use Rita Charon's words (2006). What this means is that we have to listen closely to all aspects of a patient's story. In the case of Kira Johnson, we would need to link a Black woman's social story to her medical narrative. Had her doctors factored in race as a social story, Kira Johnson might not have passed away: doctors might have been more sensitive to the way in which race affects both a Black woman's pregnancy – with the possibility of pre-existing conditions – and the way that they were listening to her story. In other words, if narrative medicine sets out to teach medical practitioners to interrogate and reflect critically on how they listen, Kira's doctors might have wondered whether, due to implicit bias, they were listening differently to Charles Johnson when he alerted them to the fact that his wife did not seem to be recovering from the C-section.

After his wife's death, Charles Johnson went on to tell his story to lawmakers across the country, eventually testifying before Congress with his own narration of the way that the colour blindness of medicine may ultimately have cost his wife's life. In order to achieve the eventual goal of colour blindness, he argued, medicine had to be colour-conscious first (Williams 1998). It had to look into how social difference might curb Black women's access to medical care. In a congressional hearing, Charles Johnson told his own story in these words:

> You know, this has been the most challenging experience [pauses] that I've… more challenging than anything I could even comprehend. That being said, the true blessing is the two tremendous gifts that Kira has left us, and that's my son Charles and my son Langston. They really are what keeps myself, my mother who's sitting right behind me, all of us going. And, you know, it's difficult as they mature and, as they now turned two and four, their ability to process and understand the absence of their mother evolves. And like I said, you know, you talk to a two-year-old, and he wants to know why his mommy is not coming home. And you explain to him, well, your mother's in heaven and she's doing important work with God. And he tells you, I want to go to heaven, too. There's nothing that I could prepare for, there's nothing that I can do, to fix that and I hope that over time – I'll be completely honest with you, it's… I'm proud to be here representing these families, but at the end of the day I'm just a father whose heart aches for his sons and a husband

> that misses his wife desperately. And every day I search for answers how to support these amazing gifts, what I am clear about is that what I have to do is that although there's nothing I can do to bring Kira back, I have to do anything that I can whenever I can to make sure I send other mothers home with their babies. If I can prevent another father from going through this, if I can prevent another child from having to understand why his mother isn't showing up at school. And I'll share this with the community, something I haven't even shared with my family, is when a three-year-old asks you, "Daddy, is mommy mad at me? I want mommy to come home. Why won't she come home?" And I've never shared that with anyone because it's just too painful for me to articulate, but I'm clear that the work we're doing here is going to prevent this continuing to happen to other women and it's going to make sure that other women get to go home with their babies.[4]
>
> (Subcommittee on Health 2018, 01:27:07–01:29:49)

In 2021, the US senate approved bill H.R. 3407, the so-called 'MOMMA's bill'. The bill was designed to allocate significant funding in order to look into maternal mortality and the possibility of racial bias in the US healthcare system. More explicitly, these are the central aims of the MOMMA's bill: 'The bill requires the Department of Health and Human Services to provide grants to all 50 states to establish state-based maternal mortality review committees to determine why women are dying from pregnancy-related deaths'.[5] Through the methodology of narrative medicine, the bill might well be said to engage in a practice of close reading: exploring the conditions under which non-White women may be listened to differently than White women in the context of maternal care. Where the bill was such a landslide victory is that it implicitly acknowledged that the ideal of colour blindness in American medicine may be just an ideal rather than a reality. Rather than simply dismissing Charles Johnson's story – and myriads of other stories very much like it – as an accident related to contingency in healthcare, the Senate acknowledged that it had to be colour-conscious first, that is, it had to listen specifically to the needs of Black women and other women of colour.

The story of Charles and Kira Johnson is thus not only an individual narrative. Rather, it is a question of how the story of medicine, because of the universalist tenets at its core, can shape the way in which healthcare providers may listen to some stories more closely than others. For Charles and Kira Johnson, this universalism resulted in the doctors' failure to listen to a story that was also related to race. What was at stake was not the violence of the cure but the colour blindness inherent in the notion of cure. However, this concept, which is at once medicine's ideal, turned out to be a form of violence, a failure to listen to a Black woman's story in the fullest sense.

In order to live up to its own ideal, medicine may need to interrogate its own universalism. The MOMMA's bill that Congress passed in 2021 may testify to the fact that in order to provide equal care for all, medicine needs to listen to social stories, not just to medical ones. It is in so doing that it may be self-reflective in the fullest sense of the term – it may look at itself not just as medical practice, but as social practice; and it may even be open to the fact that, because of implicit bias through the failure to listen to some stories as opposed to others, it may sometimes end up doing violence even when it intends to cure.

## Notes

1 In this contribution, I am specifically concerned with US healthcare. While this is not to suggest that these questions do not apply to healthcare systems elsewhere in the world, even if some of these issues may also be found in other national contexts, it is important to be context-specific because race (like other differences contributing to social inequality) is defined differently in different national imaginaries.
2 As Tina Campt has suggested, such forms of 'close listening' can also be applied to images. See her study on photography *Listening to Images* (2017).
3 Transcribed by the author.
4 Transcribed by the author.
5 Mothers and Offspring Mortality and Morbidity Awareness Act.

## References

Bambra, Clare, Ryan Riordan, Johan Ford and Fiona Matthews. 2020. "The Covid-19 Pandemic and Health Inequalities." *Journal of Epidemiology and Community Health* 74: 964–968.

Campt, Tina. 2017. *Listening to Images*. Durham, NC: Duke University Press.

Charon, Rita. 2006. *Narrative Medicine: Honoring the Stories of Illness*. Oxford: Oxford University Press.

Charon, Rita, Sayantani DasGupta, Nellie Herman, Craig Irvine, Eric R. Marcus, Edgar Rivera Colón, Danielle Spencer and Maura Spiegel. 2017. *The Principles and Practice of Narrative Medicine*. Oxford: Oxford University Press.

Charon, Rita. 2017. "Introduction." *The Principles and Practice of Narrative Medicine*, edited by Rita Charon, Sayantani DasGupta, Nellie Herman, Craig Irvine, Eric R. Marcus, Edgar Rivera Colón, Danielle Spencer and Maura Spiegel, 1–8. Oxford: Oxford University Press.

Crenshaw, Kimberlé, Neil Gotanda, Gary Peller and Kendall Thomas (eds.). 1996. *Critical Race Theory: The Key Writings that Formed the Movement*. New York: The New Press.

Cunningham, Brooke A., and Andre S. M. Scarlato. 9 August 2018. "Ensnared by Colorblindness: Discourse on Health Care Disparities." *Ethnicity & Disease* 28(Suppl 1): 235–240.

HealthIssues.org. 2016. "Dr. Joia Crear-Perry discusses the Crisis of the Black Maternal Mortality Rate in the US." 18 October. Accessed November 7, 2022. https://youtu.be/utHa0udAssQ.

Ledbetter, Carly. 2018. "Serena Williams: 'Doctors Aren't Listening' So Black Women Are Dying." *Huffington Post*, 8 May 2018. Accessed November 7, 2022. https://www.huffpost.com/entry/serena-williams-black-women-health-care_n_5aa156fce4b002df2c61c6aa.

Lister, Rolanda L et al. 2019. "Black Maternal Mortality-The Elephant in the Room." *World Journal of Gynecology & Womens Health* 3(1): 10.33552/wjgwh.2019.03.000555. https://doi.org/10.33552/wjgwh.2019.03.000555

Messling, Markus. 2019. *Universalität nach dem Universalismus. Über frankophone Literaturen der Gegenwart*. Berlin: Matthes & Seitz.

Niang, Mame-Fatou, and Julien Suaudeau. 2022. *Universalisme*. Paris: Anamosa.

Silverstein, Jason. 2013. "I Don't Feel Your Pain. A Failure of Empathy Perpetuates Racial Disparities." *Slate*, 27 June. https://slate.com/technology/2013/06/racial-empathy-gap-people-dont-perceive-pain-in-other-races.html.

Subcommittee on Health. 2018. "Hearing on 'Better Data and Better Outcomes: Reducing Maternal Mortality in the US'." 27 September. Accessed November 7, 2022. https://www.youtube.com/watch?v=-_5mw0w5lyY

Villarosa, Linda. 2018. "Why America's Black Mothers and Babies Are in a Life-or-Death Crisis." *New York Times Magazine,* 11 April 2018. https://www.nytimes.com/2018/04/11/magazine/black-mothers-babies-death-maternal-mortality.html.

Wegemer, Christoph, and Luise von Keyserlingk. 2022. "Dual Pandemics of COVID-19 and Systemic Racism: The Roles of Perceptions of Inequities, Civic Values, and Conservatism in Mask-Wearing Behavior." *Analyses of Social Issues and Public Policy* 22: 66–88.

Williams, Patricia. 1998. *Seeing a Color-Blind Future: The Paradox of Race*. New York: Farrar, Strauss and Giroux.

# Part 1

# Medical histories and biopolitics

# 1 Touching matters of care

## A visual approach to care and violence in Dr Marie Stopes' birth control campaign

*Nora Heidorn*

Care and violence can co-exist ambivalently, woven together in the same stories, objects, or personalities. I learnt this after setting out to find material things that speak to how the marker of race has historically impacted the broad field of sexual reproduction. I undertook this research as part of a practice-led PhD in collaboration with Birth Rites Collection, a unique contemporary art collection focused on the theme of childbirth. The British-based collection featuring international artists speaks to a range of experiences – mostly maternal – of fertility, pregnancy, birth, and parenthood. In my eyes, the interdisciplinary field of study and artistic work around sexual reproduction require an intersectional approach that goes beyond the traditional focus of white feminisms on gender. It is particularly crucial to address how other identity markers such as race, class, and ability impact experiences of sexual reproduction and healthcare provision in the wake of the MMBRACE studies of recent years, which consistently found staggeringly different rates of postpartum maternal mortality for Black, Asian, and white women in the UK's public health system (MMBRACE-UK 2019, 2020).

As a researcher and writer with a background in curating contemporary art, I knew that my inquiry would depart from existing material things that instruct and direct my learning about this field. An initial search for the terms 'reproduction' and 'race' in the online catalogue of the Wellcome Collection, an interdisciplinary gallery about health and medicine in London, returned an image of the 'Prorace' cervical cap, a barrier contraceptive from the 1920s (*'Prorace' cervical cap, England, 1915–1925* n.d.). The cap was trademarked by Dr Marie Stopes, instigator of the birth control movement in Britain, a feminist pioneer as well as an ardent eugenicist – hence the trademark 'Prorace'. Over the next months, this object taught me about the concomitance of care and violence.

The 'Prorace' cervical cap is a small, brown rubber object that is easily overlooked in its display case in the vast Medicine Galleries at the Science Museum in London, where many of the Wellcome Collection's holdings are on long-term loan (Figure 1.1). The mass-produced barrier contraceptive of rubber, used to cover the cervix to prevent pregnancy, is similar to the diaphragm.[1] Being aesthetically and materially rather uninteresting, the cap is not an obvious candidate for a research practice that works with visual and artistic strategies. And yet, the 'Prorace' cervical cap raises crucial questions about an eugenic agenda in a white

DOI: 10.4324/9781032660165-4

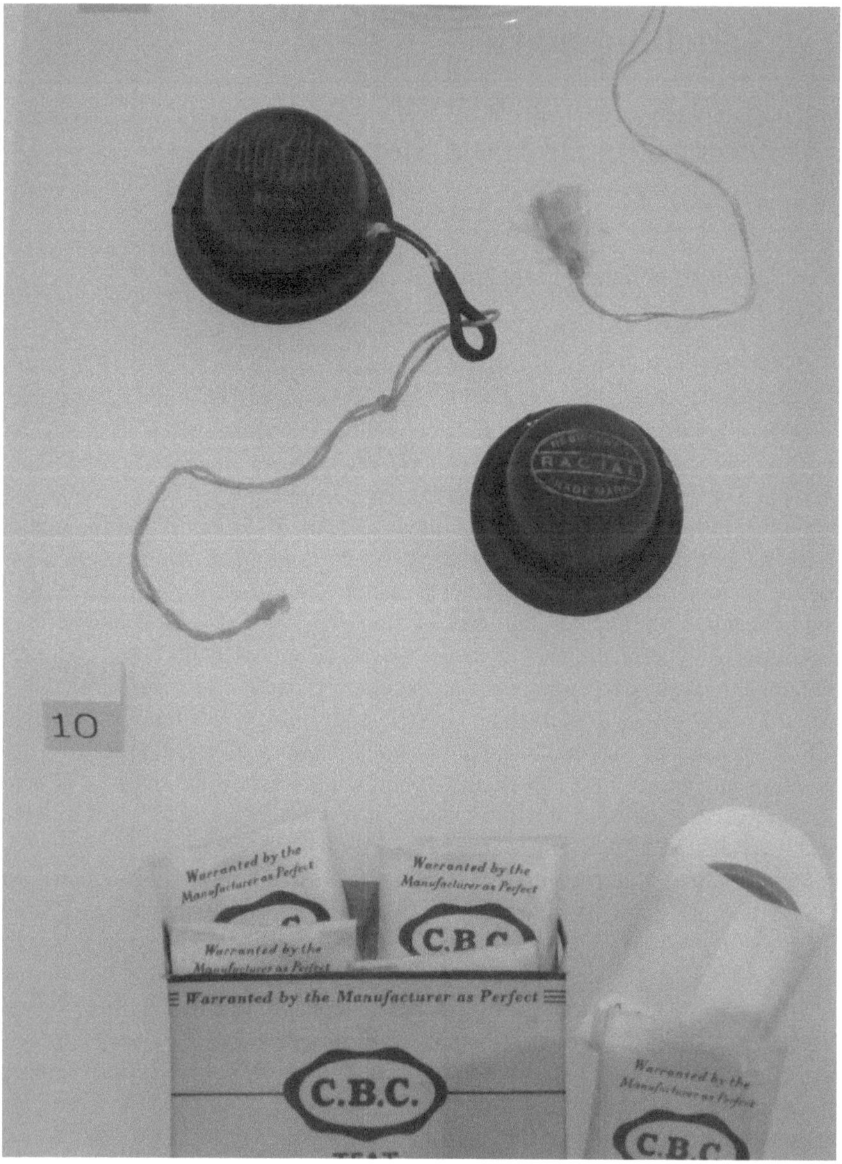


*Figure 1.1* 'Prorace' and 'Racial' brand cervical caps and condoms associated with Marie Stopes' Society for Constructive Birth Control (CBC) on display in the Medicine Galleries, Science Museum, London. Photograph by the author.

feminist struggle for reproductive healthcare and female sexual pleasure in Britain's burgeoning modernity, and more broadly, about how ideology is imbued in (healthcare) technologies.

My practice-research was concerned from the beginning with how to mediate the complexities of the 'Prorace' cap for other people: to ask questions about it, to start a discussion, and to encourage others beyond specialist circles care about it. Using artistic research methods and drawing upon new articulations of the experimental humanities and the critical medical humanities, I stage the 'Prorace' cap as a matter of care: a thing that exists in the world and requires critical and caring attention (Puig de la Bellacasa 2017).

Throughout this chapter, the reader will find short interjections taken from letters from working-class women and men all over the UK who wrote to Marie Stopes for advice on sexual health and contraception during the 1920s. I selected particularly poignant and emotive fragments from hundreds of letters collected in Ruth Hall's book *Dear Dr. Stopes: Sex in the 1920s* (1978).[2] These letters give a visceral sense of both public and intensely private conversations around sex, contraception, health, and maternity in 1920s Britain. They highlight that there was a desperate need for effective contraception and that access to reproductive healthcare was, above all else, a class issue.

This correspondence importantly shifts the attention from Stopes (whose complex personality and multiple feuds have fascinated biographers and preoccupied scholars) to the people who read her books and magazine columns, attended her clinics, wrote to her for advice, and were the (potential) users of the 'Prorace' contraceptives. These fragments are not used conventionally as primary sources within the academic argument; rather, they appear as glimpses of the lived realities of Stopes' working-class correspondents and contraceptive users. The letters are transcribed in Hall's book uncorrected, and I too transcribed these fragments as printed.

## Marie Stopes and the birth control campaign

Dr Marie Stopes was a highly educated upper-middle-class woman who began her birth control campaign after earning a PhD in palaeobotany. In 1918, she published the first of her books, the 'epoch-making marriage manual' *Married Love*, which was read across Britain and the Empire (Hall 1998, 108). Its practical sex instructions and insistence on female pleasure in marriage were ground-breaking. Stopes went on to found Britain's first birth control clinic in North London in 1921 and subsequently established a network of clinics across the UK through her Society for Constructive Birth Control and Racial Progress (Neushul 1998, 247). The clinics provided contraceptives and sexual health advice to married women of all classes.

*Your book came up for discussion in our psychology class and the Dr said it was a very good thing to have in the hands of Drs and Scientists but he strongly advised none of us to read it which of course made us all very keen*

The cervical cap was Stopes' contraceptive of choice, which was promoted throughout her birth control campaign and represents perhaps the most important material artefact remaining from her legacy. Stopes did not herself invent new methods of contraception but collected data about the efficacy of different contraceptives in her clinics and made improvements on the design of the cap. The cervical cap was an ancient method that the German gynaecologist F.A. Wilde had revived in the early nineteenth century (Neushul 1998, 255). The historian of science and technology Peter Neushul notes that users found the cervical cap difficult to use (in comparison with the more straightforward diaphragm), and that it required familiarity with the anatomy of the vulva and cervix, which many women lacked (Neushul 1998, 248, 252).

*I cannot understand how to place this cap inside to make it safe and firm fitting*

It is important to note that when Stopes first started, the medical professions in Britain and the USA had little knowledge of or interest in contraception, so she 'had no medical model on which to base her clinics and no established body of literature on birth control technology' to draw on (Neushul 1998, 247). The historian of medicine Claire Jones explains that at this time before WWII, 'the medical, charitable, and commercial sectors involved in birth control occupied the hinterland of respectability and the lines between business, charity work and medicine were often blurred' (Jones 2020, 9–10).

Throughout her campaign, Stopes emphasised the use of contraception as a modern and scientific solution to both personal and societal problems, advocating for 'joyous and deliberate motherhood' (Society for Constructive Birth Control and Racial Progress n.d.). She believed that access to contraception would make mothers happier and healthier, and improve marriage, childhood, and family life – strengthening the family as the integral unit of the nation. She made special efforts to reach working-class mothers, whom she believed needed access to contraception most, to limit their number of pregnancies for economic and health reasons.

*I am wonderfully surprised at the homely unobjectionable manner your pamphlet deals with the subject*

Today, Stopes is primarily known as a feminist pioneer whose work improved the reproductive choices of British women, but her campaign was also motivated by an eugenic agenda to improve the 'fitness' and genetic makeup of the population. Her eugenic beliefs are apparent in works such as *Wise Parenthood* (1918), where she introduces lay audiences to the 'racial and national necessity' of contraception for 'the greatest of the steps humanity can take in its next evolution' (Stopes 2007, 35). Here, she explains to married couples that 'the world needs the products of sound and beautiful love', but not 'children from unsound stock' (Stopes, 2007).

*I think that I have done my duty to my Country having had 13 children 9 boys and 4 girls and I have 6 boys alive now and a little girl*

Historian Philippa Levine explains that in the early twentieth century, 'anxieties over depopulation *and* overpopulation became associated with an eugenics movement concerned that the "wrong" people were reproducing most and that the quality of ruling elites might be degenerating' (Levine 2018, 490). Questions around the health, strength, and vigour of populations were tied to prevalent nationalist and colonial interests. Scientists became preoccupied with how states could manage the overall 'fitness' of their populations by applying 'scientific eugenics'. The discourse of population efficiency, which applied ideas and vocabularies from animal breeding, was also adopted by social reformers and birth control advocates, such as Stopes or the American family-planning campaigner Margaret Sanger (Wilmot 2018).

## 'Prorace': Branding, ideology, and biopolitics

Scholars working on Stopes often make clear that she was an eugenicist but focus their studies on a different aspect of her work. For example, Peter Neushul's paper examines the establishment of Stopes' clinics and her preference for the cervical cap over other contraceptive technologies, Claire Jones' book investigates the commercial aspects of the birth control movement, Paul Peppis' article is concerned with language and modernity in Stopes' writing, and Susanne Klausen's chapter studies Marie Stopes' influence across the British Empire, in particular in South Africa (Neushul 1998; Klausen 2002; Peppis 2014; Jones 2020). My research on the 'Prorace' cap, branded as it is with the eugenicist trademark, required a more in-depth study of Stopes' ideology and how she used the contraceptive as a means of disseminating her message alongside the more traditional communication channels of books, pamphlets, and advertising.

The 'Prorace' brand creates in the user's mind an immediate association between contraception and the theories of eugenics. Not only is the trademark stamped onto the dome of each cap as an ideological loading of the product, it can even be considered a very condensed instruction for users. I believe that Stopes intended it to act in a practical sense as a reminder, especially for women, of their responsibilities as reproducers, not just towards their own families but also as 'citizen-mothers' whose 'civic responsibilities were tied to motherhood' (Levine 2018, 496). The trademark was not only ideological but also pedagogical in function, much like Stopes' books, articles, and plays on sex, marriage, and contraception.[3]

## *I am under notice to leave my house owing to my large family*

As a white feminist living in Western Europe, I had no prior knowledge of a connection between feminist activism and eugenics in the early twentieth century. In fact, it seemed incongruous to me at first that this suffragette and advocate of female sexual pleasure was also an eugenicist. Writing about Stopes' American counterpart Margaret Sanger, historian of science Alison Bashford (2018, 507) clarifies that feminism and eugenics were not at odds: 'although often assessed as conflicting ideologies, feminism and eugenics [...] were easily and widely reconciled as programmes for progressive human transformation, at individual and population levels'. This agenda of 'progressive human transformation' also inspired Stopes' campaign and the trademark 'Prorace'.

Stopes' Society for Constructive Birth Control and Racial Progress used a birth control slogan that invoked the notion of race: 'JOYOUS AND DELIBERATE MOTHERHOOD – A SURE LIGHT IN OUR RACIAL DARKNESS' (Society for Constructive Birth Control and Racial Progress n.d.). The eugenic narrative lifted motherhood out of social and economic invisibility and from the private to the political realm, casting it as a noble task of crucial importance to the evolution of the human species. This slogan simultaneously idealises the mother figure and burdens her with the impossible responsibility of birthing and rearing ever more perfect and productive humans. The racially loaded metaphors of light and dark are employed to create a contrast between a bright, wholesome future for motherhood and the vague invocation of 'racial darkness', the perceived threat of population decline.

*if I have any more it might prove fatal my inside is quite exhausted*

Stopes set her ideal of an eugenic maternity being under the control of women against the harsh reality of involuntary motherhood, a common result of the lack of contraception and abortion care: 'Slave mothers have produced in the past, and are producing to-day, myriads of weak, inefficient, diseased and miserable lives' (Stopes 1925, 4). For her, it was evident that weary, overburdened, and poor mothers invariably produced wretched babies (whom she feared would have to be reared at the expense of taxpayers), not the 'splendid babies' that would advance 'the race' (Stopes 1925, 4). Through her promotion of the cervical cap prescribed in the vast majority of cases in her clinics and the emphasis on women and mothers in her propaganda, it becomes clear that Stopes saw that the responsibility for 'eugenic evolution' lay with women.[4]

*The health visitor was disgusted with me when I asked her about it ... she said it was very wrong to do any thing to stop yourselves from having children*

The 'Prorace' cervical cap was not only a technology to manage fertility. It was also intended as a biopolitical technology that would act on a population-wide scale. Like other technologies, it served users' needs but also shaped their subjectivities. The science historian Maria Rentetzi's (2011, 377) work shows how healthcare products can act as 'tools that discipline patients'. Furthermore, the philosopher Paul B. Preciado's (2013, 191–211) analysis of the contraceptive pill invented in the 1960s shows how contraceptives and pharmaceuticals can condition, choreograph, and even *produce* the very user they are designed to serve. Similarly to how the compliance package of the pill in the 1960s was designed to remind the user of her daily intake, the 'Prorace' cervical cap was intended to remind users in the 1920s and 1930s of their eugenic responsibilities to the nation. The eugenic trademark communicated to users that whether to have babies or not, and how many, were political choices tied to ideas of citizenship and anxieties around the strength of the nation state and Empire. Whether she is swallowing the pill or inserting a branded cervical cap into her vulva, the user literally internalises the loaded technology; she absorbs the object with its ideological dimension into her body. The cap, then, was a necessary cure to the problem of unwanted pregnancy – access to contraception is now a human right according to the United Nations charter – as well as an object inscribed with the violence of eugenic classism, racism, and ableism.

*Its wicked to bring children into the world to Practicly starve and be a burden to the ratepayers*

## Staging a matter of care

My work on the cervical cap as both a technological and visual artefact is informed by Dr Fiona Johnstone's Visual Medical Humanities, which embraces ambiguity and the suspension of certainty in the interdisciplinary field of the medical humanities. Johnstone (2018) writes that whilst ambiguity is 'often particularly evident in the case of the art object, it is also suggested by visual forms less obviously open to subjective interpretation, such as clinical objects, medical records or other purportedly documentary or evidentiary materials'. Taking inspiration from this approach and using photography, collage, and interactive digital design, I sought to develop a project that would stage the historical 'Prorace' contraceptive as a complex artefact, which sits ambiguously between feminist emancipation and the violence of eugenic ideology, between care and violence.

My thinking about the re-presentation of the 'Prorace' cap as a 'Matter of Care' is framed by María Puig de la Bellacasa's care ethics. Her 'Matters of Care' departs from Bruno Latour's concept of 'matters of concern', a philosophy of paying attention to the ethical and socio-political dimension of things often considered neutral, such as scientific findings or technologies (Puig de la Bellacasa 2017). Where Latour's being concerned can remain passive, Bellacasa calls for the more active verb 'to care'. She argues that caring for things (as a scholar, an activist, an artist, a consumer, etc.) requires us to *do* things: 'advocating for care complements the respect for things or Matters of Care with an ethical *doing*: the practical responsibility to take care…' (Puig de la Bellacasa 2011, 90). The Science and Technology Studies context of her care ethics is coherent with this investigation of the contraceptive cap, but all kinds of objects and artefacts – 'things' – could become Matters of Care through caring and critical attention to what they represent and what they do in the world.

*We would like a little pleasure out of life before it is too late*

With my background in curating contemporary art, it particularly struck me that Bellacasa uses the terms 'to stage', 'expose', 're-present', and 'exhibit' when describing what it takes to *make* Matters of Care (Puig de la Bellacasa 2017, 92, 94, 99). This vocabulary – borrowed from theatrical production and exhibition-making – implies that Matters of Care require being made public in considered ways. Taking care extends to re-presenting things 'in a way that makes others care for their existence' (Puig de la Bellacasa 2011, 91). This form of active responsibility was the practical task at hand: to stage the 'Prorace' cap beyond specialist discussions on the history of contraception or eugenics.

## Touch, proximity, and hygiene

The images of the 'Prorace' cap that have been made by the Science Museum and the Wellcome collection are uniform, professional, and purportedly neutral: the cap was always photographed sitting on its rim with the dome facing up, on its own in front of a grey or white background. In a 3D scan that is available on the Science Museum's website, it is set in empty black space like a lone planet in the universe (*'Prorace' cervical cap | Science Museum Group Collection*, n.d.). The more time I spent with these images of the cap, the more the neutral photographic backdrops and identical positioning of the object began to bother me – this standard museological professionalism seems to create a hygienic zone around the object that implies a matter-of-fact neutrality for the thing itself.

A similar effect is created by museum displays that group objects of the same kind. This taxonomising logic allows easy comparison but forecloses contact with other types of things and their meanings. I felt a desire to disturb the neutral emptiness around the 'Prorace' cap in the museum's photographs. Following this affect, I considered how I might visually put the object in contact with other things, complicating its representation and highlighting the contradictory ways in which it speaks to both care and violence. Would different images of the 'Prorace' cap prompt other people to care about this unattractive, easily overlooked thing enough to want to find out what it is, what it means?

*They told me I must have no more children, and yet when I ask them how I could prevent it they just shrug their shoulders and smile*

A different vitrine in the Medicine Galleries at the Science Museum is more interesting than the one holding my object of study. Its display combines a wooden model of a sailing ship, a yellow-and-black flag signalling quarantine, a respiratory mask used in plague times, and a full-body hazard suit used during the 2014 Ebola outbreak. Without purporting to be comprehensive or even geographically or temporally coherent, this assemblage tells stories about colonialism and trade, about contact and contamination, and about disease and the anxieties around purity I recognised from my research on eugenics in the early twentieth century (Figure 1.2).

After collecting materials on Stopes' clinics and the cervical cap in the Wellcome Library and photographing displays in the Science Museum, I began to combine these visual research materials by collaging. For example, the hazard suit with thick rubber gloves from the display reminded me of a guide I had been given in the Wellcome Library, which features photographs of archivists' hands in purple latex gloves, demonstrating how to handle rare books, photographs, and documents. I used these ready-made images of disembodied gloved hands to hold and handle other visual fragments in my research-collages.

Through this visual research practice, touch emerged as a strategy to at once highlight and disrupt the concept of hygiene that was so central to eugenic ideology. Irving Fisher, president of the Eugenics Research Association, explicitly made this connection in 1921:

> Hygiene and Eugenics should go hand in hand. They are really both hygiene – one individual hygiene and the other race hygiene – and both eugenics – one indirectly through safeguarding the quality of the germ plasm, and the other directly through breeding.
>
> (Cogdell 2004, 188)

*It is through my weakness of body that I become pregnant every single time we submit to Marital Rights*

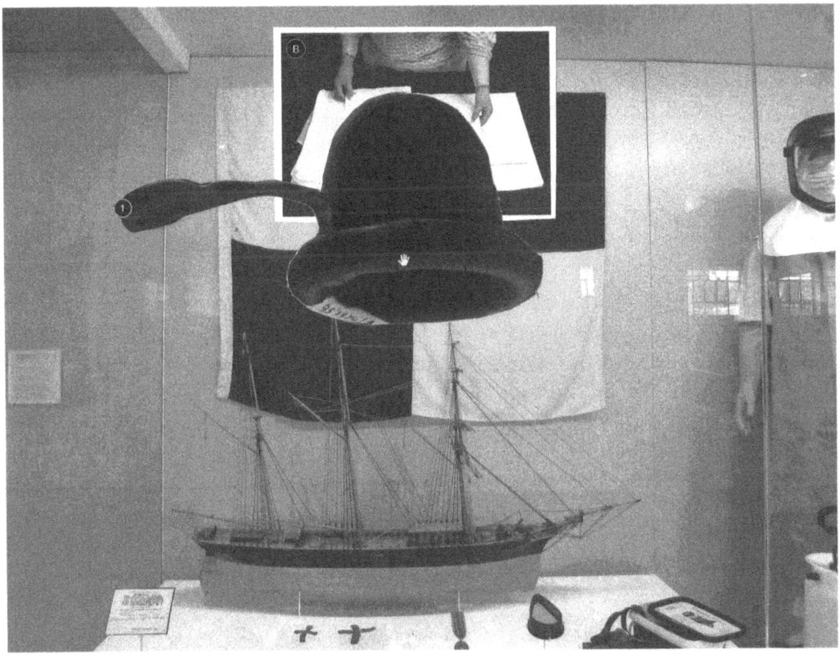

*Figure 1.2* Nora Heidorn, research-collage, 2021.

Anxieties about contact and contagion were in the air during my work on this project – after all, it began during the COVID-19 pandemic. Through the protocols that regulate touch, symbolised by latex gloves, I was able to create a visual link between the clinical spaces of Stopes' birth control centres and the places in which I encountered what was left of them: the museum and the archive. The gloved archivists' hands in my research-collages came to stand for the practical *doings* that it takes to make Matters of Care, a purposeful recontextualising to make things matter to others.

The emphasis of the resulting research-collages on the haptics of archival work echoes my desire to metaphorically touch my research object through my work, to reach for what the artist Onyeka Igwe describes as 'critical proximity' with the object and its associated archives, to become involved with it rather than to study it from a supposedly objective distance, and to embrace the partiality of the research and allow the knowledges of affect and instinct to guide this process (Igwe 2020).

*You can imagine my horror when I felt a movement in the body*

It was important to me that the visual re-presentation of the object should not resolve its complex relationship to care/violence and emancipation/oppression. It should not instruct the viewer in what to think about the 'Prorace' cap or Stopes' legacy but rather propose them as questions to critically consider and care about in the first place.

## Touching matters of care

Following an invitation from Birth Rites Collection as part of their initiative to commission digital works, I made the interactive digital project *Touching Matters of Care ('Prorace' cervical cap, 1915–1920)* that is freely available to use online.[5] It appropriates the Science Museum's 3D scan of the 'Prorace' cervical cap to stage this object and its attendant history of eugenic feminism as a Matter of Care, a complex thing that speaks of both care and violence, requiring our careful attention.

> *My husband who is a Catholic does not believe in stopping life by any means when I say I do not want any more he gets very nasty with me*

Working with the 3D scan of the cap was a natural choice since this online resource was how I had initially approached the object. I began this research in late 2020 during the COVID-19 pandemic, when the Science Museum, where it is on display, was closed. When the museum reopened, it was not possible for me to travel to the UK with any guarantee that I would be able to return home. During this period, my engagement with my research object was purely virtual, which initially seemed like a disadvantage. However, I soon realised that the touch simulated by the interactivity of the 3D scan allowed me a proximity to the object that I did not have when I observed it in its vitrine in the museum.

Moreover, navigating the 3D scan allows for a playful manipulation of the object, such as by flipping and spinning it. Touching or moving the object around would, of course, not be possible at the museum, where artefacts are only handled by certain staff under controlled conditions for reasons of conservation. The interactive digital work thus acts as an invitation for others to become proximate to the 'Prorace' cap by digitally handling it. One is invited to touch, spin, swivel, and flip it, with the movement mediated by the mouse, touchpad, or touchscreen of one's device (Figure 1.3).

*Figure 1.3* Scan this QR code to enter *Touching Matters of Care ('Prorace' cervical cap, 1915–20)*, interactive digital object, 2022. It may take a few seconds to load.

## *I really cant give the children all they should have to make them fine and Healthy*

When thinking about how to respond to Birth Rites Collection's commission, I initially worried about highlighting the 'Prorace' cap online, as it is a context where I would have less control over its reception, mediation, and dissemination than in a gallery setting. What if the wrong crowd became interested in the work for the wrong reasons? To my relief, this has not happened since the project has been available online. I decided to proceed with making the project when I realised that, obviously, photographs and the 3D scan of the 'Prorace' cap were already in the public sphere on the Wellcome Collection's and Science Museum's websites. My intervention is not one of making-public; rather, it proposes a different experience of the object online, another type of encounter. Whilst both museum catalogues present it with a one-paragraph blurb in a very matter-of-fact manner, I wanted to provide more context and highlight the complexities of the object, to make it a Matter of Care in a way that both institutions had not (*'Prorace' cervical cap | Science Museum Group Collection*, n.d.; *'Prorace' cervical cap, England, 1915–1920*, n.d.).

I made three interventions on the original 3D scan, which were executed by the creative technologist Jinia Tasnin: first, the arrow pointer indicating the cursor location was replaced with a humanoid hand covered by a latex glove, a nod to the hygienic protocols of both the clinic and the archive (see Figure 1.4). Through digitally mediated touch, the user can explore the 'Prorace' cap playfully, but they also come into a direct contact that somewhat implicates them. The playfulness that the digital work invites is intended to create interest, engagement, and (quite possibly) an uncomfortable proximity between users and the object. I hope that this

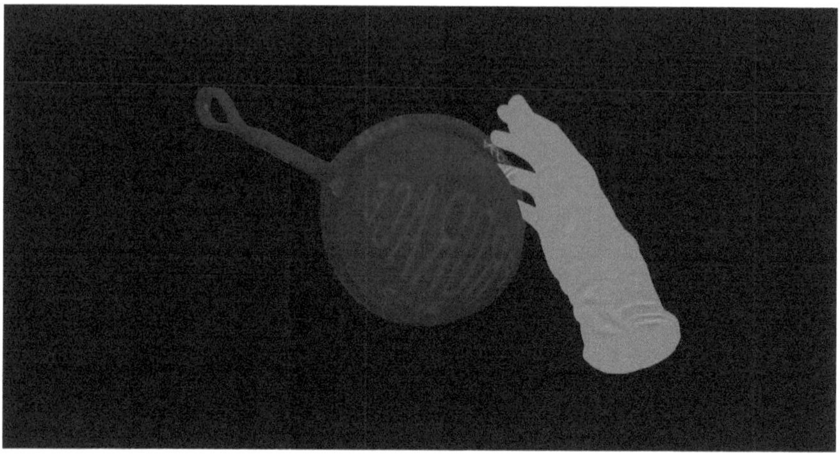

*Figure 1.4* Still from Nora Heidorn, *Touching Matters of Care ('Prorace' cervical cap, 1915–20),* digital object, 2022. Courtesy of Birth Rites Collection.

contact will lead to critical questioning of the meanings of this historical artefact. From my perspective, the exploratory character of the engagement does not negate the seriousness of the cap's entanglement with eugenics. Instead, it is designed to lower the threshold for engaging with that very history.

*I feel it a great injustice and unchristian like to think that rich women should have this knowledge and a poor woman should live in ignorance of it*

My second intervention is a backdrop that appears at certain viewing angles, filling the empty black space (Figure 1.5). The plane behind the cap creates spatial depth and a theatrical effect, reminiscent of a stage set. It is covered in historical anatomical drawings: pelvic bones, pregnant bellies, skin peeled back to reveal the reproductive anatomy. As previously mentioned, in every image of the 'Prorace' cap I found, it is shown sitting on its rim, with the dome and logo facing up (Figure 1.6). But within the anatomy of the vulva that it was designed for, the cap would be the other way around: the shape of a cup rather than a dome. In fact, the

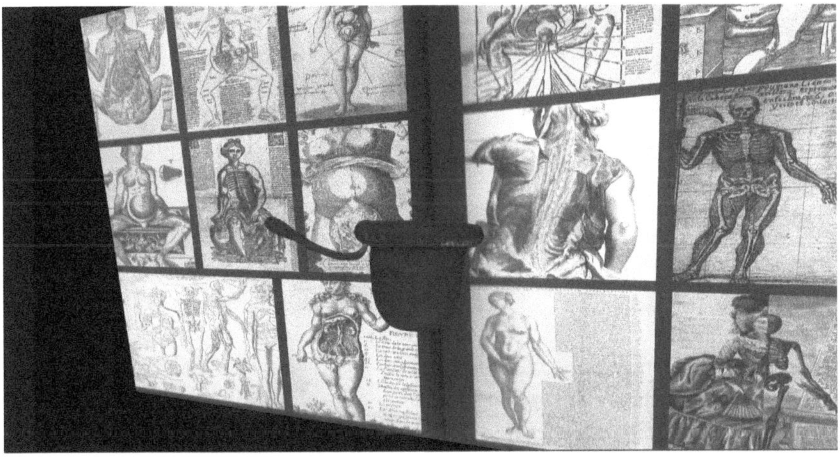

*Figure 1.5* Still from Nora Heidorn, *Touching Matters of Care ('Prorace' cervical cap, 1915–20),* digital object, 2022. Courtesy of Birth Rites Collection.

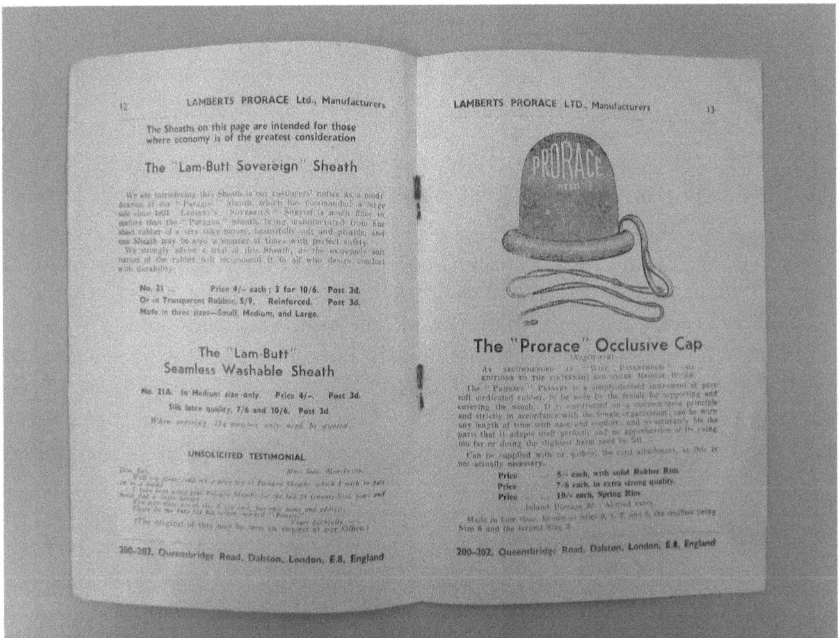


*Figure 1.6* Latest price list of approved contraceptive appliances. Lamberts Prorace Ltd, 1946. Accessed at the Wellcome Library, London. Photograph by the author.

standard representations of the contraceptive, from 1920s sales pamphlets to contemporary photographs and displays made by the museum, abstract the object from its relationship with the user's body. Within the 3D space, the user can flip the cap into its functional position inside the body. The anatomical apparitions make an explicit link between the brown dome and reproductive bodies.

My third intervention is to embed on the web page that hosts the digital project fragments of letters from people across the UK who wrote to Marie Stopes for advice on sexual health and contraception. Some of these fragments have appeared in the margins of this chapter, and I have contextualised them in the introduction. In relation to the digital work, I included them because for me, reading Ruth Hall's book of compiled letters and leafing through some of them in the archive boxes at the Wellcome Library gave me a much more well-rounded understanding of the meanings of contraception for people in the 1920s and 1930s.

*I do not like to be used for his pleasure and then abused when I am pregnant*

The letters taught me that, in particular for working-class and poor people in Britain, the availability of modern contraceptive technologies was intimately connected to many aspects of their lives. Apart from the obvious domain of sexuality, relationships, and family planning, the (lack of) availability of contraception was brought into relation by the many writers with precarious socio-economic situations (income, housing, mobility, healthcare), with spiritual, moral, and religious considerations, and with the unique and embodied experiences that shaped their lives (disability or ill health, or specific issues and situations in their families or marriages). My insights gained from these most intimate letters crucially contributed an affective and embodied dimension to my research about the 'Prorace' cap and eugenic feminism in the early twentieth century. It is this dimension of the discussions around contraception that I hope to convey, at least a little, through the letter fragments in the margins.

## Becoming affected

I chose to work on the 'Prorace' cap due to its complexity: the object speaks ambiguously to both care *and* violence, to emancipation *and* oppression, in experiences of sexuality and reproduction. It acts as a nexus from which to unpack histories spanning reproductive healthcare, feminism, eugenics, and social conditions, and how these specifically affected women, in 1920s Britain. The interactive digital work *Touching Matters of Care ('Prorace' cervical cap, 1915–20)* invites the user to explore the stories that the object holds.

*I have had 9 and 6 are boys, I don't think I have done so bad*

Rather than presenting a single, authoritative interpretation of the 'Prorace' cap, I employ artistic research to contribute to making it a Matter of Care: a thing that we should consider with critical attention. Avoiding a didactic mode typical of interactive museum screens, this project hopes to engage users to grapple with the historic object's entanglements.

Touch is both a method and a metaphor in this work, which complicates the representations of the 'Prorace' cap and questions Marie Stopes' legacy. The imagery of gloved hands refers to eugenic anxieties about the contamination of individual bodies and populations through sexual reproduction. Touch and its attendant risk of contamination resist the eugenic obsession with hygiene.

This practice of researching/touching/writing/image-making hopes to, as Puig de la Bellacasa (2011, 98) writes, 'trouble the critical distance typical of scholarly work' in order to 'transform the affective charge of things, challenging our relationship with the 'objects' of research'. It is about 'transforming things into matters of care [as] a way of relating to them, of inevitably becoming affected by them, and of modifying their potential to affect others' (Puig de la Bellacasa 2011, 99).

*To the men who condemn you, I would like to give one month as a mother in a working man's home... You wouldn't have an enemy, they would all commit suicide*

With this interactive work and other forms of public engagement with my research, I test artistic research methodologies in the emerging field of the experimental humanities and perform a translation and re-presentation of the 'Prorace' cap between different disciplines and bodies of knowledge. By addressing the uncomfortable history of 'eugenic feminism', this project also performs a caring critique of white feminist legacies. More widely, it aims to challenge the feminism of the 'art of birth' (Winant 2016), which is deeply focused on questions of gender and reproductive labour, to think more intersectionally about how race, class, and ability impact experiences of sexual reproduction.

## Acknowledgements

*Touching Matters of Care ('Prorace' cervical cap, 1915–1920)* was commissioned in 2022 by Birth Rites Collection with support from Arts Council England, and it was made with creative technologist Jinia Tasnin. It was developed out of my Collaborative Doctoral Award at the Royal College of Art, funded by the London Arts and Humanities Partnership. The original 3D scan of the 'Prorace' cap was produced by the Science Museum, London, where the object is on display. The cap is owned by the Wellcome Collection, London. With thanks to Helen Knowles and Hermione Wiltshire for encouraging and accompanying this project and to Gemma Blackshaw for her critical-caring comments on this chapter.

## Notes

1 Whilst the diaphragm is wider, the cervical cap fits snugly around the cervix. It is slightly more difficult to place in exactly the correct position to effectively prevent pregnancy, which is one of the reasons it is no longer commonly in use.
2 The letters are referenced in a separate index after the bibliography for this chapter.
3 For an analysis of Stopes' 'explicitly pedagogic' plays, see Freshwater (2009, 36).
4 Other methods of contraception, such as condoms and sponges, were also available. Stopes tended to only recommend the use of condoms—a male method of contraception—if she suspected venereal disease. The less effective sponges were given to the poorest of women, who could not afford the cap. See Stopes (1925); Neushul (1998, 254–256).
5 The interactive digital work was turned into an NFT (non-fungible token) on the Ethereum blockchain by the Birth Rites Collection. It is available for sale on an NFT platform, but it can be accessed and used online without the need to purchase it. The Birth Rites Collection's NFT commissioning programme comes out of its 2021 Blockchain Feasibility Study. Commercial and environmental aspects of the NFT technology are important to consider but beyond the scope of this article. Any proceeds from sales are shared between the Birth Rites Collection, myself, and the British charity Black Mothers Matter. For further information, see Birth Rites Collection (2022).

## References

Bashford, Alison. 2018. "World Population from Eugenics to Climate Change." In *Reproduction: Antiquity to the Present Day*, edited by Nick Hopwood, Rebecca Flemming, and Lauren Kassell, 505–520. Cambridge: Cambridge University Press.

Birth Rites Collection. 2022. "Blockchain Feasibility Study and NFTs." https://www.birthritescollection.org.uk/noraheidorn.

Cogdell, Christina. 2004. *Eugenic Design: Streamlining America in the 1930s*. Philadelphia: University of Pennsylvania Press.

Freshwater, Helen. 2009. "The Representation of Reproduction: Marie Stopes and the Female Body." In *Theatre Censorship in Britain: Silencing, Censure and Suppression*, 35–48. Basingstoke and New York: Palgrave Macmillan.

Hall, Lesley. 1998. "Heterosexuality, Marriage and Sex Manuals." In *Sexology Uncensored: the Documents of Sexual Science*, edited by Lucy Bland and Laura Doan, 107–108. Cambridge: Polity Press.

Hall, Ruth (ed.). 1978. *Dear Dr. Stopes: Sex in the 1920s*. London: Andre Deutsch.

Igwe, Onyeka. 2020. "Being Close to, With or Amongst." *Feminist Review* 125(1): 44–53.

Johnstone, Fiona. 2018. "Manifesto for a Visual Medical Humanities." *Medical Humanities*, 31 July. Accessed October 22, 2020. https://blogs.bmj.com/medical-humanities/2018/07/31/manifesto-for-a-visual-medical-humanities/.

Jones, Claire L. 2020. *The Business of Birth Control: Contraception and Commerce in Britain before the Sexual Revolution*. Manchester: Manchester University Press.

Klausen, Susanne. 2002. "The Imperial Mother of Birth Control: Marie Stopes and the South African Birth-Control Movement, 1930–1950." In *Colonialism and the Modern World: Selected Studies*, edited by Ralph C. Croizier, Martin P. Bunton, and Gregory Blue, 182–199. Armonk, NY and London: Sharpe.

Levine, Philippa. 2018. "Imperial Encounters." In *Reproduction: Antiquity to the Present Day*, edited by Nick Hopwood, Rebecca Flemming, and Lauren Kassell, 361–374. Cambridge: Cambridge University Press.

MMBRACE-UK. 2019. "MBRRACE-UK 2019: Mothers and Babies: Reducing Risk through Audits and Confidential Enquires Across the UK 2015–17." The National Perinatal Epidemiology Unit. https://www.npeu.ox.ac.uk/mbrrace-uk/reports.

MMBRACE-UK. 2020. "MBRRACE-UK 2020: Saving Lives, Improving Mothers' Care - Executive Summary." The National Perinatal Epidemiology Unit. https://www.npeu.ox.ac.uk/mbrrace-uk/reports.

Neushul, Peter. 1998. "Marie C. Stopes and the Popularization of Birth Control Technology." *Technology and Culture* 39(2): 245–272.

Peppis, Paul. 2014. "Rewriting Sex: Sexology and Sentimental Modernism in Marie Stopes's Married love and Mina Loy's Songs to Joannes." In *Sciences of Modernism: Ethnography, Sexology, and Psychology*, 148–194. Cambridge: Cambridge University Press.

Preciado, Paul B. 2013. *Testo Junkie. Sex, Drugs, and Biopolitics in the Pharmacopornographic Era*. New York: The Feminist Press.

*"Prorace" cervical cap | Science Museum Group Collection*. n.d. *Science Museum Group*. Accessed January 27, 2022. https://collection.sciencemuseumgroup.org.uk/objects/co96336/prorace-cervical-cap-cervical-cap.

*"Prorace" cervical cap, England, 1915–1925*. n.d. *Wellcome Collection*. Accessed March 2, 2023. https://wellcomecollection.org/works/ee34g3fr.

Puig de la Bellacasa, María. 2011. "Matters of Care in Technoscience: Assembling Neglected Things." *Social Studies of Science* 41(1): 85–106.

Puig de la Bellacasa, María. 2017. *Matters of Care: Speculative Ethics in More Than Human Worlds*. Minneapolis: University of Minnesota Press.

Rentetzi, Maria. 2011. "Packaging Radium, Selling Science: Boxes, Bottles and Other Mundane Things in the World of Science." *Annals of Science* 68(3): 375–399.

Society for Constructive Birth Control and Racial Progress. n.d. "The Mothers' Clinic for Constructive Birth Control."

Stopes, Marie Carmichael. 1925. *"The First Five Thousand": Being the First Report of the First Birth Control Clinic in the British Empire, "The Mother's Clinic' for Constructive Birth Control*. London: J. Bale, Sons, & Danielsson, Ltd.

Stopes, Marie Carmichael. 2007. "Wise Parenthood" (1918). In *Marie Stopes: Feminist, Eroticist, Eugenicist: Essential Writings*, edited by William Garrett, 33–48. San Francisco, CA: Kenon Books.

Wilmot, Sarah. 2018. "Breeding Farm Animals and Humans." In *Reproduction: Antiquity to the Present Day*, edited by Nick Hopwood, Rebecca Flemming, and Lauren Kassell, 397–412. Cambridge: Cambridge University Press.

Winant, Carmen. 2016. "The Art of Birth." *Contemporary Art Review LA*, 21 July, 5: 9–12.

***Index of fragments from letters to Stopes***

The fragmentary interjections throughout this chapter are taken from letters sent to Marie Stopes and her clinics. They were collected in *Dear Dr Stopes: Sex in the 1920s*, edited by Ruth Hall (1978). In the index below, the page number on the left refers to the page in this chapter, followed by the initials of the sender's name, the year the letter was written, and the place from which it was sent. This information is not available for some of the letters, which were taken from a compilation of correspondence from working-class women requesting help, published by Stopes in 1926 under the title *Mother England*. Stopes did not include any identifiers about the senders. The bracketed number on the far right of each line refers to the page number in Hall's book where the letter appears.

p. 29 Mrs L, 1923, Kettering (25)
p. 30 Mrs M, 1923, Stockport (25)
p. 31 Mr GC, 1926, Northumberland (30)
p. 31 Mrs RGH, 1921, South Wales (17–18)
p. 32 Mr LE, 1924, Surrey (27)
p. 33 Mrs NG, 1922, London (19)
p. 33 Sender not identified (41)
p. 34 Mrs NG, 1922, London (19)
p. 35 Mrs BR, 1923, Kent (22)
p. 36 Sender not identified (42)
p. 36 Sender not identified (40)
p. 37 Sender not identified (38)
p. 38 Sender not identified (41)
p. 39 Sender not identified (40)
p. 40 Mrs GA, 1923, London (20)
p. 42 Mrs SE, 1921, Norfolk (19)
p. 43 Sender not identified (40)
p. 44 Mrs RM, 1923, Bolton (21)

# 2 Politics in the time of cholera

## COVID, table manners, and bio-politics

*Federico Dal Bo*

The 2020-2023 global COVID-19 pandemic has profoundly influenced – I cannot think of a more appropriate idiom – international political discourse. Political power has increasingly been measured in terms of the ability of states to exercise social control over the lives of citizens, their bodies, and their biology. In other words, the pandemic has had an impact on political discourse, demonstrating how contemporary sovereignty has tended to be defined in strongly biopolitical terms. This complex intersection between politics and biology has sometimes resulted in a discriminatory language propagated by mass media and social media – television, Twitter, and Facebook.

This was particularly the case with some Italian, US, and Israeli politicians who initially reacted to the emerging pandemic in racist and conspiratorial, but also messianic terms. Some indulged in racism, using the pandemic as an opportunity to discriminate against all those who were supposedly alien to civilisation: the Chinese, the Democrats, and the Jews. In their monograph *'I Know Who Caused COVID-19': Pandemics and Xenophobia* (2021), Zhou Xun and Sander L. Gilman have shown that the act of blaming people for COVID-19 reinforced the boundaries between collective social groups and their respective minorities, such as the Chinese, ultra-orthodox Jewish communities, African Americans, British blacks, Asians, and so on. The discourse used during the COVID-19 pandemic was similar to that used in the past, when disease was often used as an excuse to reinforce hegemony and discrimination. In this way, societal divisions based on racial, class, sexual, ethnic, religious, national, or political identity were reinforced, and animosities between groups already labelled as 'different' in terms of hegemonic patterns were intensified (Xun and Gilman 2021). Surprisingly, as I will discuss in detail later in this chapter, this attitude has not even spared prominent progressive intellectuals – such as the famous Italian philosopher Giorgio Agamben (Salzani, forthcoming 2025) – who were misinformed and then astonishingly indulged in stereotypes when they also argued against state intervention in matters of public health. In this respect, the COVID-19 pandemic has demonstrated once again that public health is never a neutral matter of well-being but instead mobilises several political tropes:

> In the current pandemic, public health scientists often make the claim that their science is not politics but of course it always is. For public health is

DOI: 10.4324/9781032660165-5

> by definition a translational field, not from laboratory to clinic, but from laboratory or fieldwork to policy. The consequences of all policy in a pandemic/epidemic are political, beyond the field of science, as they rest upon the presuppositions of the society in which such claims are made.
>
> (Xun and Gilman 2021, 41)

In this chapter, I will examine some racist remarks made by a centre-right Italian politician who argued that an alleged lack of hygiene among the Chinese people was the real cause of the pandemic. I will then elaborate on the underlying 'Orientalist' stereotypes and examine their deeper ramifications in contemporary political discourse in Italy, the United States, and Israel. In particular, I will argue that the pandemic has provided an opportunity to mobilise several bio-political issues that are not necessarily progressive but can be discriminatory, if not reactionary. The pandemic has also shown that bio-politics is ambivalent, appealing to both the right and the left. Therefore, its ambiguous nature should be taken into account while engaging in rigorous critical thinking.

## 'Of mice and men': A bio-political concern regarding public health

During the first weeks of the COVID-19 pandemic in Italy, the centre-right Italian politician Luca Zaia, in his capacity as president of the Venetia region, was interviewed during a live television broadcast on the regional channel Antenna 3-Nord Est (Zaia 2020). At the time, Zaia was still convinced that the pandemic would ultimately spare Italy in general and Venetia in particular. Zaia argued in exquisite biopolitical terms, claiming that the Italian people adhered to higher hygienic and culinary standards than the Chinese. Somehow inspired by his own nationalistic fervour, Zaia went so far as to make a singular claim:

> Do you know why, after one week, we have [only] 116 positives [for coronavirus], of which 63 have no symptoms, and we have only 28 [sick people] in hospital? Do you know why? Because the hygiene that our people, the Venetians [and] Italian citizens have, the cultural education (*formazione culturale*) that we have, is to shower, to wash, to wash our hands often, a regime of personal cleanliness (*un regime di pulizia personale*) that is particular… even the diet, the cleanliness, the hygiene standards, the fridge, the expiration dates of food… You say, but what does that have to do with it all? It has something to do with it because it is a cultural thing (*un fatto culturale*). I think [that] China has paid a lot (*abbia pagato un grande conto*) for this epidemic they have had, because we have all seen them eating live mice (*mangiare topi vivi*) or other things like that. You know, it's also an incidental fact (*un fatto di corredo*), isn't it? Because the virus doesn't have to find an environment that becomes a substrate (*un sostrato*) The virus has to find cleanliness (*pulizia*), almost like in a hospital. We are a bit manic (*maniaci*) about this.
>
> (Zaia 2020, 00:04–01:02)[1]

Zaia's argument is quite elementary and follows some typical traits of traditional Orientalism. On the one hand, there are 'the Venetians [and] the Italians', who adhere to a political 'regime' and specific hygienic and culinary habits; on the other hand, there is 'China', which has 'paid dearly' for the chaos caused by the lack of 'cultural education' or, rather, by a specific 'cultural fact' that leads it to indulge in abhorrent culinary practices – 'eating live mice'. This lack of hygiene is described, with a kind of Aristotelian twist, as a 'substrate' for the spread of disease. I will return to this point later. For now, it is sufficient to highlight the key words used by Zaia in his interview: 'hygiene', 'regimen', 'culture', 'education', 'raw', 'substrate', and 'cleanliness'. Taken together, these are a series of concepts that are mobilised to construct a specific biopolitical texture: the pandemic is not simply a biological reality, but it is fuelled by a lack of hygiene, marking a poor level of civilisation.

Zaia's comments caused a great deal of international outrage. Newspapers, television programmes, and social media have harshly critiqued his words. Zaia was urged to retract his statement, and he said he had been misunderstood. The Embassy of the People's Republic of China reacted with great composure, praising the help of the Italian people during the emergency, without mentioning Zaia by name:

> At a crucial time like this, when China and Italy are facing the epidemic side by side, an Italian politician has not refrained from slandering the Chinese people. These are gratuitous slanders that leave us astonished. We are comforted by the fact that many Italian friends disagree with such remarks and even strongly criticise them. We are convinced that the words of a single politician in no way represent the common feeling of the Italian people, a civilised people and our friend. The new coronavirus is a common enemy that requires a common response. In such a difficult moment, it is necessary to put aside arrogance and prejudice and to strengthen understanding and cooperation in order to protect the common safety and health of all humanity.
>
> (Ambasciata della Repubblica Popolare Cinese 2020)

This brief exchange does not, however, exhaust the biopolitical issue that was inadvertently and recklessly introduced by Zaia. On the contrary, it is further complicated by an additional, no less astonishing statement. A few months before this interview, Zaia had published a post on his official Facebook page about a famine that struck the northern parts of Venice in 1917 – also known in Venetian as *l'an de la fam*, 'the year of the famine'. Zaia also commemorated the event with a photo – an 'extraordinary image' – of several dead rats hung out to dry:

> Rats left to dry in Belluno during 'l'an de la fam', the year of hunger. This extraordinary image, together with many others, is on display in the extraordinary documentary, iconographic and multimedia exhibition on Belluno during the First World War, which has just been inaugurated at Palazzo Crepadona.
>
> (Zaia 2018)[2]

At first sight, it is surprising, if not contradictory, that Zaia should praise the consumption of dried rats in Italy during the First World War while at the same time stigmatising the use of live mice in Chinese cuisine. Interestingly, no one bothered to check whether Chinese cuisine indeed includes a dish with live mice, probably because it could be argued that this question would be offensive in itself. How could anyone believe that such an ancient and civilised people as the Chinese could eat live mice? The question itself was self-explanatory: civilised people would never do such a thing, unless they were in a state of emergency, such as during a famine. Besides, even the 'civilised' Italians did it during the famine of 1917.

## 'The raw and the cooked': A question of civilisation

The omission about the actual existence of a dish with live mice in Chinese cuisine was not accidental, as it followed the same biopolitical principle to which Zaia had instinctively adhered: a special relationship between civilisation and cuisine, civilisation and hygiene, and civilisation and food. In this context, no one dared to ask whether Chinese cuisine involves culinary practices that would be considered extreme in the West, because the Chinese people are unquestionably civilised. Therefore, such a dish cannot exist. And yet one cannot help noticing that this reticence is not simply epistemological but reflects the same biopolitical paradigm that argues for a link between civilisation and specific culinary habits. In other words, there is no need to ask whether Chinese cuisine can include this peculiar dish precisely because the Chinese people are civilised and therefore can only have certain culinary habits that conform to civilised standards. On the contrary, only 'barbarians' would eat such a thing. In this respect, the simple fact that no one even bothered to check whether there is a Chinese dish that involves the consumption of 'live mice' is not simply and unquestionably respectful or epistemologically redundant. More subtly, it is also paradigmatic of a specific 'Orientalism' that is actually a circular argument: a Chinese person should not normally eat 'live mice' because he is 'civilised', and he is 'civilised' because he does not normally eat 'live mice'. The question underlying this disturbing issue is even more disturbing, but also more subtle – how would eating dried rats in Italy be different from eating live mice in China?

On closer inspection, the issue is not the consumption of rat meat but its preparation. The obvious difference between eating dried rats and eating live mice is that the former are dead and somehow cooked, while the latter are clearly alive and raw. Beyond his simple-minded intentions, Zaia was referring to a well-known trope about the consumption of cooked or raw food – famously introduced by Levi-Strauss in his seminal 1964 book *Le Cru et le Cuit*. In a passage from this important study of the myth of the cooking fire in Brazilian indigenous cultures, Lévi-Strauss (1964, 336) elaborates on fire, 'whose normal function is to mediatize the conjunction of the raw product and the human consumer, and whose operation thus has the effect of making sure that a natural creature is at one and the same time cooked and socialized'. In this respect, it is not really the consumption of a particular type of meat – however repugnant it may be – that is being discussed here, but rather its culinary preparation in relation to a socialised group. The question of preparation allows us not only to appreciate the underlying tension between nature and culture, but also to qualify the position of a social group between them. Since 'cooking brings about the cultural transformation of the raw' (Lévi-Strauss 1964, 142), the consumption of raw meat – or, in its most extreme form, live mice – can only evoke the suggestion that those who consume raw food are somehow inferior and remain 'imprisoned in nature and rawness, and perhaps even destined to decay' (Lévi-Strauss 1964, 338). In this respect, if we follow Zaia's implicit argument and extend Lévi-Strauss's point, the Chinese people would somehow be doomed to decay precisely because they indulge in culinary practices that ultimately reject culture – here symbolised by the cooking fire and its ability to extract nourishment from the natural world and transform it into food.

On the other hand, the consumption of disgusting meat can only be justified in special circumstances. Finally, it should be noted that Zaia himself had proudly claimed that during the famine of 1917 the Venetian people had eaten rat meat in a true 'state of emergency'.[3] In this respect, the famine emergency of 1917 would justify – in every sense of the word – the consumption of dried rat meat. Such meat would still be abhorrent, but it would be far removed from the gruesome dimension of rawness and somehow closer to the standard of decently cooked meat. It was probably with this in mind that Zaia gave the photo of the dried rats a rather telling hashtag: *#VenetoDaAmare* ('Venetia to love'). In this case, the horror of eating rat meat was mitigated by not eating them alive – and therefore raw – but by drying them, thus taking them out of the rather vague category of 'raw' and somehow including them in that of 'cooked'. In Zaia's implicit argument, the culinary exception of eating 'cooked' rat meat should even be celebrated as a symbol of resilience in times of famine. Conversely, the consumption of 'raw' meat of live mice would only be an abomination, the ultimate consequence of which would be the spread of a pandemic.

Interestingly, Zaia argued that the 'lack of hygiene' among the Chinese people was a 'substrate' for the virus. He used the term 'substrate' in a rather unclear, if not misleading, way. He seemed to be suggesting that the 'lack of hygiene' provided the conditions for the virus to spread. Although it is impossible to verify that this was the actual meaning of his slightly inappropriate expression, one cannot help but elaborate on this phenomenal philosophical term and take it very seriously. What, then, is a 'substrate'?

The term 'substrate' is a calque from the Latin *substratum*, which in turn translates the Greek term *hypokeimenon* and designates what lies beneath the surface and, by extension, what underlies a change – its 'matter' (*hyle*). This traditional understanding of 'substrate' is usually projected against a cosmological background. According to this, the four basic 'elements' (*stoikeia*) – air, fire, earth, and water – can be transformed into each other by a kind of 'primordial matter' (*he prote hyle*), which is not exactly identifiable but more primitive than those elements. In this respect, the 'underlying' matter at first appears to be 'neutral' in the sense that it is neither (*nec*) one nor (*uter*) another of the four elements. Moreover, the 'neutrality' of the 'substrate' is also reflected in the neutral gender of the term itself, both in the Greek (*hypokeimenon*) and in the Latin (*substratum*). Accordingly, Aristotle typically conceived of a 'substrate' for elemental change as a kind of 'ungendered' matter: a neutral, basic form of existence that is indeterminate but at the same time not really devoid of some basic 'essential' characteristics. Otherwise, it could not support being 'impressed' by any of the four elements. Accordingly, the substrate must be 'disembodied' (*asomatos*), 'formless' (*aneidos*), and 'without figure' (*aschematistos*) (see, e.g., Arist. *Metaph.*, 1092 a, 2–7; see also Cohen 1984).

Against this traditional reading (the ramifications of which cannot be explored in the present context), the feminist Italian-American philosopher Emanuela Bianchi has recently argued that the notion of 'substrate' is actually gendered and 'enformed by the masculine'; thus, the substrate 'in fact possesses and is capable of producing its own form of motion, aleatory motion, a motion that has effects, identifiable retroactively through observation and thought, but unknowable and invisible to the scientist or philosopher seeking first causes, the why of things' (Bianchi 2014, 82). Consequently, the polarisation noted above should be reformulated more precisely as a contrast between the lack of hygiene, which is 'Oriental', 'natural', linked to 'matter' and therefore fundamentally 'feminine', and the hygienic (i.e., the hygienic that is proper to the West), cultural, and masculine. I would still insist that this biopolitical link between food and culture has the effect of obscuring the deeper ideology of Zaia's argument.

## 'Man is what he eats': Health and power

There is no doubt that Zaia spoke as carelessly as he was misinformed, if not prejudiced, against the Chinese people. And yet no media outlet has bothered to check whether Zaia was telling the truth about the consumption of live mice and, if so, whether this strange culinary practice is culturally accepted by the Chinese or other peoples of Asia.

It is rather disturbing to read that some historical sources, as well as some modern footage, suggest that traditional Chinese cuisine includes a unique dish eloquently called 'Three Screaming Mice' (Sān jiào shǔ) (三叫鼠) or 'Three Squeaks' (Sān zhī er) (三吱儿) (Wikipedia 2022). This traditional dish, which involves the consumption of live newborn mice, is first briefly described in the third chapter on food in the historiographical work *The Classified Anthology of Qing Anecdotes* (Qīng bài lèi chāo) (清稗類鈔) (Wikisource 2019). The name of this strange dish probably reflects the rather gruesome way in which mice are eaten alive. In particular, the 'three squeaks' would indicate that the mice squeak when they are placed on the plate, when they are dipped in the soy sauce, and when they are placed in the mouth before being eaten. In the present context, the question of whether this unique dish is merely legendary, still served in some local Cantonese restaurant, or banned in China altogether is not relevant. The more subtle question is that this dish – whether or not it actually exists – has stirred up a powerful narrative with important theological and political ramifications.

This is particularly evident in the writings of the Tibetan activist Khenpo Tsultrim Lodrö, who is considered an important Tibetan scholar and lama. In some of his highly polemical writings, Khenpo Tsultrim Lodrö specifically refers to the category of 'barbarism' (*dmu rgod*) and 'savagery' (*gdug spyod*) to describe some extreme Chinese culinary practices.[4] Khenpo Tsultrim Lodrö specifically mentions three dishes that prove the ruthless nature of the Chinese people: a fish fried half-alive, live monkey brains, and, finally, newborn mice eaten alive (Mkhan 2004, quoted in Gayley 2017, 267; see also Barstow 2018).

It cannot be overlooked that this kind of accusation also resembles some media representations of the Far East in Western films, which either humorously or polemically use cinematic tropes and offer a bizarre, if not vulgarised, representation of 'Oriental' cultures. Perhaps the most notorious examples in modern cinema are the infamous monkey brain-eating scene in John Alan Schwartz's controversial horror film *Face of Death* (1978) and its parodic but no less controversial reference in Steven Spielberg's second instalment of the Indiana Jones saga, *Indiana Jones and the Temple of Doom* (1984). The infamous banquet scene features a gruesome meal of snakes, fried bugs, eyeball soup, and monkey brains. Spielberg originally intended this horrific meal to illustrate the evil of a death cult that was oppressing a colonial Indian village. But in the end, this construction would only repeat the tired trope of an 'Oriental' population unable to free itself, waiting for the 'white' archaeologist Indiana Jones to finally destroy the evil cult and restore peace (see Boulin 2017; Hurst 2015).

The actual existence of a dish with monkey brains should also be further investigated. While it is possible that someone may have actually eaten such a dish in some peculiar circumstances, it cannot be dismissed that the existence of this dish may have been caused by disinformation and manipulation of sources. Indeed, it is plausible that this horrific dish is nothing more than an ordinary, if not innocent, vegetarian dish in Chinese cuisine, which uses as its main ingredient the edible mushroom 'Lion's Mane' (*Hericium erinaceus*). This mushroom is also known by its Chinese name *hóu tóu gū* (猴头菇) ('monkey head mushroom') because of its resemblance to a mammal's brain (see Arjana 2015, 142–145; Schreiber 2002; Fujita 1940, 27–30). In this respect, the idea of eating a real monkey brain would only be a distortion of a vegetarian dish. Therefore, either by misinterpreting or manipulating actual information, the legendary but non-existent dish – eating an actual monkey brain, rather than a mushroom shaped like a monkey brain – would have emerged as a sinister myth to serve the purpose of defaming the Chinese people by attributing to them cruel and disgusting eating habits.[5] Moreover, we cannot ignore the gendered implications of meat consumption, if not the consumption of flesh, as recently pointed out by Paul Beatriz Preciado, who has studied the relationship between the visible and meat and its ecofeminist implications. In particular, it has been noted that 'the feminine body is meat and animal meat is a body that has been feminized by the normative heterosexual gaze. [There] is [a] cannibal chain and its biocultural links of blood relations, desire, power and violence' (Preciado 2014, 32).[6]

In her well-informed study of Lodrö's advocacy of vegetarianism, Holly Gayley eloquently comments on the difficult distinction between a legendary dish and a modern culinary practice. She goes on to explore the biopolitical ramifications of Lodrö's assumptions:

> It is unclear whether the revulsion invoked by such descriptions would effectively translate into Tibetans giving up everyday meat consumption.

> Another way to read his argument in [the book called] *Timely Advice* is as an anti-assimilationist message directed at urban Tibetans, who frequent Chinese restaurants and may be exposed to unusual fare. In exoticizing and demonizing the excesses of the Han banquet, Tsultrim Lodrö tacitly cautions against the uncritical imitation of Han customs and capitulation to the terms of Chinese modernity. I refer to this strategy as "reverse orientalism" since it turns the tables on the civilizing project of Han-centered state discourse and policy toward minorities in China.
>
> (Gayley 2017, 43)

Again, the question of food takes on a bio-political significance: the occupation of Tibet is as cruel as these typical Chinese dishes. The obvious assumption is that anyone who can consume such a cruel dish can only support an equally ruthless regime and its accompanying imperialism. Conversely, a vegetarian would be more inclined to follow the path of peace. Gayley allows us to understand the deep logic in Lodrö's argument, that a culinary practice lies at the intersection of nature and culture, as Lévi-Strauss argued in his *Le Cru et le Cuit.* The implication is that certain dishes can reflect either an uncivilised or a civilised attitude towards food and, by extension, towards animals and human beings in general. Anyone who indulges in cruel culinary practices and eats in a 'merciless, savage manner' – without killing animals before cooking or eating them – is barbaric and somehow more inclined towards nature than culture. Such a person would certainly be less likely to be persuaded by reason and civilisation. In this respect, one can agree with Zaia's and Lodrö's reflections on Chinese cuisine – the lack of compassion for animals, the strange culinary practices, and the lack of hygiene – and conclude that this recklessness could lead to a catastrophic event, such as a global pandemic. It may not necessarily be true that certain practices caused a pandemic in the strict sense of the term. On the other hand, the rhetorical argument used by both Zaia and Lodrö is that the pandemic resulted from certain culinary, hygienic, and therefore political choices.

## Conclusion: A question concerning technology

The questionable link between hygiene, culture, and politics was also suggested by some other observers, who were eager to conclude that the incipient pandemic was a symptom – in every sense of the word – of a more general disease: globalisation. Consider, for example, an inspired tweet by the prominent and controversial young Italian philosopher Diego Fusaro, who first wrote some monographs on Italian Marxism, arguing for a deeper theoretical connection between the Italian communist Antonio Gramsci and the fascist neo-idealist philosopher Giovanni Gentile (see Fusaro 2005, 2021).[7] Fusaro has gradually moved from the left to the far right, while claiming that this political distinction is obsolete in the face of globalisation, emphasising similar arguments proposed by his mentor, the Italian philosopher Costanzo Preve.[8] At the same time, Fusaro has made a name for himself as a prominent opinion-maker in the Italian media. Due to his geopolitical views and his acquaintance with the Italian neo-fascist movement Casa Pound, the Russian neo-fascist philosopher Aleksandr Dugin, and the far-right American media executive and political strategist Steve Bannon, Fusaro is usually described with the Italian neologism *rossobruno* ('red-brown colour') in reference to his political ambiguity between left and right (see McAdams 2022, 3; Broder 2020, 298–300; Zúquete 2018, 426). In his typically caustic and radical style, Fusaro linked the pandemic to globalisation:

> With its ruthlessness (*spietatezza*), the Coronavirus teaches us that if we lived in the borderless and unregulated world so dear to the financial overlords and their fuchsia guards, we would all be dead long ago.
>
> (Fusaro 2020)[9]

The grotesqueness of this tweet cannot be overlooked, as it humanises the virus, an almost non-living entity, by attributing 'ruthlessness' to it. In the same vein, a few days later, Casa Pound repeated the same assumption in an epigrammatic, effective, and violent tweet: 'patient zero is globalization (*il paziente zero è la globalizzazione*)' (Casa Pound 2020).[10] There is no need to point out that these two statements are inherently false. Anyone with a modest school education knows very well that borders have never stopped a pandemic. Historical examples abound: the Black Death pandemic, the Spanish flu pandemic, and so on. Borders between states were closed, sealed, or fought over in the case of COVID-19, but this did not prevent a pandemic from spreading around the world. In this respect, the quasi-biological nature of a virus and the pandemic it caused is less important than its symbolic power and ability to associate a transgression of hygienic, culinary, legal, and cultural standards with fears of loss of national purity and political integrity.

And yet the intersection between the pandemic and the political also involved 'progressive' intellectuals: two exponents of so-called 'Italian thought', Giorgio Agamben and Roberto Esposito, and the French 'deconstructionist' Jean-Luc Nancy. These three scholars publicly debated the nature of the pandemic and the danger inherent in the social measures already taken to prevent it (Nancy 2020; Agamben 2020a, 2020b; Sotiris 2020; Esposito 2020). The debate began with Agamben's publication of a one-sided and polemical piece entitled 'The Invention of a Pandemic'. His starting point was that the pandemic was merely an 'invention' (*invenzione*), and that it had been invented for the sake of social control. After meticulously examining the 'emergency measures' (*misure di emergenza*) already taken by the Italian state, he described them as 'frenetic, irrational and completely unmotivated' (*frenetiche, irrazionali e del tutto immotivate*). He concluded his astonishing contribution with another surprising remark:

> The disproportion to what the [Italian] National Research Council says is a normal flu (*una normale influenza*), not very different from those that recur every year, is striking. One could say that, having exhausted terrorism as a cause for exceptional measures (*causa di provvedimenti d'eccezione*), the

> invention of an epidemic (*l'invenzione di una pandemia*) could provide the ideal pretext (*il pretesto ideale*) to extend them beyond all limits.
>
> (Agamben 2020c)

One cannot underestimate the seriousness of this incredibly reckless contribution. Agamben uses specific legal vocabulary to justify his uninformed opinion about the nature of the impending pandemic. He thereby emphasises how 'normal' this disease actually is (since it does not require extreme measures) and how 'disproportionate' any extreme measure necessarily is.

Unfortunately, within a few weeks Agamben was quickly disproved by the course of events. Italy witnessed a tragic, exponential growth of the epidemic, which claimed the lives of over a thousand people within a month of his rash statement. And yet this fact – one might even say this material evidence – did not cause Agamben to retract, or even to revise, his previous statements. On the contrary, he reaffirmed his position in a second post. He even introduced an additional element: the traditional figure of the 'spreader of the plague', informally designated with the Italian term *untore* (literally, 'greaser'). According to Agamben, this figure is alien to the principles of Hippocratic medicine and thus implicitly far removed from Greek rationality. By implication, he argues that Italy was experiencing a similar irrational sentiment, as public measures were being taken to prevent any carrier of the virus from contaminating others.

In a second paper, published under the title 'Contagion' – eerily reminiscent of Soderbergh's homonymous and prophetic 2011 film – Agamben argued that there was an 'analogy' (*analogia*) between the measures taken to control the pandemic and those taken to control terrorism.[11] More specifically, he wrote:

> The most recent measures (taken by the government in decrees which we hope—but it is an illusion—will not be confirmed by Parliament in laws within the prescribed time limit) de facto turn every individual into a potential spreader of the plague (*trasformano di fatto ogni individuo in un potenziale untore*), just as those on terrorism de facto and de jure considered every citizen to be a potential terrorist (*consideravano di fatto e di diritto ogni cittadino come un terrorista in potenza*).
>
> (Agamben 2020b)

Again, the recklessness of this contribution cannot be underestimated. Agamben argues that the Italian state manipulated the nature of the COVID-19 disease for a conspiratorial purpose: to provide false information in order to justify 'exceptional' measures whose aim would not be to prevent a pandemic but rather to repress the Italian population, as happened during incidents of Italian terrorism.

In a polite reply to his colleague, Nancy did not dispute Agamben's theoretical principle that certain conditions can be exploited for a political agenda. Nevertheless, he elaborated on the link between the pandemic and globalisation:

> Giorgio notes that governments are appropriating all sorts of pretexts to establish permanent states of exception. But he fails to see that the exception

> is in fact becoming the rule in a world in which technical interconnections of all kinds (relocations, transfers of all kinds, exposure or diffusion of substances, etc.) are reaching an unprecedented intensity and are growing in step with the population. The multiplication of the latter, even in rich countries, means that life expectancy is increasing, as is the number of elderly and generally vulnerable people. There is no doubt that a whole civilisation is being called into question. There is a kind of viral exception – biological, informatic, cultural – that is pandemising us (*il y a une sorte d'exception virale – biologique, informatique, culturelle – qui nous pandémise*). Governments are only the sad actors, and to pick on them seems more like a diversion (*manœuvre de diversion*) than a political reflection (*réflexion politique*).
> (Nancy 2020)

The point raised by Nancy is particularly important. He criticises, contextualises, and develops the notion of a 'state of emergency' that would characterise contemporary society and allow for almost extra-legal procedures. Nancy does not deny the exceptional nature of these measures, nor, despite appearances, the grim reality that the current epidemic is very serious. Rather, he suggests something more interesting: that the government is reacting in this way not because it lacks a political agenda but because it is relying exclusively on technological devices that take the place of politics.

In this respect, Nancy seems to agree with Zaia on the question of technology. While Zaia argued that the Chinese people were responsible for the spread of the pandemic because of their lack of hygiene and their failure to conform to the technological standards of the West, Nancy argued that the pandemic destabilised Western societies precisely because it irreparably disrupted political life and showed that technology was outstripping politics – here understood as the interplay between biology and political science – in containing the pandemic. Perhaps the most interesting outcome of the early confrontation with the emergence of the pandemic is the subordination of ordinary politics to biopolitics.

## Notes

1 The transcription, translation, and clarifications are mine. Due to the extemporaneous nature of this interview, Zaia's Italian is not always clear or idiomatic.
2 English translation mine.
3 I use this expression with a clear reference to Carl Schmitt's *Die Dikatur* (1921) and *Politische Theologie* (1922), as well as Giorgio Agamben's *Lo stato d'eccezione* (2003). These two scholars conceive of the 'state of exception' (*Ausnahmezustand*) as an exceptional circumstance that allows for transgressing an established norm.
4 In particular, the Tibetan expression *dmu rgod* was adopted by the Mongols and predates the Mongol empire with the early Bon. This expression describes the earliest tribes of Tibet who had not yet been exposed to Buddhism, and by implication a malevolent spirit. The expression *gdug spyod* generally refers to 'bad behaviour'. See Das (1997, 983, 660); Martin (1994, 77). I would like to thank Dr Albion M. Butters (University of Turku) for helping me with these expressions.
5 This form of deforming habits from a different culture by subtle (mis)reading of actual data is widespread in every society. For instance, Christian scripture frequently uses this

strategy to stigmatise the non-Jewish surrounding cultures. See Buber and Rosenzweig 1994, 88; Dal Bo 2013, 60.

6 I owe this suggestion to Nora Heidorn.

7 On the connection between Gramsci and Gentile from another perspective, see Dal Bo (2020, 112–117).

8 Costanzo Preve (1943–2013) was a prominent Italian post-Marxist philosopher who also discussed the obsolescence of the distinction between left and right. See, e.g., Preve (2021); Bravo (2021). See also Dal Bo (2025).

9 English translation mine.

10 English translation mine.

11 For an exploration of Soderbergh's film, which unfolds the grim scenario of a global flu turning into a pandemic, in relation to Agamben's problematisation of surveillance methods and Queer Studies, see Sikora (2021).

## References


Agamben, Giorgio. 2020a. "Clarifications." *European Journal of Psychoanalysis*. https://www.journal-psychoanalysis.eu/coronavirus-and-philosophers/.

Agamben, Giorgio. 2020b. "Contagio." *Quodlibet*, Una voce. Rubrica di Giorgio Agamben, 11 March. https://www.quodlibet.it/giorgio-agamben-contagio.

Agamben, Giorgio. 2020c. "L'invenzione di una pandemia." *Quodlibet,* Una voce. *Rubrica di Giorgio Agamben*, 26 February. https://www.quodlibet.it/giorgio-agamben-l-invenzione-di-un-epidemia.

Ambasciata della Repubblica Popolare Cinese (@AmbCina). Twitter post, 28 February, 9:03pm. https://twitter.com/AmbCina/status/1233482854778261506?ref_src=twsrc%5Etfw.

Arjana, Sophie Rose. 2015. *Muslims in the Western Imagination*. Oxford: Oxford University Press.

Barstow, Geoffrey. 2018. *Food of Sinful Demons: Meat, Vegetarianism, and the Limits of Buddhism in Tibet*. New York: Columbia University Press.

Bianchi, Emanuela. 2014. *The Feminine Symptom: Aleatory Matter in the Aristotelian Cosmos*. New York: Fordham University Press.

Boulin, Katherine. 2017. "Indiana Jones Must Retire: Archaeology, Imperialism and Fashion in the Digital Age." *Everyday Orientalism*, 22 August. https://everydayorientalism.wordpress.com/2017/08/22/indiana-jones-must-retire-archaeology-imperialism-and-fashion-in-the-digital-age/.

Bravo, Salvatore. 2021. *Pratica filosofica e politica in Costanzo Preve*. Pistoia: Petite Plaisance.

Broder, David. 2020. "(Post)fascists, the Constitution, and the Defense of the Italian Nation." In *Back to the '30? Recurring Crises of Capitalism, Liberalism, and Democracy*, edited by Jeremy Rayner, Susan Falls, George Souvlis, and Taylor C. Nelms, 293–306. Cham: Palgrave Macmillan.

Buber, Martin, and Franz Rosenzweig. 1994. *Scripture and Translation*. Bloomington: Indiana University Press.

Casa Pound. 2020. (@CasaPoundItalia). Twitter Post, 27 February 27, 11:25 am. https://twitter.com/CasaPoundItalia/status/1232974997494300674?s=20.

Cohen, Sheldon. 1984. "Aristotle's Doctrine of the Material Substrate." *The Philosophical Review* 93(2): 171–194.

Dal Bo, Federico. 2013. *Massekhet Keritot. Text, Translation, and Commentary*. Tübingen: Mohr Siebeck.

Dal Bo, Federico. 2020. *Il linguaggio della violenza. Estremismo e ideologia nella filosofia contemporanea*. Bologna: Biblioteca Clueb.
Dal Bo, Federico. 2025. "A Marxian Political Theology of Nihilism: Costanzo Preve and Domenico Losurdo on Marx's Historical Materialism." *The Resistible Crisis of Italian Thought. Between Politics and Metaphysics*, edited by Federico Dal Bo and Carlo Salzani. New York: SUNY (in print).
Das, S. Chandra. 2004. *A Tibetan-English Dictionary, with Sanskrit Synonyms*. New Delhi-Madras: Asian Educational Services.
Esposito, Roberto. 2020. "Curati ad oltranza." *Paradoxia epidemica, Antinomie. Scritture e immagini*, 28 February. https://antinomie.it/index.php/2020/02/28/curati-a-oltranza/.
Fujita, Dennis K. 1940. *Chinese Dinner*. General Directorate of Railways: South Manchuria Railway Company.
Fusaro, Diego. 2005. *Antonio Gramsci: La passione di essere nel mondo*. Milano: Feltrinelli.
Fusaro, Diego. 2020. (@DiegoFusaro), Twitter post, 23 February 23 10:29 pm. https://twitter.com/DiegoFusaro/status/1231511269351600128?s=20.
Fusaro, Diego. 2021. *Bentornato Gramsci*. Milan: La Nave di Teseo.
Gayley, Holly. 2017. "The Compassionate Treatment of Animals: A Contemporary Buddhist Approach in Eastern Tibet." *Journal of Religious Ethics* 45(1): 29–57.
Lévi-Strauss, Claude. 1964. *The Raw and the Cooked. Introduction to a Science of Mythology I*, translated by Sander L. Gilman. New York: Harper & Row.
Hurst, Anna Sophie. 2015. "Discourse: Orientalism and Indiana Jones." *Analyzing Film and Media Theory*, 21 November. https://annahurstfmstheory.wordpress.com/2015/11/21/discourse-orientalism-and-indiana-jones/.
Martin, Dan. 1994. *Mandala Cosmogony. Human Body Good Thought and the Revelation of the Secret Mother Tantras of Bon*. Wiesbaden: Harrassowitz.
Mazzoni, Alana. 2020. "Disturbing Footage Shows Diner Calmly Dipping a Baby Mouse in a Bowl of Sauce before Eating it Alive as Part of Banned Chinese Delicacy Known as 'Three Squeaks'." *Mail Online*, 25 January. https://www.dailymail.co.uk/news/article-7927747/Asian-man-dips-baby-mouse-bowl-sauce-eating-ALIVE.html.
McAdams, A. James. 2022. "Introduction." In *Contemporary Far-Right Thinkers in the Era of Liberal-Democratic Crisis*, edited by A. James McAdams and Alejandro Castrillon, 3–24. London: Routledge.
Mkhan po Tshul khrims blo gros. 2004. *Dus su bab pa'i gtam lugs gnyis gsal ba'i me long. In Yang dag lam gyi 'jug sgo blo gsar yid kyi dga' ston,* 2 vols. Hong Kong: Fojiao cihui fuwu zhongxin.
Nancy, Jean-Luc. 2020. "Eccezione virale." *Paradoxia epidemica, Antinomie. Scritture e immagini*, 27 February. https://antinomie.it/index.php/2020/02/27/eccezione-virale/.
Preciado, Paul (credited as Beatriz). 2014. "The Phantom Limb: Carol Rama and the History of Art." In *The Passion According to Carol Rama*, 13–33. Barcelona: Museu d'Art Contemporani.
Preve, Costanzo. 2021. *Destra e sinistra. La natura inservibile di due categorie tradizionali*. Pistoia: Petite Plaisance.
Salzani, Carlo. forthcoming 2025. "The Crisis of a Paradigm. Agamben's Misunderstanding of the COVID-19 Pandemic." In *The Resistible Crisis of Italian Thought: Between Politics and Metaphysics*, edited by Federico Dal Bo and Carlo Salzani, in press. New York: SUNY Press.
Schreiber, Mark. 2002. "Debunking Strange Asian Myths: Part II." *The Japan Times*, 8 August

Sikora, Tomasz. 2021. "Queer Epidemics." *Interalia* 16: 12–32.
Sotiris, Panagiotis. 2020. "Against Agamben: Is a Democratic Biopolitics Possible?" *Critical Legal Thinking*, 14 March. https://criticallegalthinking.com/2020/03/14/against-agamben-is-a-democratic-biopolitics-possible/.
Wikipedia. 2022. "三叫鼠" *Wikipedia*, Wikimedia Foundation, December 14, 2022, 2:26 pm: https://zh.wikipedia.org/wiki/三叫鼠.
Wikisource. 2019. "清稗類鈔", *Wikisource*, Wikimedia Foundation, September 1, 2019, 7:53 am, https://zh.wikisource.org/wiki/清稗類鈔/107#粵人食鼠.
Xun, Zohu, and Sander L. Gilman. 2021. *'I Know Who Caused COVID-19.' Pandemics and Xenophobia*. Chicago, IL: Chicago University Press.
Zaia, Luca. 2018. Facebook post, 26 November. https://www.facebook.com/zaiaufficiale/posts/1048419028693345.
Zaia, Luca. 2020. "Zaia: 'Grazie all'igiene dei veneti solo 116 positivi, i cinesi? Li abbiamo visti tutti…'." 28 February. https://youtu.be/aqKPFtH3eDE.
Zúquete, José-Pedro. 2018. "From Left to Right and Beyond. The Defence of Populism." In *Routledge Handbook of Global Populism*, edited by Carolina de la Torre, 416–434. London: Routledge.

# 3 Bio-story

## Michel Foucault and the history of social medicine

*Xenia Chiaramonte*

### Introduction

A profound understanding of the medical encounter necessitates an exploration of the intertwined dynamics of violence, care, and cure. These elements, deeply entwined with our individual and collective needs, intricately shape the fabric of our experiences within the realm of healthcare. We all need this art we call medicine, while at the same time fearing its potentially harmful effects, hasty and erroneous diagnoses, and authoritarian tendencies.

For this reason, we need sophisticated, complex, yet honest analyses that start from a simple yet crucial piece of information: the history of medicine is social and political. It is not only a kind of knowledge that passes through the individual exchange between doctor and patient but a knowledge that 'forms part of a historical system'. As such, 'it is not a pure science, but is part of an economic system and of a system of power' (Foucault 2004, 19). Michel Foucault clarified this point in October 1974, when he gave three lectures in Rio de Janeiro on the archaeology of the cure. The first two – which I will comment on in this piece – were published a few years later in France with the original titles *Crise de la médicine ou crise de l'antimédicine?* and *La naissance de la médicine sociale*. It is on this occasion that Foucault introduced the concept, or rather the prefix, 'bio' in his analysis, and it is here – as my reflections intend to demonstrate – that we may trace the original meaning of a term that today seems rather abused, and find a valuable analytical framework for a cogent approach to the relationship between medicine and power dynamics.

As is well known, the issue of biopolitics or biopower was, beginning with a series of research endeavours by the French philosopher,[1] employed by many interpreters and in various disciplines, especially philosophy. The concept of biopolitics, defined as politics taking charge of life,[2] or perhaps more drastically as the right of death and power over life,[3] continues to be called into question for different purposes by diverse parties, with greater or lesser reference to the overall reading of Foucault's *oeuvre*.

To avoid entering into a debate that would be difficult and too onerous to reconstruct here, I do not intend to address the age-old theme of biopolitics in its entirety, but to limit myself to sketching the phases of 'bio-history'. This purpose, however,

DOI: 10.4324/9781032660165-6

is not based solely on a practical necessity. This piece argues that we shall look at the crossroads of medicine and society to recover the depth of what 'bio' implies.

Bio-history is the term Michel Foucault (2001a, 134) initially uses – in the second lecture – to refer to what he defines as 'the effect of medical intervention at the biological level, the imprint left of human history [...] by the strong medical intervention that began in the eighteenth century'. As we can see, this is a definition that is both more specific and more complex than what Foucault will elsewhere provide under the prefix 'bio'. Bio-history is a specifically political history in which we are still fully involved. Hence, it is worth retracing the steps of this history to understand where we are today. I intend to show the ambiguities that have been circulating for some centuries around the matter of medicine, and its interconnection with legal and police matters, which can lead to various consequences – just as, in the past, they have led equally to the 'glorious' years of the welfare state and to authoritarian medicalisation. This proposition is rooted in the core idea that we are currently experiencing a scenario where specific occurrences have resulted in a crisis. These occurrences, according to Foucault (2004, 18) have remained largely unchanged since the eighteenth century, a period when the concept of a political economy of health emerged. This era saw the introduction of widespread medicalisation and mechanisms related to the intersection of biology and history providing the main features to a system of thought and practices that constitutes a history of the present.

## A somatocracy?

As Foucault (2004, 7) underlines,

> we live in a regime that sees the care of the body, corporal health, the relation between illness and health, etc. as appropriate areas of State intervention. It is precisely the birth of this somatocracy, in crisis since its origins, that I am proposing to analyze.

We live in an era that considers the body, its health, and its disease to be crucial. It is not just the generic right to life that is at stake here, but the more specific and complex problematic that has taken the name of the right to health. Let us start by sketching the legal history of this protection.

With the well-known Beveridge plan, a system of reforms of English social welfare (Hills et al. 1994) – from which Foucault's first intervention begins – we see the establishment of a model that will make history and become the basis of various national constitutions, as well as the Universal Declaration of Human Rights (United Nations, Paris, 10 December 1948) and a ruling by the World Health Organization (1948).

In particular, the report *Social Insurance and Allied Services*, originally commissioned by Winston Churchill in 1939 but first circulated on 1 December 1942, radically changed the social security system in the United Kingdom. The commission chaired by Beveridge drew up a program based on the universality of public assistance. The establishment of the National Health Service aimed at guaranteeing the improvement of the physical and mental health of people through the prevention, diagnosis, and treatment of diseases, a program based on certain principles: the universality of access financed through general taxation.

Article 25 of the Universal Declaration of Human Rights, which was deeply influenced by the British NHS, states that

> Everyone has the right to a standard of living adequate for the health and well-being of himself and of his family, including food, clothing, housing and medical care and necessary social services, and the right to security in the event of unemployment, sickness, disability, widowhood, old age or other lack of livelihood in circumstances beyond his control.

According to Foucault, this is a crucial turning point: an old logic, according to which a healthy individual was at the service of the state, inverts its polarity. Here, 'the concept of the healthy individual in the service of the State was replaced by that of the State in the service of the healthy individual', thus comprising 'not only a question of a reversal of rights, but also of what might be called a morality of the body' (Foucault 2004, 6).

Healthcare now enters the field of macroeconomics and becomes a decisive factor for statistical studies. In other words, the human body becomes the object of a story. Yet, it is not just the human body alone but the human as a species among living beings, including its very relationship with other living beings. Admittedly, Foucault (2004, 11) writes that

> The history of man and life are profoundly intertwined. The history of man does not simply continue life, nor is it simply content to reproduce it, but to a certain extent renews it, and can exercise a certain number of fundamental effects on its processes.

Once healthcare has become central, and the state begins to serve a healthy population, authoritarian intervention also becomes possible through procedures such as mass screening or vaccination campaigns. In other words, taking care also means exercising control over individuals and, above all, over the 'population', a concept that has a special place in the history of systems of thought, starting from the possibility of its management in hygienic-sanitary terms.

A population is the collective entity that allows the frequency with which disease spreads to become visible. The population facilitates knowledge of morbidity rates and becomes a statistical field divisible by age, lifestyle, social position, and the coordinates of space and time. The population is the field in which dangers manifest and the basis on which one understands how to act at the level of their government. In other words, it is through the population that criteria of normality (and therefore, obviously, normalisation) can be elaborated.[4]

According to Foucault (2004, 13), in the eighteenth century, four major processes characterise the consolidation of medicine: the emergence of 'a medical authority, which is not restricted to the authority of knowledge' but that 'can make decisions concerning a town, a district, an institution, or a regulation'; medicine becomes a 'field of intervention' not only for diseases but with regard to the consequences of such things as 'air, water, construction, terrains, sewerage'; the birth of the hospital, as earlier 'the hospital was not an institution of medicalisation, but of aid to the poor awaiting death'; and finally, the 'introduction of mechanisms of medical administration: recording of data, collection and comparison of statistics, etc.' This set of factors produces what Foucault calls the political economy of health. This means that, in contrast to the order of things before the eighteenth century, it was no longer enough to just provide for the health of individuals as a workforce, whether for reproductive or economic purposes. There is in fact a further step, which changes the role of medicine. Its connection with the economy certainly remains but becomes, in a certain sense, more complex. It is necessary that medicine is not only functional vis-à-vis the reproduction of the workforce but that it positively produces well-being. Well-being henceforth acquires market value; it becomes a capitalisable asset. Indeed, Foucault highlights:

> Health becomes a consumer object, which can be produced by pharmaceutical laboratories, doctors, etc., and consumed by both potential and actual patients. As such, it has acquired economic and market value. Thus the human body has been brought twice over into the market: first by people selling their capacity to work, and second, through the intermediary of health. Consequently, the human body once again enters an economic market as soon as it is susceptible to diseases and health, to well being or to malaise, to joy or to pain, and to the extent that it is the object of sensations, desires, etc.
>
> (Foucault 2004, 16)

## The quarantine plan

The centrality assumed by the body implies that the technologies of power do not act only on a 'mental' level – a split between mind and body that now, as ever, holds little analytical value – and nor do they function as a kind of propaganda.

> Society's control over individuals was accomplished not only through consciousness or ideology but also in the body and with the body. For capitalist society, it was biopolitics, the biological, the somatic, the corporeal, that mattered more than anything else. The body is a political reality; medicine is a biopolitical strategy.
>
> (Foucault 2001a, 137)

The model that has been in place since the eighteenth century is more specifically the model of the plague, one no longer based on exclusion – like that of leprosy (see also Foucault 1977) – but on permanent registration, detailed analysis, and constant inspection. In cases of plague or other types of epidemics, the ideal form of organisation and control is the quarantine, based on an 'emergency plan' (Foucault 2001a, 144–145) and the loose concept of 'measure' (see Napoli 2009). In general, Foucault identifies three models in the history of social medicine: state medicine (Germany), urban medicine (France), and labour-force medicine (England). Let us dwell on the French and the English models.

Foucault defines the French model of social medicine in relation to urbanity. Urban medicine administered burial places and controlled and reduced the dangers that corpses posed, making air and hygienic conditions a fundamental stage of its 'development'. It is important to note, however, that these kinds of changes are not to be read exclusively with an eye towards the ethical. Foucault shows how cataloguing, the control of circulation, and a new economy of the living and the non-living simultaneously took place alongside these processes. Consider this crucial example: in the eighteenth century, humans started dealing with death. It was not a matter of Christian respect for death and the corpse – this is precisely the ethical prejudice we need to avoid – but rather the emergence of a norm of public hygiene and a new political-health ideal that took into account the living. Air quality and distance from town were the basic factors calculated by an urban and political restructuring that led to the 'first medical and urban policing sanctioned by the banishment of the cemeteries' (Foucault 2001a, 147).

Urban medicine focused more on things than people: air, water, and the general state of health. Healthiness is precisely not people's health; it rather refers to the concept of the environment. The French constituent assemblies of 1870 and 1871 conceived of public health on the basis of this latter concept. Here poverty was not yet taken into consideration in terms of danger and fear. It is the English model that would produce this break in the second half of the nineteenth century, with the organisation of a public health plan that, to guarantee the reproduction of the bourgeoisie, will result in mechanisms for the control and care of the poor: vaccination control, obligatory immunisations, the registering of epidemics (and possible indicators of contagious diseases to come), the location of unhealthy places, etc. The controlling tendencies of this national Health Service 'campaign' were so tangible that there was no shortage of forms of rebellion – which, paradoxically, those same public actions were aiming to avoid or radically eradicate. With the Poor Law Amendment Act, approved by the English Whig government in 1834, workhouses were established where, as is well known, the poor were systematically exploited. These actions, then, were certainly not a matter of protecting human rights – a framework that did not yet exist – but a matter of defending a utilitarian cause (healthy environmental conditions to improve the health of the workforce and consequently increase the productivity of factories) and result (a happier, healthier, more productive, and ideally docile proletariat). According to Foucault, it is on the basis of the developments of the British model that our contemporary model of medicine – comprising medical assistance, control of the workforce, management of dangers, data collection, population screening, and mass vaccination campaigns – was formed (see Engels 1973; Szreter and Mooney 1998).

## The politics of health

A few years later, in 1976, Foucault returned to the issue, in a certain sense recapitulating what he had said more broadly in the Rio de Janeiro conferences. I refer now to *La politique de la santé au XVIIIe siècle*,[5] a short text that nevertheless clarifies important implications that his previous lectures had left unelaborated. In particular, Foucault (2001b, 92) explained that *nosopolitics* – literally a politics of the disease – had not been a set of top-down strategies since the eighteenth century, when they were vertically imposed on the population.

The general plan was not so much to take care of needy people through assistance – although this was certainly also the case – but something more radically innovative. The political and sanitary problem of the time revolved around the following issue: 'how to raise the level of health of the social body as a whole', while the proposed solution was based on standards of 'physical well-being, health, and optimal longevity' (Foucault 2001b, 94). The practice required to obtain these three key principles of the new health policy was carried out by the 'police'.[6] Hence, the question was how to defend the 'newborn' society, this social body affected by diseases and susceptible to epidemic contagion? Medical care and police control were ultimately born together. Here, Foucault situates the birth of medicine as the intersection of an economy of assistance and a *police* of health. Once the diseases of the poor have been included in the more general problem of the health of the population, we move from the ethical and charitable hypothesis of medical aid to a form of 'medical police'.

It is crucial to understand the enabling conditions of this fundamental transformation. According to the French philosopher, the answer lies in the 'accumulation of men' and the 'demographic upswing in Western Europe', which made it necessary to develop 'finer and more adequate power mechanisms' for managing a growing population. At the same time, this population was taking on the appearance of an 'object of surveillance, analysis, intervention, modifications' (Foucault 2001b, 95). In this new technology of power, the family assumes a central role and becomes the 'target for a great enterprise of medical acculturation' (Foucault 2001b, 97), which is located in the interstices between private and public, keeping alive the private ethics of health, healthy reproduction, and moral responsibility towards the child. Part of medicine is clearly practised in the hospital institution, but it is also convenient for the market to maintain a domestic form of hospitalisation. In other words, public health is more a general technology, which takes charge of forms of life and existence (including sexuality, reproductive capacity, and the risk of epidemic contagion), than a 'simple' ethics of care. Quoting Nikolas Rose, an important interpreter of Foucault, especially in the field of medicine, we might say that 'the vital politics of our own century' is, in fact, 'neither delimited by the poles of illness and health, nor focused on eliminating pathology to protect the destiny of the nation'. The current phase of public health and social medicine can be rather described as a *politics of life itself*, that is based on 'our growing capacities to control, manage, engineer, reshape, and modulate the very vital capacities of human beings as living creatures' (Rose 2007, 3).

But what do we mean by *life*? We shall comprehend what life really means and, therefore, how a bio-story can be advanced. Perhaps, it is from this very assumption of life itself that the double-edged weapons intertwining with the concepts of violence, care, and cure can emerge today. As always, considering a critical and genealogical standpoint, the issue is not about distinguishing the positive from the negative. Instead, it involves comprehending how the breadth and consequences introduced by the notion of life can act as a conduit for both aspects.

## Living in and with a new form of life?

Let us now go back a few years, to the lectures in Rio de Janeiro in 1974. I would like to pause on two passages, in particular, to draw some important conclusions that this notion of bio-history can offer us in the present. The first excerpt, from the beginning of the second conference, contains an invitation: 'it would be interesting to study the evolution of relations between humanity, the bacillary or viral field, and the interventions of hygiene, medicine, and the different therapeutic techniques' (Foucault 2001a, 135). The second passage is taken from the first conference and recalls an event that took place in the zoological field, among non-human animals: 'One must not forget that the first major epidemic studied in France in the eighteenth century and which led to a national data gathering was not really an epidemic but an epizootic' (Foucault 2004, 16).

Reading these two passages together, it seems clear that Foucault had grasped and intended to comprehend in the concept of bio-history a way of conducting archaeology that should not remain within the confines of the events that bind human animals together. On the contrary, he sought to suggest the usefulness of an approach that would take into consideration all living beings. In the world of life, he seems to also include – certainly well in advance – viral forms of life (*le champ viral*). This aspect is extraordinarily original if we consider that in the contemporary field of biology, there is an open debate about whether viruses are part of the tree of life or not. When the coronavirus pandemic began, that debate was resumed, and new contributions were published. This time, an emergent consensus, which had the potential to enter the order of discourse, had begun to see the virus as a living form. Before, the virus had been considered a parasite that only exploited the life of others.[7] This is just an example of the 'social' nature of the sciences, of their status as both historical and political, being coterminous with power and change according to the contingency of events. From this methodological approach, we might analyse what happens in this conflictual field of knowledge and see what kind of hygienic norm it might lead to, how preventive and therapeutic techniques might change, and where the ensuing global data-gathering might bring us.

To say that medicine is a social, historical, and political matter, always linked to power, is to confirm what Rudolf Virchow himself – one of the 'fathers' of social medicine (and thus perhaps of biopolitics) – said: 'Medicine is a social science, and politics is nothing more than medicine in larger scale' (quoted by Waitzkin 2006, 7).[8] As always, we need to understand what politics can be invented and what new institutions we can forge to give that 'bio' one sense or another. 'We move in a world of perpetual strategic relations. Every power relation is not bad in itself, but it is a fact that always involves danger' (Foucault 1990, 168).

The archaeology of care is certainly useful for looking, with a gaze that is not too shrouded by ethics, at the events in which we inevitably participate. This awareness must also prevent idealising a hypothetical past that never existed, an Eden that the world has never known (Haraway 1992), where people lived in harmony with so-called nature. A hypothetical 'type of natural hygiene or paramedical bucolicism', writes Foucault, offers 'alternatives' that 'do not make sense' (Foucault 2004, 18). As Foucault claims,

> A series of phenomena, like the radical and bucolic rejection of medicine in favour of a non-technical reconciliation with nature, themes of millenarianism and the fear of an apocalyptic end of the species, represent the vague echo in public awareness of this technical uneasiness that biologists and doctors are beginning to feel with regards to the effects of their own practice and their own knowledge.
>
> (Foucault 2004, 12)

The vision of science as a kind of exact knowledge is still widespread and seems to be founded on the teleology of progress. What should be dismissed instead is precisely this (exclusively human) epic based on development (Stengers 2015). Indeed, with Latour, it is worth mentioning that

> After a hundred years of socialism limited just to the *redistribution* of the benefits of the economy, it might now be more a matter of inventing a socialism that contests *production itself*. Injustice is not just about the redistribution of the fruits of progress, but about the very manner in which the planet is *made fruitful*.
>
> (Latour 2020)[9]

We are also in global mourning, but at the same time we are in a system of thought that struggles to conceive the inevitable risk contained in life: illness and death.[10] 'Life is what is capable of error' – this is what Foucault (1991, 22) writes in the introduction to the most important work by his master Georges Canguilhem, *The Normal and The Pathological*. Illness is not measured as a deviation from pre-established norms; it is a change in the quality of life. We need medicine because we are sick, which implies that medicine cannot arise from physiology but necessarily from pathology. And pathology calls normality into question

> The consciousness of biological normality includes the relation to disease, the recourse to disease as the only touchstone which this consciousness recognizes and thus demands. [...] In order for the normal man to believe himself so, and call himself so, he needs not the foretaste of disease but its projected shadow. [...] health is an equilibrium which he redeems on inceptive ruptures. The menace of disease is one of the components of health.
>
> (Canguilhem 1991, 285–287)

## Conclusion

A life lived under protection is also a life that surrenders itself, which is dependent on a certain idea of security, possibly expecting the realisation of this security from the national state, and therefore inevitably falling under the conditions set by the state itself. In this regard, Foucault (1990, 172) pointed out in *Un système fini face à une demande infinie* (1983) that we need to know 'how people are going to accept being exposed to certain risks without being protected by the all-providing state'. What Foucault did not have the opportunity to see completely – leaving this world prematurely, precisely because of a virus – is that healthcare has undergone an epochal turning point, in a neoliberal sense, in which centrality is given to the reason of the market.[11] However, the approach he proposed remains fundamental, as it provides us with a perspective for grasping the ambiguity of medicine: 'what allows medicine to function with such force is that, unlike religion, it is inscribed in the scientific institution' (Foucault 2001c, 76).[12] Or, in other words

> One of the great functions of medicine [...] has been precisely to take the place of religion and reconvert sin into illness, to show that what was, what is sin, of course, may not be punished there, but will certainly be punished here.
> (Foucault 2001d, 1249)[13]

Foucault always intended to pause in the ambiguity, the complexity of the intertwining between knowledge and power, as in the following methodological warning: 'We cannot simply designate the disciplinary effects of medicine. Medicine can work well as a mechanism of social control; it also has other functions, technical and scientific' (Foucault 2001c, 76).[14] In other words, when we attempt to separate the authoritarian aspects from those of care, there is a risk of encountering a dichotomy that fails to capture the political and social complexity of healthcare. This does not imply hiding the more or less visible violence within the medical space. Nor does it suggest that medicine can exist independently of the web of power dynamics and market dominance. However, alternative paths in this field, as in others, offer the possibility of experimentation, creating new and unexpected connections.

It is on the basis of this complexity that the possibility of inventing new institutions and building new practices is always open, ensuring the duplicity of advances in techniques and their parallel potential for control. Foucault's reflections constitute a valuable compass for our practice

> We have to transform the field of social institutions into a vast experimental field, in such a way as to decide which taps need turning, which bolts need to be loosened here or there, to get the desired change; we certainly need to undertake a process of decentralization, for example, to bring the decision-making processes, thus avoiding the kind of grand totalizing integration that leaves people in complete ignorance of what is involved in this or that regulation. What we have to do then is to increase the experiments [...]

> bearing in mind that a whole institutional complex, at present very fragile, will probably have to undergo a restructuring from top to bottom.
>
> (Foucault 1990, 165–166)

## Notes

1 In *Society must be Defended*, Foucault (2003, 242) defines biopower as a concentration of interest that, starting from the second half of the eighteenth century, emerges as a technology of power that is exercised not on the man-body 'but in the direction of man-species'.

2 See Foucault (2003), in particular the lecture of 17 March 1976.

3 See Foucault (1978): in particular Part V.

4 Foucault dwells on the concept of population in several lessons in *Security, Territory, Population* and *The Birth of Biopolitics*. But above all, see *The Politics of Health in the Eighteenth Century*, the version translated by Richard A. Lynch (2014, 117), in which he states that 'an element appeared at the center of this materiality, an element whose importance unceasingly asserted itself and grew in the seventeenth and eighteenth centuries: it was the *population*, understood in the already traditional sense of the number of inhabitants in proportion to the habitable area, but equally in the sense of an ensemble of individuals having between them relations of coexistence and constituting therefore a specific reality. The "population" has a growth rate; it has its mortality and morbidity; it has its conditions of existence, whether a question of the necessary elements for its survival or of those which permit its development and improvement. In appearance, it is a question of nothing but the sum of individual phenomena; nevertheless, one observes there constants and variables which are proper to the population; and if one wishes to modify them, specific interventions are necessary'. See also Pandolfi (2006).

5 Here I refer to the English translation included in *Power: The Essential Works of Foucault, 1954–1984, Vol. 3*, translated into English by Colin Gordon. There are two similar versions under the same name of this text; the two texts appeared originally in volumes also bearing the same title, *Les machines à guérir* ['Curing Machines'].

6 As we know, the modern concept of 'police' does not name a unitary institution but a set of activities: economic regulation, measures of public order, rules of hygiene, etc. In other words – at least in French history – the police have embodied the administration of the social *body*: 'The police, as an institutional ensemble and as a calculated modality of intervention, was responsible for the "physical" element of the social body: the materiality, in some sense, of this civil society, about which in the same period, moreover, it was attempted to conceive the juridical status and forms' (Foucault 2014, 117). For a study on the ambiguity of the 'police' that historically develops this question and charts a Foucauldian approach, see Napoli 2003.

7 On this debate, see Moreira and López-García (2009), where the authors express ten reasons to exclude viruses from the tree of life; Claverie and Ogata (2009), on the contrary, propose ten reasons to include viruses in the evolutionary picture. This debate has recently arisen again. See, for example, Harris and Hill (2021), who reconsider 'a place for viruses on the tree of life'.

8 See Virchow (1957, 1958).

9 He adds that 'this does not mean de-growth, or living off love alone or fresh water. It means learning to select each segment of this so-called irreversible system, putting a question mark over each of its supposed indispensable connections, and then testing in more and more detail what is desirable and what has ceased to be so' (Latour 2020).

10 In *The Birth of the Clinic*, Foucault (1976, 146) states, 'Behind the doctor's back, death remained the great dark threat in which his knowledge and skill were abolished'. As he explains (1976, 145), 'it is at death that disease and life speak their truth: a specific,

irreducible truth, protected from all assimilations to the inorganic by the circle of death that designates them for what they are'.

11 Various scholars have focused on how the eclipse of the concept of the right to health runs parallel to the WHO's loss of a leading role in international health policy, to the benefit of the World Bank. In fact, in 1987, the World Bank published its first document on health: *Financing Health Services in Developing Countries: An Agenda for Reforms*. Its recipe is well known, advocating for: introduction of user fees (direct payment of services) in order to promote insurance programs, the privatisation of health services, and the decentralisation of health care. In this era of health (and its complex legal concept), new problems arise, mainly linked to the fact that the market has become the protagonist of our history of medicine. Vaccination campaigns follow the course of choices, clearly aligned with the profit motive, that pharmaceutical corporations establish. See the works of Howard Waitzkin, namely, *Medicine and Public Health at the End of Empire* (2011) and *Health Care Under the Knife: Moving Beyond Capitalism for Our Health* (2018). In the journal *Lancet*, Julian Tudor Hart, a visionary general practitioner who set up preventive health care in a Welsh mining community back in 1971, wrote an article entitled *Inverse Care Law*. Here, Hart (1971, 405) explains, 'The availability of good medical care tends to vary inversely with the need for it in the population served. This inverse care law operates more completely where medical care is most exposed to market forces, and less so where such exposure is reduced. The market distribution of medical care is a primitive and historically outdated social form, and any return to it would further exaggerate the maldistribution of medical resources'.

12 My translation of 'ce qui permet à la médecine de fonctionner avec une telle force, c'est que, contrairement à la religion, elle est inscrite dans l'institution scientifique' (2001c, 76).

13 My translation of 'l'une des grandes fonctions de la médecine […] a été précisément de prendre le relais de la religion et de reconvertir le péché en maladie, de montrer que ce qui était, ce qui est péché bien sûr ne sera peut-être pas puni là-bas, mais sera certainement puni ici' (2001d, 1249). See the reflection of Agamben (2020).

14 My translation of 'On ne peut se contenter de désigner les effets disciplinaires de la médecine. La médecine peut bien fonctionner comme mécanisme de contrôle social, elle a aussi d'autres fonctionnements, techniques, scientifiques' (2001c, 76).

## References


Agamben, Giorgio. 2020. "Medicine as Religion." Translated by Adam Kotsko, 2 May. https://itself.blog/2020/05/02/giorgio-agamben-medicine-as-religion/. Originally in https://www.quodlibet.it/giorgio-agamben-la-medicina-come-religione.

Canguilhem, Georges. 1991. *The Normal and the Pathological*. New York: Zone Books.

Claverie, Jean-Michel, and Hiroyuki Ogata. 2009. "Ten Good Reasons Not to Exclude Viruses from the Evolutionary Picture." *Nature Reviews Microbiology* 7(8): 615.

Engels, Friedrich. 1973. *The Condition of the Working Class in England in 1844*. Moscow: Progress Publishers.

Foucault, Michel. 1976. *The Birth of the Clinic: An Archaeology of Medical Perception*. Abingdon: Routledge.

Foucault, Michel. 1977. *Discipline and Punish: The Birth of the Prison*. New York: Random House.

Foucault, Michel. 1978. *The History of Sexuality Volume I: An Introduction*. New York: Pantheon.

Foucault, Michel. 1990. "Social Security." In *Politics, Philosophy, Culture: Interviews and other Writings, 1977–1984*, edited by Lawrence Kritzman, 159–177. Abingdon: Routledge.

Foucault, Michel. 1991. "Introduction." In *The Normal and The Pathological*, edited by Georges Canguilhem, 7–24. New York: Zone Books.

Foucault, Michel. 2001a. "The Birth of Social Medicine." Translated by Colin Gordon. In *Power: The Essential Works of Foucault, 1954–1984*, Vol. 3, edited by James Faubion, 134–156. Chicago, IL: New Press.

Foucault, Michel. 2001b. "The Politics of Health in Eighteen Century." Translated by Colin Gordon. In *Power: The Essential Works of Foucault, 1954–1984*, Vol. 3, edited by James Faubion, 90–105. Chicago, IL: New Press.

Foucault, Michel. 2001c. "L'extension sociale de la norme." In *Dits et Écrits, 1954–1988,* Vol. II, edited by François Ewald and Daniel Defert, 173, 74–79. Paris: Gallimard.

Foucault, Michel. 2001d. "Les grandes fonctions de la médicine sociale dans notre société." In *Dits et Écrits, 1954–1988*, Vol. I, edited by François Ewald and Daniel Defert 110, 1248–1250. Paris: Gallimard.

Foucault, Michel. 2003. *'Society Must Be Defended': Lectures at the Collège De France, 1975–76.* Paris: Picador.

Foucault, Michel. 2004. "The Crisis of Medicine or the Crisis of Antimedicine?" *Foucault Studies* 1: 5–19.

Foucault, Michel. 2014. "The Politics of Health in the Eighteen Century." Translated by Richard A. Lynch. *Foucault Studies,* 18: 113–127.

Haraway, Donna, 1992. "The Promises of Monsters: A Regenerative Politics for Inappropriate/d Others." In *Cultural Studies*, edited by Lawrence Grossberg, Cary Nelson, and Paula A. Treichler, 295–337. New York: Routledge.

Harris, Hugh M. B., and Colin Hill. 2021. "A Place for Viruses on the Tree of Life." *Frontiers in Microbiology* 11: 1–16.

Hart, Julian T. 1971. "Inverse Care Law." *Lancet* 297: 405–412.

Hills, John, John Ditch, and Howard Glennerster. (eds). 1994. *Beveridge and Social Security: An International Retrospective.* Oxford: Clarendon Press.

Latour, Bruno. 2020. "What Protective Measures Can You Think of So We Don't Go Back to the Pre-Crisis Production Model?" http://www.bruno-latour.fr/node/853.html. Originally in *AOC* https://aoc.media/opinion/2020/03/29/imaginer-les-gestes-barrieres-contre-le-retour-a-la-production-davant-crise/.

Szreter, Simon, and Graham Mooney. 1998. "Urbanization, Mortality, and the Standard of Living Debate: New Estimates of Life at Birth in Nineteenth Century British Cities." *Economic History Review* 51: 84–112.

Moreira, David, and Purificación López-García. 2009. "Ten Reasons to Exclude Viruses from the Tree of Life." *Nature Reviews Microbiology* 7: 306–311.

Napoli, Paolo. 2003. *Naissance de la police moderne. Pouvoir, normes, société.* Paris: La Découverte.

Napoli, Paolo. 2009. "Misura di polizia: un approccio storico-concettuale in età moderna." *Quaderni Storici* 44: 523–547.

Pandolfi, Alessandro. 2006. "La 'natura' della popolazione." In *Governare la vita. Un seminario sui Corsi di Michel Foucault al Collège de France (1977–1979)*, edited by Sandro Chignola, 91–116. Ombre Corte: Verona.

Rose, Nikolas. 2007. *The Politics of Life Itself. Biomedicine, Power, and Subjectivity in the Twenty-First Century*. Princeton, NJ: Princeton University Press.

Stengers, Isabelle. 2015. *In Catastrophic Times: Resisting the Coming Barbarism.* New Jersey: Open Humanity Press.

Virchow, Rudolf. 1957. *Werk und Wirkung.* Berlin: Rutten & Loenig.

Virchow, Rudolf. 1958. *Disease, Life, and Man.* Stanford, CA: Stanford University Press.

Waitzkin, Howard. 2011. *Medicine and Public Health at the End of Empire.* Abingdon: Routledge.

Waitzkin, Howard. 2006. "One and a Half Centuries of Forgetting and Rediscovering: Virchow's Lasting Contributions to Social Medicine." *Social Medicine,* 1: 5–10.

Waitzkin, Howard. 2018. *Health Care under the Knife: Moving Beyond Capitalism for Our Health*. New York: NYU Press.

### *Legislation*

Beveridge, William. Report: *Social Insurance and Allied Services*. London: HMSO, 1942.

The Poor Law Amendment Act: 14 August 1834.

The United Nations. Article 25. *Universal Declaration of Human Rights*. Paris, 1948. https://www.un.org/en/about-us/universal-declaration-of-human-rights.

World Health Organization. *Constitution*. Geneva: World Health Organization, 1948. https://apps.who.int/gb/bd/pdf_files/BD_49th-en.pdf#page=6

# Musing 2

## Counteracting psychiatric violence through critical heritage studies and cooperation

*Elisabeth Punzi, Helen Johansson and Annica Engström*

Within psychiatry, many forms of violence exist: for example, epistemic, chemical, juridical, and physical. Physical violence, including compulsory care, coercion, and isolation rooms, represents obvious forms. There are also slow forms of violence. One example is the prevalent idea that people who experience severe mental distress are inherently dysfunctional and lack agency (see, e.g., Bentall 2009). Such a perspective ignores the connections between mental distress and violence, abuse, trauma, and neglect. It also ignores that we often do not know why people experience severe distress, along with the fact that each person who experiences severe distress is unique, having personal values, capabilities, and wishes.

Throughout the history of psychiatry, different diagnostic systems have competed for superiority and have replaced each other, and different diagnoses have had their names changed or their thresholds lowered (Horwitz 2021). There is currently increasing criticism towards psychiatric diagnostic systems and interventions among researchers, patients, their relatives, and professionals (see, e.g., Moncrieff 2015, 204; Russo and Sweeney 2016, 2–5). Simultaneously, we live in a society in which we tend to perceive our distress, and the distress of our loved ones, as expressions of underlying psychiatric conditions (Brinkmann 2014, 122; Rose 2018). The degree of criticism towards diagnostic procedures, interventions, and psychiatry itself varies. Some researchers, patients, and professionals are outspokenly critical and want to abolish psychiatric diagnoses and interventions, and even the whole discipline, altogether. Others are more doubtful about psychiatry as a discipline, as well as its diagnoses and methods, and sense that things could and need to be changed for the better. Even we writing this chapter do not agree on everything. But we find common ground, enjoy each other's company and perspectives, and work together, and this is meaningful and important to us.

A diagnosis can be connected to various forms of support: for example, one's personal finances or living conditions. A diagnosis, however, also opens the question of *mentalism*. The term 'mentalism', coined by psychiatric survivor Judi Chamberlin (1979), connotes how categorising persons in accordance with psychiatric disorders puts them in inferior positions, which means that professionals are assumed to know what is best for them. At worse, the patient is treated as a 'pawn' in a game of chess, forced to be complicit with what professionals say (Every-Palmer et al. 2021, 247). Since others know better than the patients themselves, and since mental

DOI: 10.4324/9781032660165-7

distress is perceived as a life-long brain disorder, any intervention, regardless of how violent or dangerous it is, may be seen as legitimate. Many patients become complicit and learn to 'play the game'. They are not in a position to protest, and if they do, they may be misunderstood, and violence may erupt or increase.

Therefore, we need to acknowledge that patients within psychiatric in-patient care are utterly dependent on the professionals they encounter, especially if they are in compulsory care. The relationships between the patient and the professionals become inherently complex, as those who hold the power to restrain, coerce, and control are also the ones who provide care and interventions that may be supportive. This leaves a mark, not least when the staff members whom the patient has learned to trust also must take part in interventions that are violent. Some questions that we would like to raise include, what kinds of marks does this leave, not only in the relationship to staff members but also in other relationships? How can these marks be avoided, and how can the scars they leave be healed?

Amid all this, we want to acknowledge all those professionals who encounter patients in supportive and respectful ways in systems that do not always provide the conditions to do so. Such professionals have witnessed violence and abuse towards patients, in the present and throughout history.

Paternalism, violence, and denial of agency are often portrayed as history, not happening here or now. In museums and exhibitions, the history of psychiatry is nearly almost portrayed as a success story (Yahm 2014, 204). Violence and mistreatment tend to be presented as historical errors that are understandable, since the striving was to cure the disorder. Thereby, psychiatry and psychology are excused for their former wrongdoings. This shows the power of epistemic violence.

Still today, when stories about patients are presented in psychiatric museums, they may be portrayed as dangerous, passive, or exotic (Punzi 2022, 289–290; Rodéhn 2020, 206). There is seldom a focus on patients' memories, experiences, and narratives, and seldom are patients involved in establishing the museums or the exhibits. Subtle forms of violence, such as epistemic violence, paternalism, and violence in the name of a cure, are often downplayed, while obvious forms of physical violence, such as lobotomy, are exhibited and marvelled at. When violence is understood in terms of excusable historical errors and connected to old institutions, ongoing violence may be obscured and thereby perpetuated, rather than scrutinised and ended.

We strive to contribute to a thoughtful remembrance of the past and to decreased violence and oppression in the present through a grassroots initiative called Mad Heritage and Contemporary Arts. This is an association by and for artists, patients, professionals, researchers, survivors, and museum and heritage workers. We arrange exhibitions and workshops, collect memories and narratives, and have our own website in Swedish and English (madheritage.se). We have also published a book *Mad studies, kulturarv & konst* ('Mad studies, heritage & the arts', Engström & Punzi 2022).

Our work has three aims, which are somewhat overlapping. The first aim is to strive for thoughtful and respectful remembrance of patients' past, and to present alternatives to mainstream historical representations. The second aim is to shed light on what needs to be changed today (e.g., through discussing how the past can be understood to change the present and the future). The third aim is to focus on the meaning of the arts. We present visual arts, stories, handicrafts, and poetry made by members of our association and by people in our network. Through this, we show the power of the arts to express agency, criticism, distress, and personally held values, and to engage in meaning-making, change, and creative joy. The violence one has been exposed to can be handled through the arts, and through a long and painstaking process the marks the violence has left can be processed into something meaningful and beautiful (Wandt 2022, 133). We also seek to show the richness of creative works that people who have been patients in psychiatry have produced throughout history. Their works become a form of resistance to violence and attempts to exclude their voices. It should be remembered that these artworks were created by people who were often deemed incapable and at times exposed to restraints, mentalism, and physical abuse by the very persons who were supposed to care for them. We argue that patients' memories and objects should be approached as a form of heritage that is worth being preserved and valued. To perceive and present the memories, narratives, and objects of former patients in thoughtful ways means to recognise and honour them (Demke 2022, 59–61). Thereby, remembrance can become a form of delayed apology. Such an apology could inspire a more human rights-based and non-violent approach to patients within psychiatry today. Violence should not be seen as a solution or necessary evil but something to be avoided (Broberg et al. 2020; Puras and Gooding 2019).

In summary, we sense that it is easy to condemn what people did in the past. Therefore, we should all make sure that we do anything we can, right now, so that the future will not condemn us.

## References

Bentall, Richard. 2009. *Doctoring the Mind. How Psychiatric Treatments Fail*. New York: New York University Press.

Brinkmann, Svend. 2014. "Psychiatric Diagnoses as Semiotic Mediators: The Case of ADHD." *Nordic Psychology* 66(2): 121–141.

Broberg, Emma, Agneta Persson, Anna Jacobson, and Anna-Karin Engqvist. 2020. "A Human Rights-Based Approach to Psychiatry: Is it Possible?" *Health and Human Rights Journal* 22(1): 121–131.

Chamberlin, Judi. 1979. *On Our Own. Patient-Controlled Alternatives to the Mental Health System*. New York: McGraw-Hill.

Demke, Elena. 2022. "Mad Pride." In *Mad Studies, kulturarv & konst* ('Mad Studies, Heritage & the Arts'), edited by Annica Engström and Elisabeth Punzi, 59–61. Vimmerby: Trapart.

Engström, Annica, and Elisabeth Punzi. 2022. *Mad Studies, kulturarv & konst* ('Mad Studies, Heritage & the Arts'). Vimmerby: Trapart.

Every-Palmer, Susanna, Leah Kininmonth, Giles Newton-Howes, and Sarah Gordon. 2021. "Applying Human Rights and Reducing Coercion in Psychiatry following Service User-led Education: A Qualitative Study." *Health and Human Rights* 23(2): 239–252.

Horwitz, Allan. 2021. *DSM. A History of Psychiatry's Bible*. Baltimore, MD: John Hopkins University Press.

Madheritage.se. Mad heritage and contemporaru arts. https://madheritage.se/
Moncrieff, Joanna. 2015. "Antidepressants: Misnamed and Misrepresented." *World Psychiatry* 14(3): 302–303.
Punzi, Elisabeth. 2022. "Långbro Hospital, Sweden – From Psychiatric Institution to Digital Museum: A Critical Discourse Analysis." *Space and Culture* 25(2): 282–294.
Puras, Dainius, and Piers Gooding. 2019. "Mental Health and Human Rights in the 21st Century." *World Psychiatry* 18(1): 42–43.
Rodéhn, Cecilia. 2020. "Emotions in the Museum of Medicine. An Investigation of how Museum Educators Employ Emotions and what these Emotions do." *International Journal of Heritage Studies* 26(2): 201–213.
Rose, Nikolas. 2018. *Our Psychiatric Future. The Politics of Mental Health*. Cambridge: Polity Press.
Russo, Jasna, and Angela Sweeney. 2016. *Searching for a Rose Garden. Challenging Psychiatry, Fostering Mad Studies*. Monmouth: PCCS Books.
Wandt, Marta. 2022. "Ett Stilla Resonerande" (A restful reflection). In *Mad Studies, kulturarv & konst* ('Mad studies, Heritage & the Arts'), edited by Annica Engström and Elisabeth Punzi, 132–141. Vimmerby: Trapart.
Yahm, Sara. 2014. "Oregon State Hospital Museum of Mental Health." *The Journal of American History* 101(1): 203–208.

Part 2

# Unsettling and working through practices and languages of cure

# 4 The 'interpretation workshop' as artistic research

## A methodological approach to original biographical national socialist writings

*Lena Ditte Nissen*

### Introduction

The research material of the overall inquiry of my PhD project within the field of *artistic research* consists of two types of historical texts by two National Socialist women to whom I am related. On the one hand, I look at autobiographical texts by my grandmother Camilla Nissen (née Conti 1902–1993): memoirs written in the years between 1969 and 1971 and a diary written between April and July of 1945. These writings were originally intended only for the immediate family. On the other hand, I examine the writings of her mother, my great-grandmother, Nanna Conti (1881–1951). She was the *Reichshebammenführerin* in the *Third Reich* and published numerous articles and commentaries in the *Deutsche Hebamme* ('German Midwife') magazine, of which she was the chief editor. From the very beginning, these texts were intended to reach a wider audience. In this chapter, I will focus on describing the process analysis and creative rendering of the biographical texts by my grandmother.

Many of the approaches within the German 'culture of remembrance' (*Erinnerungskultur*) are embedded at an institutional, factual level. They undertake the important work of documenting the National Socialist regime and its victims. The cultural discourse of remembrance has increasingly also included the perpetrators.[1] In my opinion, however, the psycho-social level of remembrance is often neglected in the remembrance of National Socialism, the Shoah, and the Second World War, especially when it comes to investigating biographies and the actions of perpetrators in one's own family.

For this reason, confronted with the National Socialist, antisemitic, racist, and eugenic texts of my own ancestors, I ask: *How can I use the example of my own family history to make the emotional affects, often arising from intergenerationally inherited emotions, in confrontation with Nazi crimes of family members visible and perceptible through artistic research? How can I use an ethnopsychoanalytic method, the 'Interpretation Workshop', in this investigation? What kind of aesthetic renderings emerge from it when they are transferred into artistic products?*

In describing the methodological research process and the decisions that informed it, I will argue for the use of the Interpretation Workshop as an appropriate method and an action of care in order to reveal and discuss the emotional

DOI: 10.4324/9781032660165-9

affectedness of confronting perpetrators of National Socialism within the family in the context of the German-speaking former *German Reich* (Germany and Austria). My PhD with artistic research is not a therapeutic project, and it does not aim to present any form of *cure* through which the ambiguities of memory of family members who were perpetrators during the time of National Socialism could be resolved. Rather, I propose to use the Interpretation Workshop and its possible adaptations to cultural products as one tool in a toolbox of many in order to approach the complexities of remembering perpetrators within the family, and my project as an example of a template of what this might look like.

## Methodology

I approach my textual research material by using and adapting one method: the depth-hermeneutic Interpretation Workshop (*Deutungswerkstatt*), which originates from the field of ethnopsychoanalysis.[2] The methodological approach was developed by Prof Emeritus Maya Nadig in the 1990s as a conversational method for groups of researchers to examine the individual emotional entanglement of a researcher with her field. Nadig, who taught European Ethnology and Cultural Sciences and worked as a psychoanalyst as well, argues to define and understand the transferences and counter-transferences between her and her field in the research process as knowledge generated as part of the research results. In Nadig's (2009) own words, 'The Interpretation Workshop aims to explore these unconscious dynamics, taking into account the social and cultural differences of the participants in the group'.[3]

For an Interpretation Workshop, a group of researchers gathers in a circle of chairs in order to discuss field material of one of the group members for about one hour. Also, a group analyst is always present to lead, intervene, and possibly question the process taking place. In the beginning, the person whose research material is being discussed will briefly explain and introduce the material in the way they find it relevant and productive for the group. After this initial introduction, the researcher does not speak anymore but remains present in the group and is allowed to take notes.

> Through the various methodological steps of the Interpretation Workshop – from the first affective reactions to the linking of these emotional irritations with concrete text passages and situations found in the research material, to the linking of the various reactions with the personal history of the individual participants – the emotional is linked to the cultural.
>
> (Nadig 2009)

The members of the group speak from their own perspectives, educational backgrounds, and personal life experiences, but they also try to reflect upon how the given material came to be, and what kinds of emotions and thoughts the researcher may have had in the process of gathering the material. Furthermore, the Interpretation Workshop is not simply a method of spoken language, where only what is said by the participants in the group is read as the outcome. In addition to the emotional and intellectual analysis of a given set of material, the dynamics that develop in the group, or between members of the group, are read as a manifestation of what is implicit in the research material and thus as part of the knowledge produced by the process. These manifestations are often pointed out by the analyst leading the group. For example, if the material is an interview, it might include an inner conflict of an interviewee, which manifests itself as a conflict between two workshop members within the conversation. Another example could be a topic in the material that is omnipresent, but no one in the group talks about it. This could be interpreted as a manifestation of the interviewee's shame about discussing a certain topic. At the very end of a session, the person bringing the material has the possibility to speak again, to reflect on what they heard and what they take from it. This last statement is most often a reflection on which questions, comments, ideas, and emotions resonated with them and their research project.

As my research project is based on my being explicitly *implicated* as a subject[4] within and around the material and the dynamics that I am investigating, using the Interpretation Workshop offers a method to dig into exactly this implication. I would like to explore three more reasons, inherent in the structure of the method, for how it is closely related to my previous professional and personal experience and, as such, is productive for my research undertaking.

In many German families there is often an unspoken rule not to talk about the Nazi perpetrators in one's own family. This is also the case in my family. An aspect of the Interpretation Workshop that I find very interesting is that I continue this ban on speaking while at the same time I break it: during the interpretation of the texts of my grandmother, I silently sit in the circle of chairs. I am not allowed to speak in this setting. In this way, the participants speak for themselves but also as representatives of me in the affective interpretation of the text material. While the participants function as a kind of distanced mirror, my silence during the conversation is representative of the silence of many; thus, in a way, it is embodied and reinscribed here. The silence remains, and at the same time it is structurally thematised in the method itself.

The question of remembering the perpetrators of National Socialism in one's own family is inevitably linked to intergenerational questions about the inheritance of emotions, or so-called *Gefühlserbschaften* in German. This can be taken into account in the group structure of the Interpretation Workshop by having the participants represent different age groups. In this way, intergenerational perspectives and dynamics are made perceivable and become part of the results of the workshops, which can be further analysed as part of the research project.

In addition, the exploratory nature of the Interpretation Workshop as experimental arrangements, the course of which remains beyond my control during the event, mirrors my previous artistic works, which were also created in consciously experimental processes. This processual nature of the method, which unfolds in the concrete passage of linear time and therefore has the character of a non-repeatable performance, corresponds to my focus on time-based artistic forms of expression – such as film, performance, and video – and in this way is also linked to my previous work.

With the aim of exploring the aesthetic properties of the methodology and their potential within the creative process of creating an artwork, the workshops in this research process are being recorded. The audio recordings are then adapted within the framework of artistic production in a second step and transformed into time-based artworks. Here, I focus on describing the process that I have already undertaken with the textual material of my grandmother Camilla Nissen: a series of Interpretation Workshops based on excerpts from her so-called *Fluchttagebuch*,

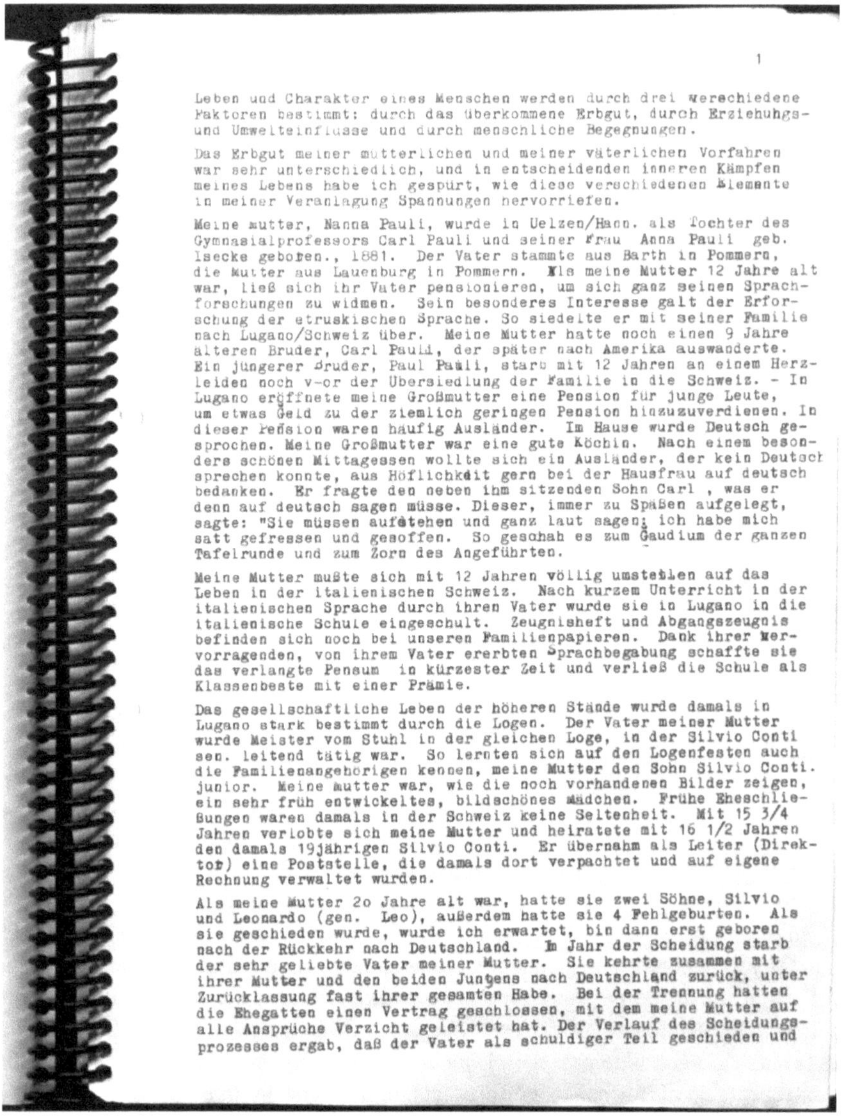

1

Leben und Charakter eines Menschen werden durch drei verschiedene Faktoren bestimmt: durch das überkommene Erbgut, durch Erziehungs- und Umwelteinflüsse und durch menschliche Begegnungen.

Das Erbgut meiner mütterlichen und meiner väterlichen Vorfahren war sehr unterschiedlich, und in entscheidenden inneren Kämpfen meines Lebens habe ich gespürt, wie diese verschiedenen Elemente in meiner Veranlagung Spannungen hervorriefen.

Meine Mutter, Nanna Pauli, wurde in Uelzen/Hann. als Tochter des Gymnasialprofessors Carl Pauli und seiner Frau Anna Pauli geb. Isecke geboren., 1881. Der Vater stammte aus Barth in Pommern, die Mutter aus Lauenburg in Pommern. Als meine Mutter 12 Jahre alt war, ließ sich ihr Vater pensionieren, um sich ganz seinen Sprachforschungen zu widmen. Sein besonderes Interesse galt der Erforschung der etruskischen Sprache. So siedelte er mit seiner Familie nach Lugano/Schweiz über. Meine Mutter hatte noch einen 9 Jahre älteren Bruder, Carl Pauli, der später nach Amerika auswanderte. Ein jüngerer Bruder, Paul Pauli, starb mit 12 Jahren an einem Herzleiden noch v-or der Übersiedlung der Familie in die Schweiz. - In Lugano eröffnete meine Großmutter eine Pension für junge Leute, um etwas Geld zu der ziemlich geringen Pension hinzuzuverdienen. In dieser Pension waren häufig Ausländer. Im Hause wurde Deutsch gesprochen. Meine Großmutter war eine gute Köchin. Nach einem besonders schönen Mittagessen wollte sich ein Ausländer, der kein Deutsch sprechen konnte, aus Höflichkeit gern bei der Hausfrau auf deutsch bedanken. Er fragte den neben ihm sitzenden Sohn Carl , was er denn auf deutsch sagen müsse. Dieser, immer zu Späßen aufgelegt, sagte: "Sie müssen aufstehen und ganz laut sagen: ich habe mich satt gefressen und gesoffen. So geschah es zum Gaudium der ganzen Tafelrunde und zum Zorn des Angeführten.

Meine Mutter mußte sich mit 12 Jahren völlig umstellen auf das Leben in der italienischen Schweiz. Nach kurzem Unterricht in der italienischen Sprache durch ihren Vater wurde sie in Lugano in die italienische Schule eingeschult. Zeugnisheft und Abgangszeugnis befinden sich noch bei unseren Familienpapieren. Dank ihrer hervorragenden, von ihrem Vater ererbten Sprachbegabung schaffte sie das verlangte Pensum in kürzester Zeit und verließ die Schule als Klassenbeste mit einer Prämie.

Das gesellschaftliche Leben der höheren Stände wurde damals in Lugano stark bestimmt durch die Logen. Der Vater meiner Mutter wurde Meister vom Stuhl in der gleichen Loge, in der Silvio Conti sen. leitend tätig war. So lernten sich auf den Logenfesten auch die Familienangehörigen kennen, meine Mutter den Sohn Silvio Conti. junior. Meine Mutter war, wie die noch vorhandenen Bilder zeigen, ein sehr früh entwickeltes, bildschönes Mädchen. Frühe Eheschließungen waren damals in der Schweiz keine Seltenheit. Mit 15 3/4 Jahren verlobte sich meine Mutter und heiratete mit 16 1/2 Jahren den damals 19jährigen Silvio Conti. Er übernahm als Leiter (Direktor) eine Poststelle, die damals dort verpachtet und auf eigene Rechnung verwaltet wurden.

Als meine Mutter 2o Jahre alt war, hatte sie zwei Söhne, Silvio und Leonardo (gen. Leo), außerdem hatte sie 4 Fehlgeburten. Als sie geschieden wurde, wurde ich erwartet, bin dann erst geboren nach der Rückkehr nach Deutschland. Im Jahr der Scheidung starb der sehr geliebte Vater meiner Mutter. Sie kehrte zusammen mit ihrer Mutter und den beiden Jungens nach Deutschland zurück, unter Zurücklassung fast ihrer gesamten Habe. Bei der Trennung hatten die Ehegatten einen Vertrag geschlossen, mit dem meine Mutter auf alle Ansprüche Verzicht geleistet hat. Der Verlauf des Scheidungsprozesses ergab, daß der Vater als schuldiger Teil geschieden und

*Figure 4.1* First page of the memoir by Camilla Nissen. Image by the author.

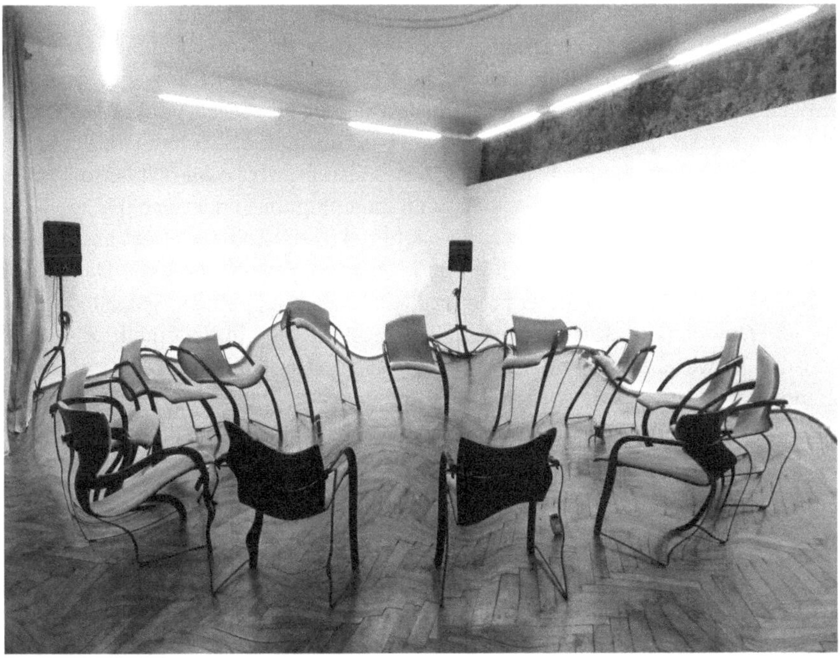

*Figure 4.2* Circle of chairs for Interpretation Workshops at Künstlerhaus Büchsenhausen, Austria, 2020. Image by the author.

or 'flight diary' (April–July 1945), and her memoirs (1969–1971). As my position within the project is strongly influenced by my family relations, I first situate my own cultural biography (Ashplant et al. 2000) within the context of this research. I then describe Camilla Nissen's textual material and outline the practical process of the Interpretation Workshops as well as the considerations that informed the aesthetic decisions during the production of a performance piece and a video installation based on the audio recordings of the sessions (Figures 4.1 and 4.2).

## Cultural biography

I would like to begin by describing why and how I entered into my research project, and how my perception of a sense of identity in relation to family memory has changed through the process so far.

My mother is Danish and my father is German. My mother grew up in a fairly poor Danish working-class household, and my father was born into a well-educated middle-class family with political power. One family seems to have had little to do with National Socialism, and one was part of the Nazi leadership. Despite growing up in Munich, Germany, at first I only really perceived my Danish family as my actual family – my Danish grandparents, cousins, aunts, and uncles were the ones we spent time with, and Denmark was the place where we went every single holiday, besides a few trips to Italy. I vaguely remember my Danish grandfather telling me about how he remembered the time when the Nazis occupied Denmark. I sadly have forgotten all the details and I do not remember any specific political statements. What I do know about him is that he started working as a construction worker at the age of 14, always voted for the Social Democrats, and had four daughters, my mother being the eldest. I also clearly recall that he sometimes referred to my father as 'the German' with an ambiguous undertone that made me feel uncomfortable. At times, I was also referred to as 'German' – perhaps because I share my father's surname, while my brother carries our mother's Danish surname. My Danish grandmother never talked to me about politics; she voted for the Social Democrats as well and worked as a cleaning lady in a hospital for a while. Mostly she was a housewife and took care of the four children. Both my Danish grandparents were uneducated and their daughters grew up in poverty. My mother was the first in the family to pursue higher education. I grew up speaking both languages, Danish and German, with Danish being my true mother tongue, in the sense that my mother only spoke Danish to me from the very beginning. Although I was raised in Germany, my intuitive familial and national identification was mostly Danish until I was a teenager. This changed into a much less clear sense of national and language-based identity as I got to learn more about my German family, the family of my father.

Camilla Nissen, my German grandmother, was always described to me by my father as a loving, caring, warm, strict but fair, and hardworking person, who kept the family from being torn apart in the period after 1945. I was often told that I looked and behaved just like her. I only met her two or three times myself as a very young child before she died in 1994, so I have no memories of my own to rely on and compare those descriptions with. I lived with my father's adopted memories for many years. In ninth grade, when I was 14 years old, history classes in school focused solely on National Socialism for the whole year. In that year my father, who was born in 1935, decided to give me his mother's *Fluchttagebuch* ('flight diary'), written in 1945, in which she describes the family's situation and their flight from persecution by the Soviet Army. I remember reading it with great concentration as a teenager and feeling confused and deeply disturbed afterwards. For example, the text includes the information that my father was part of the *Hitler Jugend* ('Hitler Youth') at nine years old for a short period in 1945. In addition to this shocking fact, the writings also contain numerous racist, anti-Semitic phrases, and descriptions by my grandmother. During that time, I came to the conscious realization of my father being very old in comparison to other parents in my peer group. He was the age of my friend's grandparents, many of whom were also born before the end of the Second World War. In a way, within the process of transmission of memory, one generation is missing. My generational position is somehow misplaced, as most people with parents at the age of my father are about 30 years older than me. Today, I see this fact as one of the reasons of my consternation and, thus, my interest in the history of National Socialism in relation to my family. This somehow puts me in a position in between different generations – on the one hand, affected by a parent who grew up during National Socialism, the Second World

War, and the post-war period, and on the other hand, marked by the social, cultural, and political realities of the 1990s and 2000s.

My father gave me the *flight diary* following a half an hour conversation, after which I was told that I was not to ask any further questions, and that he did not want to discuss the topic with me anymore. So I did not ask. I did not discuss it. I also did not speak to my mother about it. Instead, I discussed it with my best friend, who to this day remembers how upset I was. I also asked her about her family history back then and what her grandparents had done or been during National Socialism, but she did not want to ask her parents out of fear of what she might find out. For me, this was the beginning of trying to make sense of the contradictory information I had been given about Camilla Nissen: my father's loving memory of her and the clearly National Socialist person who she presented herself as in her own writings. I could not bring them together or reconcile this ambivalence within me. I was suddenly no longer the descendant of a brave, warm-hearted, and strong woman, with whom I could and also wanted to identify, but a descendant of a convinced Nazi.[5] As a young teenager, I was overwhelmed by the question of how both *good* and *evil* could somehow be part of me. Had I inherited the evil? What was I, as a descendant, capable of? What was *true*? At school, we had learnt about the horrors of National Socialism, the Holocaust, and the war, but the obvious fact that my grandmother, or classmate's grandmothers and other family members, most likely were passionate Nazis was not covered in our lessons. My sense of self was disturbed and started lingering in between Danish and German, perceived by me as the *good* and the *evil* side.[6]

When I was 28 and Europe was at the height of the so-called migration crisis, my father decided to send me more of his mother's writings, namely her 200-page memoir, which she had written when looking back at her life up to 1971. Her descriptions only reinforced my opinion that she had been an ardent National Socialist. Again, I was not supposed to ask any questions, as the writings had been sent to me without comment, without an invitation to a conversation. Confronted with right-wing politics gaining new strength in Germany, I could not but compare the rhetoric of my grandmother with those by some prominent members of the PEGIDA-movement.[7] It was the same language, and I felt the need to do something, to position myself, to become more visibly politically active. I decided that one day I would have a closer look at both texts, hoping to finally understand them and to find out what meaning they might have for me. As it was unwelcome – indeed, clearly forbidden – to talk about any of this within the family, I looked elsewhere for a way and people with whom I could share my questions, and in 2018 I found the Arbeitskreis für intergenerationelle Folgen des Holocausts ('Study group for intergenerational consequences of the Holocaust') in Cologne. This is a working group that was founded in 1995 by Jewish and non-Jewish German psychologists, therapists, and analysts. Today it is organised as an association and consists of people from many different professions. As the association writes about itself:

> Our aim is to shed light on the deeper layers of the past and analyse how it still affects us today, both personally and collectively. We combine the

> intellectual and the emotional in order to address the topic of the Holocaust and the war and their intergenerational consequences in a multi-layered way. (Website PAKH)

One of the core activities of the organisation is a dialogue group. Here, the members – descendants of victims and perpetrators of National Socialism – meet once a month for informal dialogue. For me, it was the first time that I had been in an environment where the ambivalence of family memory with regard to the perpetrators of National Socialism was openly discussed. The resonance I found in this group, whose most other members were more than twice my age, was an experience of belonging and the feeling that I was not the only one disturbed and confused by the ambivalence of how memory within their family was constructed and conceived in the present. The conversations with the group made it much easier for me to define my distress and my questions and accept my implication in the very process of fabricating memory within my family.

Already before, in art school in 2014, I was introduced to *ethnopsychoanalysis* by Prof Marie Luise Angerer, and through my interest in this field I had learned about the Interpretation Workshop. The method was intriguing to me, as it resonated with my wish to start working more in collaboration with others. Later then, through my experiences with the conversations in the intergenerational study group, I came to the conclusion that using this method could give me the opportunity to invite others to read and think *with* me, and, as described in the first section of this chapter, perhaps even *for* me in some way. Since I was not allowed to talk about the Nazi history in my family, and did not take the agency to speak for so long, I was still sometimes at a loss for words. The Interpretation Workshop could allow me to take the reflection much further by including several analytical voices and perspectives in the reflective process. I hoped that it would also make the process less lonely. I was seeking to create a space and resonant group that would look more specifically at the experience and role of women during National Socialism and its reverberations within family memory, as this had already become one of my main interests. Until that point I had only theoretical knowledge of the method, so I looked to gain practical experience with the Interpretation Workshop as well and found Prof Dr Jochen Bonz, who uses this method in its original form for groups of researchers at various university institutions as well as in independently organised groups. Jochen Bonz studied with Prof Emeritus Maya Nadig, with whom he also led workshops. I became part of an interpretation group that met once a month in Bremen, in order to analyse and reflect on the participants' different research projects by reading excerpts from interviews, descriptions of participatory observations, and images collected during fieldwork. This was an interesting way of learning how the method works. It was especially intriguing to observe how facial expressions and gestures, as well as the group dynamics themselves, became part of the outcome of the workshops. The experience only strengthened my resolve to pursue my goal of facilitating a series of Interpretation Workshops based on my grandmother's writings. With his expertise, Jochen Bonz has become a collaborator in my project, leading the workshops that I facilitate within my inquiry.

As the above shows, arriving at the point of defining my research questions and an appropriate strategy for possibly answering them was not a purely intellectual journey but very much influenced by my own experience of a sense of collapsing identification within the family memory and structure, followed by the urgency of trying to reorder information and rebuild a new sense of family and national identity.

## Interpretation workshops as artistic research

The basis for the first Interpretation Workshops in my research project is the textual material of my grandmother Camilla Nissen: her flight diary from 1945 and her memoirs written between 1969 and 1971. The texts were transcribed by computer (flight diary) and typewriter (memoirs) from the original texts written in the old German script Sütterlin, and then copied for distribution within the family. These transcriptions into easier readable typography were made by the mother of the ex-husband of one of my deceased aunts. I have never seen the original writings, nor have I met or spoken to the woman who transcribed them, nor have I even met my aunt's ex-husband. By this, I want to make it clear that there is a possibility that some parts may be slightly different from the original writings, that things may have been left out, or that additional information may have been added. At the moment, it is unclear where the original Sütterlin version of both writings is stored. I scanned the transcriptions for further use and gave the group of interpreters the passages selected for the workshops in the form of PDFs sent by email.

The four Interpretation Workshops based on the writings of Camilla Nissen took place within the context of the International Fellowship for Art & Theory at Künstlerhaus Büchsenhausen in Austria. I found the participants for the series of workshops via an open call, which was distributed in Innsbruck and Tyrol with the help of the funding institution. Eleven people contacted me, and all of them eventually took part in the workshops. The group consisted of ten women and one man, ranging in age from 23 to 67, nine of whom were students or had completed academic training, and two of whom had attended art academies in Austria. All were white, with only one participant of non-Austrian origin. This is to say, the group was quite homogeneous, which is telling about the means and range of the open call for participants, as well as about those who were willing and able to take the time and energy to participate in such a process. While reacting to such a call may also have to do with whether or not someone feels they have *something interesting* to say, the reasons for the final composition of this group are only speculative. Before coming together as a group, during individual conversations, either in person or by telephone, the participants could ask questions about how I would handle the material gathered in the Interpretation Workshops, in terms of privacy, and what they could expect from the group process. They were also able to share in advance some of their concerns or uncertainties about the topic and their participation. Thus, all the participants were well informed about the methodology and agreed that I could use the audio recordings of the workshops in a transcribed and anonymised form for further use in the context of creative production. The workshops were scheduled to take place over two weekends, two workshops of 1.5 hours per day, at the end of January 2020 and again in mid-April 2020. The second weekend had to be postponed to the beginning of September 2020 due to the COVID pandemic. In total, 12 hours of conversations took place and were documented with several audio recordings.

As examples of how the method works, I will now describe how two different yet connected issues became perceivable through the use of the Interpretation Workshops, thereby informing part of the knowledge produced through the method. In reflecting on the process with and within the group of participants in the workshops, I observed that as the process began with the first conversations with the individual participants, they were all characterised by a certain uncertainty about wanting to take part in the conversations. I can only describe this from my notes, as these first phone calls and meetings were not recorded. Most of the participants felt ambivalent about exposing themselves to historical content that they knew was explicitly Nazi and anti-Semitic. And most of them linked this ambivalence to their own family history; being conflicted in their perceptions of their family's position and role in Nazism, they seemed to feel the same reluctance to label their ancestors as either victims or perpetrators of Nazism, as well as the need to do so in order to be able to *identify* either *with* or *against* their dead family members. Most of them struggled to understand and reconcile the ambivalence within themselves. Already in the individual interviews and then later in the workshops themselves, it became clear that these ambivalences were shaped by different histories, depending on the age of the participants.

The older participants (45–67 years) had mostly gone through a process similar to mine, in which the sense of a coherent family memory had been disrupted by factual knowledge about their ancestors. For some, the then-fragmented understanding of their family history as an individualised memory was still troublesome. Others had accepted the sometimes contradictory stories and historical facts about their ancestors. Most of them had found a clear positioning for themselves as descendants of perpetrators but were still emotionally charged about the issue. While the younger ones (23–38 years old) had not gone through such a process, they had always been conflicted about how to perceive their family history – as belonging to either the perpetrators or the victims. Most of them were unsure how to position their family, but emotionally they were more distant from the issue. Discussed in the Interpretation Workshops, this was explained by the generational gap and the different temporal distances of their life experiences with National Socialism. In the beginning of the second conversation, Participant A of the group stated

> I noticed something very strongly, especially with you who are younger. It seemed rather positive to me, but it seemed to me that you don't have this… you're much more distanced. It would be more a question of whether you also feel a reverberation in the family, yes – or whether for you it's already the great-grandparents, that was so long ago, and I go to university and there I can deal with it and so on. And you have a distanced view.

Two younger participants responded to this, both in a way agreeing but also explaining their more distanced way of discussing the topic in terms of different reasons: class and nationality.
Participant B

> Yes, and what it is for me as well, maybe that I perceive it differently: for me these people are rich, they live in a town, they have a maid there, they have Biedermeier furniture that they have to look after and my grandparents were still farmers. So, it is… we have no family history and there are a handful of photos, so to speak, of my great-grandmother, who should be the same age here. My grandmother didn't write anything down, so we have stories that she told orally, but the more often you remember them, the more you change them, because you didn't write them down. And that's why – even for me it's a different world with maids and all this furniture.

Participant C

> Hum… I have the feeling I have to make a confession, because your diagnosis was quite correct. I personally don't really have a connection to… neither through my family nor personally to the NS. I've been living in Austria for seven years now. I'm originally from Romania.

These reflections show the importance of having a diverse group of people as part of the workshops, as with that comes a more layered and faceted reflection on the text. For example, the issue of class had not occurred to me to be very prominent in the material, yet in the remark by Participant B it was brought up as an interesting and important aspect.

Another topic that was very prominent in the interpretations by the group – and became the main driver for the creative rendering of the conversations – was the ambivalence that the participants felt towards the author of the text.
Participant D

> …that if she had been born in a different family, she might have been a resistance fighter, but I think it's always both. Every person has individual traits and every person is unthinkably connected to their time and their environment and what comes out is a mixture of parts… the proportions vary, but of both. I think it's very difficult to separate oneself from one's socialisation. But it was precisely her lively, interested and, um, committed nature that were certainly her individual traits, but where it then led to was certainly very much the socialisation. That's how I would say it now.

Participant E responded

> Well, I can well understand that she had to burn for something, because there was so much passion behind it, but this inevitability through fate through

> socialisation, so to speak… I haven't found a way out of it yet, but it really gets to me. I then think to myself, this must not be allowed to happen.

Participant D responded again: 'It is also depressing when you break it down to this'.

One could read these lines as an excuse for my grandmother's stark National Socialist convictions, but I believe it also says something about how the group really wanted to understand her reasoning for becoming a Nazi. I would argue that this wish to understand her political and personal decisions derives from the imperative 'never again', which forms such an important part of the German-speaking *Erinnerungskultur*. For this imperative to actually be realized, it requires an understanding why most Germans within the broader society supported National Socialism. The first group consisted of individuals that decided to spend two complete weekends to reflect upon the National Socialist writings of my grandmother, a person who was unknown to them. This dedication to the issue already shows their interest and their wish to reflect and understand. On the other hand, later remarks in the same conversation appear more and more as excuses.
Participant F

> I was also thinking yesterday whether you can make a decision at all then. Apart from what the environment does to you, can you really stand up to it? Can you be so cool? So objective? That the people around you have nothing, nothing … what is good and evil, nothing to this… So whether there is an inner balance you can fall back on? […] The concept of the perpetrator's family (*Täterfamilie*) got stuck in my head. I thought to myself that it's reciprocal: you're so strongly connected to the family that you feel responsible, but vice versa, that you also try to understand it, or yes… these, these tensions… The family simply. That a young girl… what are her possibilities?

This short excerpt begins with what should be read as an excuse: that the author of the text, my grandmother, had no other choice than to become a Nazi. Later on, the participant describes very clearly the ambivalence with which the group read the text. At the same time, they describe the ambivalence that I felt – and feel – when dealing with the texts. This is an example of how an Interpretation Workshop can work: the participants both speak for themselves and make it possible to detect potential underlying issues felt by the person whose material is being analysed, as they are in the process of working with it.

## Conversational artwork

The process of translating the experience of the Interpretation Workshops into artistic practice began with the transcription of the audio recordings of the conversations, followed by a close reading of the sessions, extracting the various themes that seemed to be of the most importance to the group of interpreters, such as the two examples just described.

The decision about how to proceed from that point was influenced by an invitation from two curators to create a piece for a series of performances by a number of different artists to be held at a cemetery of Second World War soldiers in Berlin, the Standortfriedhof Lilienthalstraße in the district of Kreuzberg. The possibilities and limitations of the location and the financial framework provided by the curators significantly shaped the form and duration of the piece I created from the transcriptions. The overall form of the piece was a 60-minute performative walk through the cemetery with two actresses and a historian, with the title TAKE IT AS IT IS, which the audience followed through a space marked by old trees and simple gravestones. I rewrote excerpts from the transcripts of the workshops as dialogues and selected passages from my grandmother Camilla's original texts. These two linguistic layers, performed by the two actresses, were complemented by short presentations of biographies of female National Socialist perpetrators, which appeared as intermezzi by the historian and were interjected into the more theatrical parts performed by the actresses.

I worked with actresses Almut Zilcher and Ruth Rosenfeld. Almut is from Austria, born in 1954; her family background included National Socialists. Ruth is Jewish, born in Los Angeles; she grew up in the United States and Israel and is now in her mid-40s. They both work in German theatres, at the Deutsches Theater and the Schaubühne in Berlin. I chose them because they embody some of the tensions inherent in the subject: the notion of generation and intergenerational memory, and the complication of victim and perpetrator. These facts about Almut and Ruth were

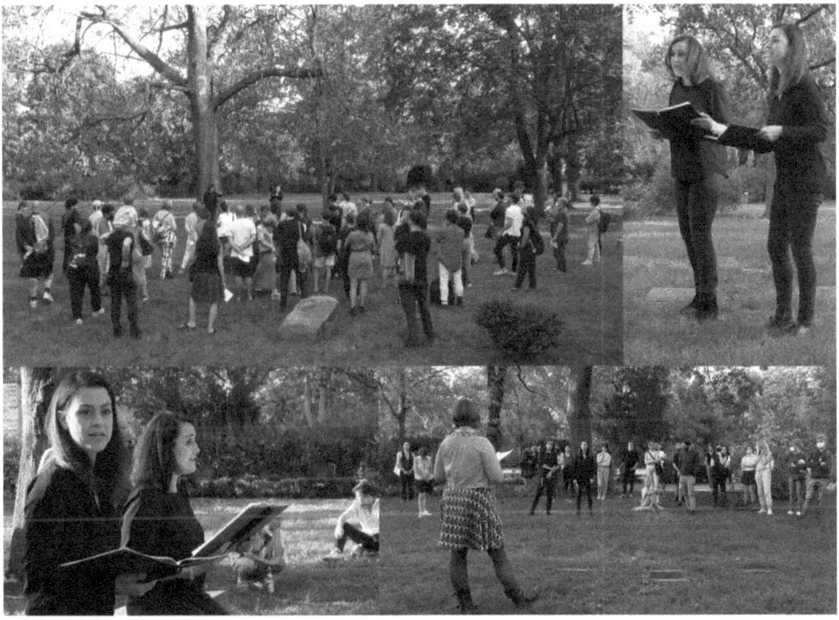

*Figure 4.3* Performance TAKE IT AS IT IS at Standortfriedhof Lilienthalstraße, Berlin, September 2020. Image by the author.

not mentioned anywhere in the announcement or description of the performance. They were a physical and embodied presence of the historical conflict that I wanted to be present in a subtle way throughout the piece. The actresses wore black trousers and blouses, with their hair loose. I wanted them to look as much alike as possible, as they would be playing Camilla Nissen partly together, quoting excerpts from her original writing as a chorus. Quoting Camilla's original texts in the same voice made clear the difference between the two different types of text – the original and the scripted dialogue – and aesthetically marked the historical quotations as such (Figure 4.3).

The historian Sandra Franz is the director of the Villa Merländer, the National Socialist documentation centre in Krefeld. I did not edit her short essays on female perpetrators, nor did I decide on a specific outfit for Sandra but left it entirely up to her how she wanted to convey these biographies with her professional background. The language in which the essays are written is therefore very different from the other two language layers. This made it even clearer that these intermezzi were historically researched and spoken with a different authority of truth and veracity. It was also written in the invitation and the description available at the performance that Sandra is a historian. It was – and is – important to me to give Camilla's writings and conversations about her texts a wider context in order to confront the problematic act of reproducing explicit Nazi content. The anti-Semitic and racist phrases of Camilla's original writings were embedded in a historical context and thus again clearly marked as quotations. Sandra Franz spoke about a number of women in her short essays, including Nanna Conti. No mention was made of the fact that she was the mother of the person whose private writings the audience was also listening to. I wanted to leave it to the visitors to make their own connections between the text of an ordinary National Socialist woman and the biographies of more well-known female perpetrators, in order to perhaps make a connection between the two – personally and with their family history.

## Conclusion

By facilitating the Interpretation Workshops as both my research method and as an experimental cultural practice, using my family narrative as well as the concrete original texts as a friction surface and mirror for the participants, I hope to create a situation in which my individual experience can become adaptable to other people and other contexts, a situation and an experience that will allow those who are part of it to question their own family narratives in a productive and careful way. Besides the creative rendering of the Interpretation Workshop into a performance, the conversations themselves could also be described as a discursive art practice. I adjusted one important parameter of the method and in doing so changed it significantly: the material I gave to the group to interpret was not a text or an image I produced during fieldwork, as the original method intended. The material is historical writing, which is my research material, written by people who are no longer alive and with whom I have a personal relationship. In this sense, I am no longer working with the original method. I would argue that one important specification of the methodology is still present: the personal involvement of the researcher in the material, namely, an emotional connection to what the group is reading and interpreting. The crucial mechanism of the method, that the conversation is a polyphonic reflection of my personal involvement as a researcher in my material, is still at work. The Interpretation Workshop*s* per se were framed as art or artistic research by the fact that they took place in an art institution and by the way that I introduced myself as an artist and filmmaker. I believe this was helpful to the process as it already shifted expectations of the participants away from institutional fact-based knowledge and towards the realm of affect, feeling, imagination, and storytelling.

The further adaptation of the audio recordings of the workshop conversations into clearly defined works of art adds to the experience and outcome of the conversations in the sense that I, as the researcher, have been able to use the group's reflections to inform further steps within my artistic practice and the artistic research process. While the workshops aim to open up the research and include the voices of a plurality of people, the reflective and creative process that follows them is a highly individual and subjective layer of the project. On the one hand, I use the conversations as textual material, and on the other, they act as a catalyst for both personal intellectual reflection on the method and intuitive aesthetic choices in the adaptation of the material through and into artistic practice. The performance becomes objects of research themselves, as I reflect on their form and content, and these reflections then inform the next steps within the research process in preparation for the Interpretation Workshops on the writings of my great-grandmother Nanna Conti.

In the concrete context of commemorative culture in Germany, the Study Group on the Intergenerational Consequences of the Holocaust in Cologne, inspired by my project, has established a practice similar to the Interpretation Workshop. The two main organisers of this group asked me to share my experience in order to help them organise their meetings, which take place online. Members bring texts from their deceased family members. The group does not follow the guidelines of an Interpretation Workshop but instead tests different methods of reading and affective analysis. Two members trained as therapists lead the group through 1-hour long conversations. Since the Study Group on the Intergenerational Consequences of the Holocaust (of which I am a member) is one of the few associations that deals with the intergenerational aspects and ambivalences of family remembrance of National Socialism in Germany, my research project is situated in this specific context of the existing culture of remembrance and memory studies. On the other hand, my project enters the discourse of contemporary art and documentary film and addresses the audience that belongs to these contexts. By framing the project as artistic research, it is also part of related academic conversations in the field of cultural studies.

## Notes

1 Some examples of this are the international Perpetrator Studies Network (http://perpetratorstudies.sites.uu.nl) founded in 2015 by Susanne C. Knittel, the *Journal*

*of Perpetrator Research* (JPR) published by the network, and volumes such as the *Routledge Handbook of Perpetrator Studies* (2020) or *Complicated Complicity: European Collaboration with Nazi Germany during World War II* (2021).

2 Ethnopsychoanalysis traces its origins to George Devereux's seminal publication 'Anxiety and Method in Behavioral Studies' (1967). Devereux argued for the application of psychoanalytic methods to ethnographic research to make the resulting insights usable in research projects. Furthermore, representatives of ethnopsychoanalysis were motivated by the thesis that it is possible to detach the psychoanalytic method from its purely therapeutic properties and instead develop methods to use it beyond the investigation of mental illness for the investigation of cultural developments and phenomena (Erdheim and Nadig 1984).

3 All translations from German into English are by the author.

4 I use the term *implicated* as introduced by Michael Rothberg in *The Implicated Subject: Beyond Victims and Perpetrators* (2019).

5 For a study of the tension within the intergenerational memory of grandparents who adhered to National Socialism, see Welzer et al. (2014).

6 As a teenager I was unaware of the many ways in which Denmark as a state and the Danish people had collaborated with Nazi Germany. Claus Bryld (1995/2008) gives an interesting auto-ethnographic perspective on this in *Hvilken Befrielse* ('What Liberation'), an account of his father who was active in the Danish Nazi Party before and during the German occupation.

7 PEGIDA is short for Patriotic Europeans against the Islamisation of the West (Patriotische Europäer gegen die Islamisierung des Abendlandes).

## References


Ashplant, Timothy G., Graham Dawson, and Michael Roper. (eds). 2000. *The Politics of War Memory and Commemoration*. London: Routledge.

Bitunjac, Martina and Julius H. Schoeps. (eds). 2021. *Complicated Complicity – European Collaboration with Nazi Germany during World War II*. Berlin/Boston, MA: De Gruyter.

Bryld, Claus. 1995/2008. *Hvilken Befrielse* (What Liberation). Copenhagen: Gyldendal.

Devereux, George. 1967. *Anxiety and Method in Behavioral Studies*. Berlin/Boston, MA: De Gruyter.

Knittel, Susanne C., and Zachary J. Goldberg. (eds). 2020. *Routledge Handbook for Perpetrator Studies*. Abingdon/New York: Routledge.

Nadig, Maya. 2009. *Einführung in eine ethnopsychoanalytische Deutungswerkstatt*. Accessed January 10, 2024. http://www.ethnopsychoanalyse.org/seiten/forschung/methoden/deutungswerkstatt_methode.html.

Rothberg, Michael. 2019. *The Implicated Subject: Beyond Victims and Perpetrators*. Stanford, CA: Stanford University Press.

Website of the *Study Group on Intergenerational Consequences of the Holocaust*. Accessed January 10, 2024. https://www.pakh.de/language/en/the-study-group-on-intergenerational-consequences-of-the-holocaust/.

Welzer, Harald, Sabine Moller, and Karoline Tschuggnall. 2014. *'Opa war kein Nazi.' Nationalsozialismus und Holocaust im Familiengedächtnis*. Frankfurt am Main: S. Fischer

# 5 'The way out is via the door'

## R.D. Laing and the cure from the family

*Janina Klement*

### Introduction

This chapter is concerned with the development of R.D. Laing's (1927–1989) psychotherapeutic practice as departing from his critical engagement with British psychoanalysis. Laing was a Scottish neurologist and psychoanalyst whose clinical practice centred on the family, for he noted that his patients were enmeshed in troubled relationships with their immediate familial network. In his first book, *The Divided Self* (1960), he already proposed that the development of schizophrenia was closely linked to disjunctive experiences in family life. In the preface to his second book, *Self and Others* (1961), Laing cited Confucius to ask: 'The way out is via the door. Why is it that no one will use this method?' Thereupon, he theorised a connection between fantasy, family, guilt, and madness, proposing that schizophrenia could arise from the fantasy of quitting the confining kinship group and a subsequent imagination of what consequences this step might impose, ranging from being perceived as ungrateful to being guilty of attempting to destroy both oneself and the family. The temporal scope of investigation are the years 1956–c. 1967, when Laing was employed as a consultant psychiatrist by the Tavistock Clinic and pursued training in psychoanalysis at the Institute of Psychoanalysis in London. The argument is that his involvement as well as his disagreements with British psychoanalysis, specifically object relations, crucially informed both the development of his social-phenomenological research into schizophrenia and his systemic therapeutic approach.

A recent acknowledgment[1] of Laing's significance for the history of human sciences appears in opposition to the still-dominant historiography that seeks to relativise what are perceived to be overly embellished self-declarations of his own achievements.[2] Those accounts focus on Laing as an 'anti-psychiatrist', a label that, according to him, has been misunderstood as a statement of the general rejection of psychiatric practices. In this chapter, I argue that Laing developed his therapeutic programme not merely in reaction to institutional psychiatric practice (in which he participated and which he helped to shape as a young doctor in Scotland) but mainly through his critical engagement with clinical psychoanalytic work. In his autobiography, he states that his colleague David Cooper (1931–1986) coined the term 'antipsychiatry' 'because he felt that psychiatry as the theory and practice

DOI: 10.4324/9781032660165-10

of medical psychiatry was and is predominantly repressive, anti-psychiatric in the sense of the science and art of mental healing' (Laing 1985a, 2). This self-perception must be taken seriously in order to trace what counter-strategies Laing proposed to deal with severe mental illnesses. At present, the hegemony of bio-chemical treatments of psychiatric diseases (Moncrieff 2013; Harrington 2019; Scull 2022) and the credibility of the Freudian talking cure (Borch-Jacobsen and Shamdasani 2011; Borch-Jacobsen 2021) are once again under scrutiny, and calls to revive and improve 1960s-style community psychiatric approaches (Editorial Board 2022), as well as calls for early intervention for anxiety, depression, and psychosis,[3] are springing up again. Also, in light of these developments, Laing's contributions deserve fresh evaluation.

Laing never published a cohesive method that would demarcate his therapy from that of other schools or set out teachable principles. In one of his last interviews, Laing reflected on his reluctance to lay out his method, explaining that it would 'immediately be subject to unbearable corruption and misunderstanding' (Mullan 1995, 316) and be used and transformed in embarrassing ways. Yet, he still considered formalising what he had done in theory and practice 'by the time I [...] re-enter things' (Mullan 1995, 316), a project he would not get around to before his sudden death in 1989. To approach the question of Laing's therapeutic contributions to the cure of psychosis, I begin by sketching out his professional development up until his psychoanalytic training and employment in London, as well the origins of his frictions with Tavistock and British psychoanalysis and his transition to largely independent research and work. By considering his studies of families with a schizophrenic member, in particular the case of the Abbott family, this chapter illuminates Laing's methodological deviations vis-à-vis psychoanalysis and the development of his social-phenomenological approach coupled with an existential analysis of action. A second case, centred around David Clark, a boy considered to be schizophrenic by his psychiatrist, traces the limits of Laing's systemic therapy and his departure from clinical psychotherapy to adopt a religious notion of camaraderie as therapy.

## Laing and psychoanalysis

Laing completed his medical degree at the University of Glasgow in 1951, specialising in neurology and psychiatry (Laing 1985a, 117). After his army service in the psychoneurotic unit at an English military hospital, he returned to Glasgow in 1953 and held subsequent placements at psychiatric and neurosurgical in-patient hospital units. During these placements, he deployed and experimented with a broad range of therapeutic interventions. He was involved in setting up an experimental group therapeutic space known as the 'rumpus room', while also using an orthodox Freudian approach to better understand the experiences of long-term psychotic patients. Occasionally he would recommend the use of electroconvulsive therapies for patients, which stands in stark contrast to his later involvement with force- and medication-free therapeutic communities, such as Kingsley Hall in East London. In 1956, he accepted a full-time position at the Tavistock Clinic in London and began a four-year training in psychoanalysis with Charles Rycroft, supervised by Donald Winnicott and Marion Milner. Laing described his analysis as 'undramatic' and Rycroft as 'an urbane, intelligent man who had no major scenario that [...] he was laying on me' (Mullan 1995, 150). Rycroft, as well as Winnicott and Milner, belonged to the 'Middle Group', an independent group of analysts in the British Psychoanalytical Society that sided with neither of the two dominant and competing camps, representing Melanie Klein's object relations and Anna Freud's child and ego psychoanalysis. With certain variations and emphases, the independents pursued both directions (Thompson 2000, 485). Laing's decision to train with the eclectic 'Middle Group' reflected his lack of ideological subscription to any specific psychoanalytic school. More than anything, the decision to train as a psychoanalyst was a strategic choice, for he thought at the time that pursuing a career in neurology would take him too far afield from his interest in understanding mental illness through the prism of relationships. To Laing, psychoanalysis appeared to represent an 'intermediary position between philosophy and phenomenology and clinical studies' (Mullan 1995, 146), the three fields that he attended to most. However, he soon began to experience frictions with the therapeutic methods taught and employed at Tavistock. In his former positions, Laing had stretched the boundaries of what was usually perceived to be an appropriate therapeutic intervention, for instance, sitting in a padded cell together with a patient and listening to him through the night, or giving a patient refuge in his family home for three months (Laing 1985a, 95, 141). The Tavistock analysts, however, had no tolerance for modifications in the makeup of the consulting room or the technical setting of the therapeutic encounter, and Laing noticed a lack of camaraderie and rapport with patients among his Tavistock colleagues (Mullan 1995, 151, 164, 346).

The completion of Laing's training analysis in 1960 coincided with the publication of *The Divided Self*, followed by *Self and Others*, and alongside his continuous employment at Tavistock, he opened a private psychotherapeutic practice in London. Undeterred by his professional successes in the UK, his gaze was directed towards France, Germany, and Switzerland, where he found phenomenological and existentialist thinkers whose work had fascinated and influenced him since his formative years in Glasgow, such as Maurice Merleau-Ponty, Jean-Paul Sartre, Martin Heidegger, Carl Gustav Jung, and Karl Jaspers (Mullan 1995, 160). Despite his psychoanalytic training, Laing had positioned himself as an interpersonal social phenomenologist. He believed that truth was best approached through detailed observations of relationship ensembles and analysis of their interpersonal communication (Feldmar et al. 2021).[4] His early acquired experience with therapeutic groups in Scotland – which he further developed at Tavistock – had contributed to drive his interest towards social relations. For this reason, Laing came to reject the epistemology of object relations theory, which he was exposed to during his training at the Institute of Psychoanalysis. Finding that it did not serve him beyond an analysis of how individuals project their internalised libidinal relations between ego and 'good' or 'bad' objects onto others, he instead sought to investigate relationship dynamics between people to gain an understanding about how reality is negotiated in the realm of the social.

In 1958, after years of immersion in group psychoanalysis following Wilfred Bion's (1897–1979) approach, Laing and his colleague Aaron Esterson (1923–1999) published their first article challenging psychoanalysis' explanatory power regarding relational experiences in therapeutic groups. They responded to Bion's observation that when two people enter into a relationship during group therapy, the basic assumption of both the group and the pair was that their connection was of a sexual nature. Laing and Esterson objected, noting that there were numerous other reasons why people might come together, and that assuming pairing was necessarily sexual was 'a defence against what is not specifically sexual at all' (Laing and Esterson 1958, 118). Ultimately, they argued, Bion's claim was reductive and the result of psychoanalysis' insufficient recognition of the structural advantages that therapeutic groups have over individual therapy. The dyadic constellation of the latter would limit psychoanalysts when it came to pointing out to the analysand when they believe he or she projects a fantasy figure onto them. The group analyst, by contrast, could observe 'the spontaneous *response* of one person to being seen by another not as he is, but as a figure in that other person's phantasy system' (Laing and Esterson 1958, 119, my emphasis). Paying attention to this process of interpersonal perception would reveal that relationships were subject to negotiations between the fantasy of oneself and the other's fantasy projection. For example, Laing and Esterson recorded that reactions to being perceived differently than how one perceives oneself can lead some, depending on their level of self-confidence, to 'quarrel in anger or [...] break off the relationship under pressure of anxiety' (Laing and Esterson 1958, 120). A common motive for pairing, for example, was a mutual testing of reality that Laing termed 'collusion'. Describing a social dimension of self-deception, he argued that collusive relationships were animated by striving to find in another a complement that helps sustain one's fantasy of self. According to Laing, the psychoanalytic notion of 'projection' failed to acknowledge precisely the demand on another to embody an object in one's fantasy: 'one person does not use the other merely as a hook to hang projections on' (Laing 1969, 111). The two major reasons Laing gave as to why individuals succumb to becoming the embodiment of another's fantasy were either guilt or the prospect of reciprocation (i.e., the other returning one's concession by embodying the fantasy one desires). In summary, Laing's point was that paying attention to the relation between perception and response helps to uncover how reality is socially negotiated. His experience with therapeutic groups gave him an impetus to argue that relationships can function to complement a fantasy of self that otherwise would not be socially maintainable.

Laing and Esterson further developed this position through an independent research project they started in the late 1950s, funded by the American institution Foundations' Fund for Research in Psychiatry. The project evolved around the families of 25 hospitalised female schizophrenic patients, yet only 11 studies were published as *Sanity, Madness, and the Family* in 1964. Their research addressed the question whether schizophrenia is more socially intelligible than had been previously assumed. The meaning of 'social' in their research did not depart from the family context. The premise of the project was to maintain total epistemological openness towards what schizophrenia is: they supposed neither bio-chemical nor psychological explanations. The study design implied that if what are usually interpreted as schizophrenic symptoms turn out to be intelligible responses to relational patterns in the patient's social environment, schizophrenic nosology would lose its relevance and therapeutic intervention would need to shift to the group level. The research was also founded on a rejection of the psychoanalytic method of inquiry. Heavily building on their objections to psychoanalytic interpretation in group therapy, Laing and Esterson criticised the status quo of the psychoanalysis of psychosis. They alleged that psychoanalysts claimed interpretative authority to give meaning to seemingly nonsensical schizophrenic language while neglecting interactions of the schizophrenic patients in their familiar environment. In the introduction to their study, they stated

> Our findings are presented with very few interpretations, whether existential or psychoanalytic. [...] The psychoanalyst frequently makes attributions about the analysand's motives, experiences, actions, intentions, that the analysand himself disavows or is unaware of.
>
> (Laing and Esterson 1971, 25)

But several remarks in *Sanity, Madness, and the Family* reveal that Laing and Esterson were still writing in conversation with psychoanalysis and with clear knowledge of appealing to a psychoanalytic readership. This is evident, for example, in a footnote to a passage outlining the reaction of one of the parents to their daughter's confessions about her sexual life:

> We are limiting ourselves very largely to the transactional phenomenology of these family situations. Clearly [...] the material we present is full of evidence of the struggle of each of the family members against their own sexuality. Maya without doubt acts on her own sexual experience [...] by way of splitting, projection, denial, and so on. Although it is beyond the self-imposed limitation of our particular focus [...] the reader should not suppose that we wish to deny or to minimize the person's *action on himself* (what psychoanalysts usually call defence mechanisms)...
>
> (Laing and Esterson 1971, 42, emphasis in original)

The focus on the family represents Laing's greatest interface with the questions posed by psychoanalysis, and it was maintained in his research collaborations with Esterson, the earliest dating back to the period from 1954 to 1959.[5] By deliberately contrasting their inquiry into family interactions with psychoanalytic models of presupposition and interpretation, Laing and Esterson aimed to establish a social-phenomenological method whose premises went beyond those of psychoanalysis. They therefore introduced spatial and methodological shifts in the therapeutic setting, which constitute conceptual deviations from psychoanalytic orthodoxies: the clinical consulting room was replaced by the private environment of the family nexus, and individual therapy gave way to phenomenological observation of communication between family members in teamwork. Their research method was to simultaneously document the interactions within the family as a relationship ensemble and to grasp each of the member's perspectives on this shared situation. To sketch a complete picture of these multi-dimensional scenarios in retrospect, Laing and Esterson tape-recorded the interviews they conducted with individual family members and with the family unit. The minutes of these tapes were transcribed by Laing and subsequently subjected to an 'existential analysis of action', the results of which were published as case studies condensed into book form.

## Laing's existential analysis of the Abbott family

Through his experience with therapeutic group work, Laing had discovered that a disjunction between how one perceives oneself and how one is being perceived by another can yield dyadic collusions of mutual self-deception – an unstable and mostly short-lived formation, in part due to hatred that is felt towards the other. But he observed that even though such '[crises] of the inter-experience' (Laing 1969, 41) occur in families, the family nexus often promises stability. Laing (1969, 40–41) hypothesised that in order to remain stable, families are bound together by a 'social fantasy system' that fulfils their need 'to find a pseudo-real experience [which only works] through the modality of phantasy', while a 'crisis in the behaviour of the nexus' can be triggered by a family member attempting to opt out of the shared reality. While this might be tolerated and treated as harmless by a lot of families, some other families will punish or label mad those who challenge the nexus' sense of reality. Consequently, the 'way out via the door' might be blocked for those who find themselves in an untenable position because of group demands that are irreconcilable with their experience. The untenable position is defined by Laing as a state of in-between, where it becomes impossible to either stay in a relationship or leave one's acquired fantasy of self and others. Concerned with the ways in which 'the agent is disclosed, wittingly or unwittingly, intentionally or unintentionally, in and through his actions' (Laing 1960, 18), Laing's existential analysis of action ultimately aims at delivering explanations for how individuals come to find themselves in untenable positions. Informed by the idea that psychosis might be a social event that is best understood 'by seeing what sort of world the family has [...] fleshed out for itself, both as a whole and differentially for each of its members' (Laing and Esterson 1971, 21), Laing and Esterson rejected the notion that schizophrenic behaviour patterns could be rendered intelligible through psychoanalytic interpretation. Instead, they proposed that what was usually seen as signs and symptoms of schizophrenia might be intelligible in relation to the social environment of the individual. Their approach can well be illustrated by the example of Esterson's patient Maya Abbott[6] and her family, representing one of the case studies published in *Sanity, Madness and the Family* (see Laing and Esterson 1971, 31–50). The evaluation of this study established that the factuality of her clinical diagnosis indeed dissolved through its remarkable intelligibility in relation to the social reality in which she lived.

At the time of investigation, Maya was 25 years old and had spent the last decade in a psychiatric hospital. Clinically diagnosed as paranoid schizophrenic, she experienced auditory hallucinations and exhibited signs of depersonalisation, catatonia, affective impoverishment, autistic withdrawal, and impulsive behaviour. The parents reported that by the age of 14, Maya began to pursue autonomous studies, wanted to take on tasks independently, and no longer sought physical closeness to them. According to Laing, Maya's developing autonomy and independence of thought and action were interpreted by her parents as alarming signs of illness. Maya's maturing sense of self led to a crisis in the family's sense of reality in which Maya had usually just '[accepted] everything' (Laing and Esterson 1971, 34–35) the parents had said and asked from her. As further conversations revealed, the parents therefore felt emotionally disregarded and rejected by Maya, and in response to the disjunction they convinced themselves that Maya could read their minds, though she possessed neither control nor knowledge of her ability. In the interviews, the parents eventually confessed that they began secret experimentations, such as mutely sitting next to Maya and concentrating on her, to test how she 'reacted' to their thoughts; however, they scoffed at Maya's developing suspicion that they were trying to influence her. Moreover, what Maya knew to report about her own life experience was outright denied or contradicted by her parents, even '*in the presence of the interviewer*' (Laing and Esterson 1971, 42, emphasis in original), based on the premise that because of her illness she did not know her own memory and experience anymore

> They spoke and acted as though they knew better than Maya what she remembered, what she did, what she imagined, what she wanted, what she felt, whether she was enjoying herself or whether she was tired…
>
> (Laing and Esterson 1971, 42)

Laing's report (Laing and Esterson 1971, 32, 34) shows that the parents' view of Maya was so estranged from how Maya experienced herself that she came to reject her own experience of herself, claiming that what she remembered was not 'true memory' and that '"voices" often did her thinking'.[7] But especially in light of the fact that the parents *did* try to influence her in experiments and believed that she read their thoughts without any intention or doing of her own, her clinically diagnosed 'auditory hallucinations' and 'ideas of influence' appear intelligible. In terms of an untenable position, it became impossible for Maya to either remain in or leave the fantasy of not thinking her own thoughts, because not only did her parents deny that Maya could trust her experience of herself but they also denied that they were *actually* doing what Maya noticed them doing, such as conducting secret experimentations or communicating through winks and gestures with each other in her presence. Her resulting difficulty of not knowing 'when to trust or mistrust her own perceptions and memory or her mother and father' (Laing and Esterson 1971, 43) could not be resolved and, in social-phenomenological language, this caused her to remain in an untenable in-between, atrophying her sense of being a person (depersonalisation), her language (autistic withdrawal), her emotions (affective impoverishment), and her movements (catatonia).

Laing and Esterson's study not only suggested that Maya's clinical symptoms were socially intelligible in the context of her family's interactions, but it also put pressure on bio-chemical explanations of psychosis. Indeed, in Laing's account, Maya's symptoms appear as understandable reactions to the confusing and manipulative behaviour in her immediate environment. Although it is not clear from the documentation whether the interviews themselves disentangled the obvious mystifications that were going on in the families and thus helped the patients in the long term, an application drafted by Laing and Esterson in 1964 asking for further funds to continue their investigation with a control group is supported by the claim that their study indeed entailed therapeutic effects:

> [Our] method of investigation is itself therapeutic, and demands further development in this direction. All our patients were able to leave hospital as a result of our investigation, of whom seventeen per cent had relapsed after one year, compared with a relapse rate of eighty per cent for similar patients treated by standard methods.
>
> (Laing and Esterson 1964, 1)

Obviously, the authors did not count psychoanalysis as a standard method for the treatment of psychosis; they refer to the clinical use of electroshocks and psychopharmaceuticals to ease psychotic symptoms. They likewise disputed the effectiveness of these methods, for their research had produced 'compelling evidence that schizophrenia is much less of an organic illness (if it is at all) than a reaction to social stress of a peculiar kind' (Laing and Esterson 1964, 1). Laing accused biological psychiatrists of failing to pay attention to the 'patient's *experience* from the patient's point of view' (Laing 1964, 190, emphasis in original) but ultimately blamed psychoanalysis for adopting a strategy with similarly poor outcomes:

> One might have hoped that psychoanalysis would step in here. But there is an abiding tendency in psychoanalysis to suppose that the schizophrenic's experiences are somehow unreal or invalid; one can make sense of them only by interpreting them; without truth-giving interpretations the patient is enmeshed in a world of delusion and self-deception.
>
> (Laing 1964, 191)

Here, psychoanalysis is portrayed by Laing as a patronising and neglectful practice that ultimately displays remarkable parallels to the recorded behaviour of Maya's parents, who, likewise, claimed knowledge of Maya's condition without having awareness of their own complicity in its construction. Laing left Tavistock in 1967 after his external funding was not renewed. His professional exit from clinical psychoanalysis allowed him to sharpen his critique of the psychoanalysis of schizophrenia. In a lecture titled 'Introduction to Phenomenology' that he delivered in 1975, he strongly criticised Wilfred Bion's documentation of a therapeutic session with his schizophrenic patient, in which he employed the analytic framework of object relations theory. Nearly in a tantrum, Laing warned against 'this type of construction [...] currently spreading like wildfire in Latin America and Japan and I don't know [...] where else' (Laing 1975, 10). Laing's opposition to the further dissemination of the psychoanalysis of schizophrenia raises the question of what he considered to be a suitable therapeutic intervention to help individuals in untenable situations.

## Therapy and camaraderie

Despite regularly seeing patients in private practice,[8] Laing's main interest was the possibility of therapeutic intervention on a social level. As noted above, his previous research on families of schizophrenics prompted him and Esterson to call for further development of the family therapy of schizophrenia. However, the follow-up funding they were granted only covered further research with a control group, stalling the desired development of new group therapeutic methods through research. It is still possible to infer from Laing's practice what he imagined a systemic therapeutic intervention to look like. The example from his practice selected for the present purpose provides information both about Laing's approach and the mental health orthodoxy within which he practised, namely, a clinic that strongly focused on child guidance, youth delinquency, and early intervention for mental illness. Via the clinical case that Laing recalled at the occasion of the Association of Family Caseworkers' Study Day in 1968, he repeated the position that derived from his past family research. Instead of an individual crisis, a social crisis could be the root cause of a call for psychiatric help, which remained unaddressed by the psychiatric standard approach, which at the time relied mostly on individual diagnoses and subsequent medical treatment. Psychiatrists would therefore be required to redefine their task to investigating what happens on a systemic level (Laing 1999, 25).

Laing was consulted for an opinion about nine-year-old David Clark, who had been visiting a child guidance clinic for three months without any improvement in his condition. The psychiatrist in charge began to suspect that David might be schizophrenic and considered recommending hospitalisation. Laing remarked that David and his mother had exclusively attended clinical appointments, a situation that occasioned him to visit their home, where he met all members of the nuclear family and derived a picture of David's living situation. He was told by David's mother that her son's problems included not listening to her, not being interested in reading and writing, and not worrying about this state of things. A subsequent private 'man-to-man chat' (Laing 1999, 27) with David confirmed his lack of interest in reading and writing, and also that he loved to draw and work with things, and often went to construction sites to help the builders. Furthermore, Laing learned from David's mother that, in her view, David took after her and ultimately his grandfather – for just like her father, *she* was often out of the house and reckless. In the opinion of her mother (David's grandmother), this was unacceptable behaviour. David's grandmother was resentful of her husband, punished her daughter with beatings, and now counselled her to '[beat] it out of David' (Laing 1999, 28) as well. In Laing's assessment, the problem causing David's poor school performance and disobedience towards his mother was not untreated schizophrenia, but that he violated the brutally enforced family-imaginary system by following his own interests and, quite literally, choosing the 'way out via the door'. Laing's conclusion was that individual therapy away from the family context could structurally deliver no results, for it failed to grasp the *a priori* (i.e., without reflection) generationally enforced phantasma of control and penalty that had now turned against David; instead of beatings, the punishment was then psychiatric consultation and diagnosis. For David, Laing instead recommended therapy sessions for David's mother and grandmother. This result requires further reflection for although Laing shifted the question of therapeutic intervention to a systemic, generational level, in practice it was simply two different family members who required therapy. As a conclusion it appears unsatisfying, especially considering the mother-blaming discourse, yet it importantly reflects the fundamental premise of Laing's psychiatric approach, which shifted the therapeutic inquiry from *How can the individual be cured from its symptom?* to *Is the calling of an individual's symptom itself a symptom of a social crisis, whose core is bypassed in attributing mental illness to the individual?* This epistemological project led Laing, at a point, to theorise that 'schizophrenia (in this sense: being tied in a knot of non-compossible intersecting sets of relations) takes at least three generations to produce. And is really inconceivable without a 3, 4, or even 5 generational model' (Laing n.d., 15).

His reading of Sartre's late work *Critique of Dialectical Reason* (1960) – culminating in the book *Reason and Violence* (1964) co-authored with Cooper – ultimately caused Laing to pose the question of the social intelligibility of schizophrenia in relation to society as a whole. Inspired by Sartre, he increasingly employed the neo-Marxist notion of 'totalisation', probing the intellectual possibility to understand the interconnectedness of all things. It was also for this reason that he co-organised an international congress titled *Dialectics of Liberation* in 1967 in London, with the aim to create a transnational network of scholars and activists to exchange ideas about the possibility of individual and social liberation. In his talk at the congress, Laing (2015) contemplated how his findings from family research could contribute to the demystification of both human and international relations in society. While his therapeutic practice so purposefully transcended the question of the individual, it had previously focused on a domestic unit that was practically still manageable. The shift of attention to the societal level can be explained by an impasse Laing encountered in his systemic intervention approach: although he found that an individual's display of schizophrenic symptoms was intelligible within the dysfunctionality of its immediate social environment, this very familial dysfunction could not be adequately explained without recourse to a macro-structure.

When faced with the absence of a more or less defined unit allowing for a practical intervention, Laing carved out the possibility for camaraderie as therapy, a form of relationship that is therapeutic but eludes any technical micro-management of the individual and cannot be systematically learned, taught, or scientifically approached. Laing believed that if a symptom of schizophrenia was a breakdown of communication, a communal experience that fostered shared joy provided a new basis for communication. Communication – that is, a lack of separateness from others – arose from the experience of communion, which to Laing bore a decidedly religious notion of sharing an experience or a meal in a celebratory fashion (Laing 1985a, 116, 1985b, 14). In a speech he gave in 1983 under the auspices of Wellspring, a religious charity in Scotland, Laing stated that the meaning he attributed to therapy went back to its early Christian roots and described 'a dedication to skilful attentiveness to others' (Laing 1985b, 13). As Miller (2012) has demonstrated elsewhere, religion and psychiatry had already been imbricated for Laing in his early professional context and continued to do so throughout his career. From around the 1950s onwards, Laing made repeat visits to the spiritual Christian community of Iona, founded by the Church of Scotland minister George MacLeod in 1938 (Miller 2012, 147). Laing also visited (at least once) and gave a talk titled 'Birth and Death' (presumably in the early 1960s)[9] at the Withymead house in Essex, a quasi-familial therapeutic community that housed severely disturbed patients and offered a range of art therapies in the Jungian tradition.[10] Through his clinical work, his regular visits to therapeutic communities, and a broader British 'communion paradigm' (Miller 2012, 148) dissolving religious life in the community since the 1950s, Laing had adopted the view that the experience of communion via a shared sense of belonging could restore relational life to individuals who had previously been considered hopeless psychiatric cases. In his autobiography, he recalls that while working in the psychiatric wards of Gartnavel Royal Hospital in Glasgow during New Year's Eve – which used to be Scotland's biggest celebration of the year – he witnessed drastic behavioural changes in even the most catatonic and mute schizophrenic patients, such as smiles, laughs, handshaking, or wishing others a happy New Year.

> The change, however fleeting, in some of the most chronically withdrawn, 'backward' patients is amazing. If any drug had this effect, for a few hours, even a few minutes, it would be world famous, and would deserve to be celebrated as much as the Scottish New Year. The intoxicant here however is not a drug, not even alcoholic spirits, but the celebration of a spirit of fellowship.
>
> (Laing 1985a, 29)

In the Wellspring talk he gave two years before publishing his autobiography, Laing specified that

> Communing with other people [...] is nothing to do with technique [...] it is a trans-personal field – a sort of force field that is not to be discovered within the investigative competence of physics or science. So I will have to call it "spiritual".
>
> (Laing 1985b, 14)

As Miller (2012) has shown, Laing's investment in the therapeutic spirit that 'exists in us and between us and that is the only healing power that exists' (Laing 1985b, 15) can be traced back to a 'theological hinterland' that affected his psychiatric practice, in the sense that Laing employed an 'incarnational, corporate Christian theology which demanded social inclusion and political justice in the name of a "Great Feast" to which all – including the mentally ill – were invited' (Miller 2012, 139). The 'abyss of difference' between schizophrenics and non-schizophrenics theorised by the phenomenologist Karl Jaspers is countered by Laing precisely through this recourse to a corporate Christian theology that insists on an unshakeable spiritual bond 'throughout the whole creation' (Laing 1985b, 15). This, of course, leaves little doubt that his own therapeutic community experiment Kingsley Hall, that opened its doors in 1965, can be attributed to Laing's confluence of psychiatric practice and religious belief.[11] Kingsley Hall was fundamentally rooted in Laing's idea of companionship: while the use of force or medications was forbidden (which often led to conflicts, as some residents harmed themselves and sometimes others as well) and residents could engage in talking therapies with the resident psychiatrists if they so wished, the leading principle was that people experiencing turmoil or a breakdown could trust that they would be attended and safeguarded by companions who were in a more stable state of mind than them. Rarely, and mostly when alluding to the Kingsley Hall resident Mary Barnes or his friend Jesse Watkins (both of whom went through psychosis without seeking medical attention at a hospital and fully recovered), Laing called these experiences a 'journey' or 'voyage'. Amplified through Barnes's (1971) own account of her life at Kingsley Hall, *Two Accounts of a Journey Through Madness*, these terms – rather than, for example, camaraderie or friendship – became dominantly associated with what Kingsley Hall was like.[12]

Ultimately, Laing's insistence on the therapeutic dimension of companionship marked his refusal to depend on therapeutic techniques operating exclusively within the confines of his empirical findings in group settings. Both the social fantasy system of the family and the collusion of a toxic relationship rely on a relational model, defined by perception-action-reaction, which Laing observed in his group therapeutic work and phenomenological family research, and which he sought to break up through systemic interventions. Laing's Christian-inspired idea of camaraderie as therapy, however, aims to reach beyond the limits of family therapy, for it no longer takes the analysis of the vicissitudes of perception as a starting point. Instead of therapeutic techniques, the focus is on recovering the schizophrenic's lost experience of fellowship.

## Conclusion

This chapter traced the development of Laing's therapeutic practice and its conflictual relationship with post-war British clinical psychoanalysis. While Laing's focus on the family signified a continuity with psychoanalytic practice, he turned away from the psychoanalytic claim to interpretation and neglected the central place of the unconscious for the therapy of schizophrenia. In its absence, a new ensemble of therapies was proposed by Laing, which I have identified as existential analysis of action, systemic intervention, and a return to commonality. The former two are rooted in Laing's observation that mutual deception (collusion) and social fantasy are the dominant relational modes through which reality is negotiated in group interactions. Laing theorised that schizophrenic expression would find its rationality when seen in the context of relational dysfunctionality, which he ultimately reduced to a collective insistence on the truthfulness of a shared fantasy. Despite finding its expression in the individual, Laing therefore proposed that schizophrenia was better grasped in terms of a crisis within the social fantasy of the family nexus that impacted its interrelations. Following his research on families of schizophrenic patients, Laing called for structural intervention into family life to prevent children especially from being initiated into a 'schizophrenic career', and he warned medical practitioners from treating an individual scapegoat of what was in fact a social crisis. As we have seen, from the early 1960s onwards, Laing began to increasingly link the question of the family nexus' dysfunctionality to broader society. Beyond his role as therapist, he found a new vocation as a public intellectual, spreading his ideas to audiences worldwide. In response, Marxist theorists like Peter Sedgwick and Russell Jacoby critiqued the tendency in Laing's work to ignore non-immediate factors in its implicit assumption that the study of group dynamics is exhausted by an empirical analysis of a situation in its immediate display of perception-action-reaction, and that the 'game' of collusion Laing describes – which seeks constant confirmation from another to sustain the self – is one practised not by all human beings but human beings who are already 'mesmerized and mutilated' (Jacoby 1997, 144). In this chapter, however, I stressed a practical turn in Laing's therapy that coincided with his theoretical turn to society. Although his lecture activity might partially suggest otherwise, the whole of society did not practically become Laing's new patients. The practice he pursued since c. 1965 was no longer exclusively based on his phenomenological findings but increasingly owed to a Christian imperative of a human community and lived social justice. At least until 1970 – when his therapeutic community Kingsley Hall dissolved – Laing belonged to a psychiatric avant-garde in Britain: his sanctuary gave refuge and offered therapies to anyone experiencing severe forms of mental distress. A comparable willingness to take in the most seriously ill schizophrenics was not present in the therapeutic communities that followed Kingsley Hall, and in which Laing no longer assumed a central role.[13] To conclude, Laing's therapy aimed at providing his patients and clients with a 'way out' of their untenable situations, while his therapeutic community was open to those alienated from social life who had nowhere else to go. Laing's work, as demonstrated through his theoretical writings and practical interventions of this period, resists reductive categorisation, combining novel analytical frameworks with eclectic therapeutic innovations. His readiness to experiment, to engage with different approaches, and to establish alternative therapeutic spaces can enrich contemporary mental health practice – showing that theoretical and practical engagement need not be mutually exclusive.

## Notes

1 See Scott and Thorpe (2006); McGeachan (2012, 2014); Miller (2004, 2009); Wall (2017); Chapman (2020, 2021); Bradshaw and Brown (2018).
2 See Ingleby (1981); Andrews (1998); Freeman (2005); Abrahamson (2007); Beveridge (2011).
3 Wellcome Trust: Mental Health Strategy. https://wellcome.org/what-we-do/mental-health.
4 See the contribution of Andrew Feldmar during the panel discussion "Psychoanalysis and Psychedelics: The Inaugural Event" hosted by the Maudsley Psychedelic Society (mins. 1:00–1:02).
5 See Esterson and Laing's *An Existential Analysis of a Schizophrenic Woman (1954–1959)*.
6 The patients' names were pseudonymised by Laing and Esterson.
7 For a discussion of the implications of schizophrenia as existential action on the self that produces madness, see Miller (2008).
8 For a discussion of the range of methods Laing employed in individual therapy, see Schneider (2000).
9 Laing's personal notebook gives evidence of this visit. See MS Laing A672, 2.
10 For a detailed account of the Withymead therapeutic model, see Hogan (2001).
11 This connection has also been suggested by Laing's son, Adrian Laing. See Laing (1997, 102).
12 For instances of this, see Guattari (1984) and Sophia Rohwetter's chapter in this volume for Franco Basaglia's perspective on Kingsley Hall.
13 I owe this reference to Sonu Shamdasani.

## References

### *Archival sources*

Laing, Ronald David. n.d. *Draft Notes Concerning Family Relationships*. Unpublished. MS Laing A663. Special Collections, Glasgow University Library.

Laing, Ronald David. n.d. *Notes/Drafts*. Unpublished. MS Laing A672. Special Collections, Glasgow University Library.

Laing, Ronald David. 1960. *The Development of Existential Analysis*. Unpublished. MS Laing A116. Special Collections, University of Glasgow Library.Laing, Ronald David. 1975. *Lecture: Introduction to Phenomenology*. Typescript. Unpublished. MS Laing A77. Special Collections, Glasgow University Library.

Laing, Ronald David, and Aaron Esterson. 1959. *An Existential Analysis of a Schizophrenic Woman (1954–1959)*. Unpublished. MS Laing A273–275. Special Collections, Glasgow University Library.

Laing, Ronald David, and Aaron Esterson. 1964. *Application for Funds by Drs A. Esterson and R.D. Laing*. Unpublished. MS Laing A627. Special Collections, Glasgow University Library.

### *Secondary Sources*

Abrahamson, David. 2007. "R.D. Laing and Long-Stay Patients: Discrepant Accounts of the Refractory Ward and 'Rumpus Room' at Gartnavel Royal Hospital." *History of Psychiatry* 18(2): 203–215.

Andrews, Jonathan. 1998. "R.D. Laing in Scotland: Facts and Fictions of the 'Rumpus Room' and Interpersonal Psychiatry." In *Cultures of Psychiatry and Mental Health Care in Postwar Britain and The Netherlands*, edited by Marijke Gijswijt-Hofstra and Roy Porter, 121–150. Leiden: Brill.

Barnes, Mary, and Joseph Berke. 1971. *Two Accounts of a Journey through Madness*. London: MacGibbon and Kee.

Beveridge, Allan. 2011. *Portrait of the Psychiatrist as a Young Man: The Early Writing and Work of R.D. Laing, 1927–1960*. Oxford: Oxford University Press.

Borch-Jacobsen, Mikkel. 2021. *Freud's Patients: A Book of Lives*. London: Reaktion Books.

Borch-Jacobsen, Mikkel, and Sonu Shamdasani. 2011. *The Freud Files: An Inquiry into the History of Psychoanalysis*. Cambridge: Cambridge University Press.

Bradshaw, Alan, and Stephen Brown. 2018. "Up Rising: Rehabilitating J.G. Ballard's High-Rise with R.D. Laing and Lauren Berlant." *Environment and Planning D: Society and Space* 36(2): 331–349.

Chapman, Adrian. 2020. "'May All Be Shattered Into God': Mary Barnes and Her Journey through Madness in Kingsley Hall." *Journal of Medical Humanities* 41(2): 207–228.

Chapman, Adrian. 2021. "Dwelling in Strangeness: Accounts of the Kingsley Hall Community, London (1965–1970), Established by R.D. Laing." *The Journal of Medical Humanities* 42(3): 471–494.

Editorial Board. 2022. "The Solution to America's Mental Health Crisis Already Exists." In *The New York Times*, 4 October. https://www.nytimes.com/2022/10/04/opinion/us-mental-health-community-centers.html.

Feldmar, Andrew, Paul Zeal, Nathan Gorelick, and Timmy Davis. 2021. "Psychoanalysis and Psychedelics: The Inaugural Event." Panel discussion hosted by the Maudsley Psychedelic Society, 2 March. https://www.youtube.com/watch?v=HsDnRkZSBII.

Freeman, Hugh. 2005. "Psychiatry and the State in Britain." In *Psychiatric Cultures Compared, Psychiatry and Mental Health Care in the Twentieth Century: Comparisons and Approaches*, edited by Marijke Gijswijt-Hofstra, Harry Oosterhuis, Joost Vijselaar, and Hugh Freeman, 116–140. Amsterdam: Amsterdam University Press.

Guattari, Félix. 1984. *Molecular Revolution: Psychiatry and Politics*, 51–59. Harmondsworth: Penguin.

Harrington, Anne. 2019. *Mind Fixers: Psychiatry's Troubled Search for the Biology of Mental Illness*. New York: W. W. Norton & Company.

Hogan, Susan. 2001. "Withymead. Britain's First Therapeutic Community Dedicated to Art Therapy." In *Healing Arts: The History of Art Therapy*, edited by Susan Hogan, 220–289. London: Jessica Kingsley Publishers.

Ingleby, David. 1981. *Critical Psychiatry: The Politics of Mental Health*. Harmondsworth: Penguin.

Jacoby, Russell. 1997. *Social Amnesia. A Critique of Contemporary Psychology.* New York: Routledge.

Laing, Adrian. 1997. *R.D. Laing: A Biography*. London: HarperCollins.

Laing, Ronald David. 1964. "Is Schizophrenia a Disease?" *International Journal of Social Psychiatry* 10(3): 184–193.

Laing, Ronald David. 1967. *The Politics of Experience and the Bird of Paradise*. Harmondsworth: Penguin Books.

Laing, Ronald David. 1969. *Self and Others*. Harmondsworth: Penguin Books.Laing, Ronald David. 1985a. *Wisdom, Madness and Folly: The Making of a Psychiatrist 1927–1957*. London: Macmillan.

Laing, Ronald David. 1985b. "Psychotherapy as Celebration." *Metamorphosis: The Journal of the Metamorphic Association* 6: 13–15.

Laing, Ronald David. 1999. *The Politics of the Family and Other Essays*. London and New York: Routledge.
Laing, Ronald David. 2015. "The Obvious." In *The Dialectics of Liberation*, edited by David Cooper, 13–33. London and New York: Verso.
Laing, Ronald David, and Aaron Esterson. 1958. "The Collusive Function of Pairing in Analytic Groups." *British Journal of Medical Psychology* 31(2): 117–123.
Laing, Ronald David, and Aaron Esterson. 1971. *Sanity, Madness, and the Family. Families of Schizophrenics*. Harmondsworth: Penguin Books.
McGeachan, Cheryl. 2012. "(Re)Remembering and Narrating the Childhood City of R.D. Laing." *Cultural Geographies* 20(3): 269–284.
McGeachan, Cheryl. 2014. "'The World Is Full of Big Bad Wolves': Investigating the Experimental Therapeutic Spaces of R.D. Laing and Aaron Esterson." *History of Psychiatry* 25(3): 283–298.
Miller, Gavin. 2004. *R.D. Laing*. Edinburgh: Edinburgh University Press.
Miller, Gavin. 2008. "Psychiatry as Hermeneutics: Laing's Argument with Natural Science." *Journal of Humanistic Psychology* 48(1): 42–60.
Miller, Gavin. 2009. "How Scottish was R.D. Laing?" *History of Psychiatry* 20(2): 226–232.
Miller, Gavin. 2012. "R.D. Laing's Theological Hinterland: The Contrast between Mysticism and Communion." *History of Psychiatry* 23(2): 139–155.
Moncrieff, Joanna. 2013. *The Bitterest Pills: The Troubling Story of Antipsychotic Drugs*. Basingstoke: Palgrave Macmillan.
Mullan, Bob. 1995. *Mad to Be Normal: Conversations with R.D. Laing*. London: Free Association Books.
Schneider, Kirk. 2000. "R.D. Laing's Existential-Humanistic Practice: What Was He Actually 'Doing'?" *Psychoanalytic Review* 87(4): 591–600.
Scott, Susie, and Charles Thorpe. 2006. "The Sociological Imagination of R.D. Laing." *Sociological Theory* 24(4): 331–352.
Scull, Andrew. 2022. *Desperate Remedies: Psychiatry and the Mysteries of Mental Illness*. London: Penguin Books.
Thompson, M. Guy. 2000. "The Heart of the Matter: R.D. Laing's Enigmatic Relationship with Psychoanalysis." *Psychoanalytic Review* 87(4): 483–509.
Wall, Oisín. 2017. *The British Anti-Psychiatrists: From Institutional Psychiatry to the Counter-Culture, 1960–1971*. London: Routledge.

# 6 'Io sono matta'

## Psychiatric violence, militant madness, and sexual difference in Alberto Grifi's 'anthropology of disobedience'

*Sophia Rohwetter*

### Introduction

In their introduction to *The Edinburgh Companion to the Critical Medical Humanities*, editors Anne Whitehead and Angela Woods (2016, 2) call to move beyond the 'primal scene' of the clinical encounter between doctor and patient and to 'explore new scenes and sites' outside the walls of medical institutions.[1] This contribution responds to this call by looking at the historical example of the Italian radical psychiatry movement of the late 1970s, showing how in its confrontation with autonomous proletarian struggles and feminist politics of sexual difference, the psychiatric scene was reconfigured as a contested social site, amplified and mediated by the artistic innovations and interventions of Italian avant-garde counterculture. In particular, this chapter looks at scenes of militant madness unfolding in the work of experimental filmmaker Alberto Grifi, who documented the anti-institutional struggle against psychiatry as a *videoteppista*[2] in what he called his 'anthropology of disobedience'. I will discuss the documentary *Lia* (1977) – 'a feminist intervention into a mass anti-psychiatric meeting' (Goddard 2021) – and the agitprop sci-fi documentary *Dinni e la Normalina, ovvero la videopolizia psichiatrica contro i sedicenti nuclei di follia militante* (1978). Both films reveal how:

> [the] project of opening the walls of the asylum to the outside brought it into contact with the rising wave of radical politics in Italy in the 1960s and 1970s to the extent that the contestation over the asylum and its deinstitutionalization became a metaphor for politics more generally
>
> (Goddard 2021)

While Grifi's films bear witness to the radical psychiatry movement extending beyond the confines of the clinic and onto the streets, they also expose the political antagonisms within the movement. These emerge, as *Lia* and *Dinni e la Normalina* powerfully show, from divergent understandings and perceptions of violence and madness and the crisis of politics arising from the practices of feminist politics of sexual difference. By enacting forms of militant madness, *Lia* and *Dinni e la Normalina* challenge the modern rationality of both the clinic and politics, revealing the inner contradictions and political limits of the radical psychiatry movement.

DOI: 10.4324/9781032660165-11

Understanding Grifi's 'anthropology of disobedience' as an artistic and political intervention into Italian radical psychiatry, this contribution seeks to demonstrate how, in the 1970s, video became a tool of political disobedience through which medical institutions and practices were contested and critiqued. Grifi's videomilitant critique of psychiatry shows how political normalisation not only works through psychiatric and psychological violence but also through state media propaganda and the control of the social imaginary, that is, through a complicity of biomedical and media power.

## It is perhaps now time to leave, once more, the clinic...[3]

When in 1794 the French psychiatrist Philippe Pinel unchained the 'madmen' of the Parisian hospitals Bicêtre and Salpêtrière, this was initially considered an act of liberation that reflected the humanist ideals of the French Revolution. However, since Michel Foucault's *Histoire de la folie* (1961), the unchaining of the mad has been figured as an ambivalent act of freedom that signifies the epistemic turning point towards modern psychiatry, marking a shift from a Christian moral dispositif to a biopolitical one in which illness assumes the role of guilt. The chains were replaced by judicial reason, which found the insane guilty of the crime of unreason. In the spirit of the Enlightenment and in opposition to the mythological demonisation of madness, in the eighteenth century emerged a rational psychiatry that classified madness as a mental illness that could be disciplined and cured.

In the 1960s and 1970s, Foucault's genealogy of modern psychiatry influenced various critical philosophical and political engagements with institutional psychiatry, often subsumed under the label 'anti-psychiatry', a term coined by psychiatrist David Cooper in his 1967 book *Psychiatry and Anti-Psychiatry.* Drawing on phenomenology, psychoanalysis, and Marxism, anti-psychiatry called into question the ontological and normative foundations of the psychiatric institution, such as scientific conceptions of mental illness and bourgeois ideas of normality, the hierarchical doctor–patient relationship, and the objectivising gaze of the psychiatrist. Within anti-psychiatry, various and partly conflicting tendencies emerged that ranged from an emphasis on the social aetiology of mental illness to the understanding of mental illness as a social construct; from the development of experimental psychiatric practices to the call for a complete abolition of psychiatry; or from divergent understandings of madness as a political weapon against social repression to a critique of a romanticised idea of madness as an expression of bourgeois ideology (see, e.g., Crossley 1998, 878; Postel and Allen 1994, 410; Roudinesco and Plon 2004, 45f.; Proctor 2016). While Thomas Szasz, following Erwin Goffman's labelling theory, negated the existence of mental illness *as illness*, R.D. Laing and David Cooper considered it in relation to repressive social and family structures (Roudinesco and Plon 2004, 45).[4] The Italian psychiatrist Franco Basaglia, indebted to the history of Marxism and communism, considered the function of psychiatry in relation to capitalist class relations, while insisting that certain forms of psychic experience were distressing and could be treated. Basaglia viewed R.D. Laing's therapeutic work with the community at Kingsley Hall as bourgeois experiments that were disconnected from the harsh reality of psychiatric institutions. He argued that these experiments misrepresented psychic pain as a transcendent freedom from social constraints and mystified psychotic and schizophrenic episodes as hallucinogen-induced, mind-expanding journeys (Foot 2015). The Italian psychiatrist Giovanni Jervis shared Basaglia's critical view of anti-psychiatry and considered it bourgeois intellectual theory that existed more 'as a tendency, a cultural direction and a critical ferment than a practical reality' (Jervis 1978, 23, my translation). In his polemical essay *Il mito dell'antipsichiatria* (The myth of antipsychiatry),[5] first published in 1976 in the political and cultural magazine *Quaderni Piacentini* that propagated the ideas of the New Left, he criticised anti-psychiatry for engaging in a mystifying romanticisation of madness that not only denies the existence of mental illness but also reprivatises and resubjectivises the experience of madness, failing to situate it within the reality of economic and social relations.

When Basaglia took over as director of the psychiatric hospital in Gorizia in 1961, at a time when Italian mental institutions were described as 'the circles of Dante's inferno' (Trivelli 2015, 120), he had all the shackles, straitjackets, bars, and wire fences removed, and developed an open therapeutic experiment that soon became known nationally and internationally for its 'avant-garde, audacious, and revolutionary techniques of "care"' (Trivelli 2015, 120), something Basaglia (2005) described as *l'utopia della realtà*. Basaglia would later gain further recognition for his contribution to the 1978 Italian Mental Health Act, which instigated significant reforms in the psychiatric system in Italy and contained directives for the closure of all psychiatric wards, leading to their gradual replacement by a range of community-based services.[6]

Critical psychiatrists like Basaglia and Jervis played a key role within Italian radical psychiatry, which, however, could only evolve into a political movement through its interactions with proletarian and feminist struggles and the audiovisual interventions of avant-garde counterculture. While most anti-psychiatry movements operated as a 'revolt from above' (Crossley 2002, 142), in Italy the struggle against institutional psychiatry turned into a more popular mobilisation, including various professional and grassroot actors who recognised a structural similarity between the violence perpetrated in psychiatric wards and other institutions, such as factories, schools, and prisons (see, e.g., Sedgwick 2015, 297; Foot 2015, 73, 89; Scheper-Hughes and Lovell 1987, 20f.; Roudinesco and Plon 2004, 69). As Basaglia's wife and colleague Franca Ongaro Basaglia (1987, xix) reflected retrospectively,

> In Italy, the struggle against the asylum was essentially a struggle against the asylum logic, founded on the expropriation and annihilation of those who are helped, hence a struggle against social marginalization achieved under the guise of treatment, therapy, protection, and rehabilitation.

## Alberto Grifi's 'anthropology of disobedience'

Italy's 'creeping May'[7] marked a time of political upheavals and social transformations. From democratic psychiatry to the women's movement, from workers' strikes to student revolts, from the Mao-Dadaism of the free radio station Radio Alice to the video-militancy of post-neorealist cinema, every aspect of society was in a state of flux. While the 1960s witnessed the eruption of wild strikes led by autonomous extra-parliamentary actors such as Lotta Continua and Potere Operaio, the Italian Left underwent a recomposition in the 1970s. On the front lines of the political revolts emerged a new generation that would come to form the movement of 1977: the exhausted figure of the worker gave way to *gli emarginati* ('the marginalised'), a collective yet heterogeneous political subject that encompassed students, hippies, proletarian youth, women, the mentally ill, drug addicts, and other *lumpen*. The experimental filmmaker Alberto Grifi followed the political uprisings of *gli emarginati* with a portable video camera and captured their demonstrations, street fights, festivals, and counter-assemblies. In this way, his 'anthropology of disobedience' was born:

> You see, at that time the prison, the factory, the asylum, had become the terrain of a common struggle and the films of those years witnessed and spread the new behaviors, the aspirations to a new life, of what we called the new political subjects; that proletarian, ragged culture, which had never had a voice and yet had so much to say.
>
> (Grifi, cited in Zanza 2004, 2f., my translation)

While Grifi's films from the 1960s and early 1970s featured experimental editing techniques and psychedelic special effects, by the mid-1970s, amidst heightened political repression in Italy, Grifi, who had himself spent two years in prison, shifted towards video activism. He transformed from a pioneer of experimental film to a *videoteppista* of counter-information, who aimed to capture the altered political sensitivity and creative strategies of the new revolutionary subjects (Licciardello 2017, 92ff.). Reflecting on this period in an interview from 2008, he explained

> After this experience, this proletarian irruption into a bourgeois salon, it seemed clear to us that, at the moment of making counter-information, it was no longer important to count and film the clenched fists that paraded through the streets […] It seemed to me that we could do something quite different, something more important and necessary: to understand what was going on in the heads of those comrades who took to the streets […] to analyze the changes in behavior within the revolutionary project, to see if the revolution was working or not, if there were real tendencies to dissolve the mechanisms established by power at the level of character structures, to dissolve the family so that the children would become the children of all, so that we could transform subjectivity into a greater political dimension where, through the political struggle, we would also become more capable of loving.
>
> (Grifi 2008, 3, my translation)

This 'proletarian irruption' also refers to the aftermath of the production of *Anna* (1975), Grifi's most well-known work and the first Italian film shot on an open-reel video recorder. The film follows the pregnant, drug-addicted, and homeless 17-year-old Anna, whom the actor and director Massimo Sarchielli met in February 1972 in Piazza Navona, the hangout spot of the Roman *lumpenproletariat*. The film was initially conceived as a re-staging of Anna's past and her 'salvation' by Sarchielli and Grifi in the style of direct cinema and Cesare Zavattini's poetics of *pedinamento* ('shadowing').[8] However, Anna's disobedience against her role as 'anthropological object' soon began to disrupt the narrative (Kushner 2012, 255). In a key shower scene, we see Sarchielli 'cleansing' Anna's naked and pregnant body in front of the camera. He scolds her for having dirty feet and makes jokes about the lice in her hair, only to realise that it is not only Anna's head that is, indeed, infested with lice – they have spread to the entire crew, including himself. Grifi (cited in Tolve 2008, 146, my translation) later reflected: 'From that moment on, we as directors could no longer manage Anna's discomfort from above with the bourgeois instrument of pity. For Anna's discomfort had passed, through lice, right over our heads'. Anna's 'proletarian lice' constituted an act of disobedience that dethroned the directors from their pedestal and, as Rachel Kushner (2012, 259) pointed out, foreshadowed the 'seeds of revolt' that would unfold in the years that followed (Figure 6.1).

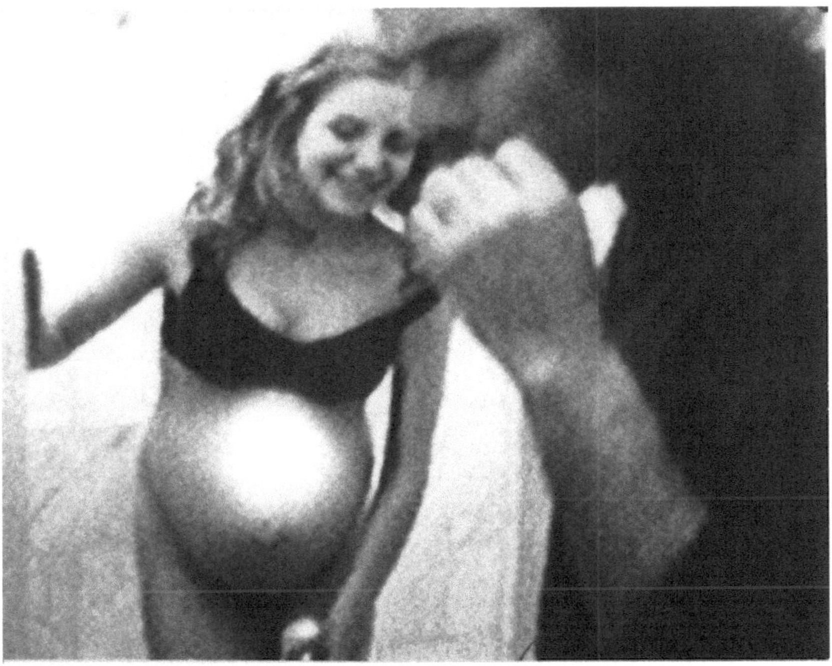

*Figure 6.1* Still from Alberto Grifi and Massimo Sarchielli, *Anna*, 1975. Courtesy Associazione culturale Alberto Grifi.

After *Anna*, Grifi focused on the subtle and subjective gestures of disobedience, intending to document the effects of the political moment at the level of subjectivity and the unconscious. Formally, his anthropology of disobedience radicalised the aims and arguments of Italian neorealist cinema: 'Let the subordinate and voiceless protagonists of history speak with no prearranged script, confer to their words the maximum power and credibility, and reinsert their cries in the chain of signification' (Barrattoni 2007, 8f.). A well-known example of this post-neorealist formula is the documentary *Matti da slegare* (Bellocchio et al. 1975) about Franco Basaglia's democratic psychiatry in Gorizia, which was edited in a collective process where every sequence and shot was discussed among the film's participants. Félix Guattari, actively involved in the anti-psychiatric efforts at the French clinic La Borde, would call *Matti da slegare* an instance of a 'cinema of combat'

> Until now, criticisms of psychiatry had come from madness 'professionals': from psychiatrists, nurses, or, less often, ex-patients. But often the language of these 'specialists' was incomprehensible to the public at large, and sometimes, it must be said, it was counterdependent upon the system itself. What is extraordinary about [*Matti da slegare*] is that it is the people involved who really get the opportunity to speak [...] children, educators, psychiatrists, militant groups; they always give the best of themselves. It's a small miracle; for once one does not have the feeling one is being presented with another 'documentary'; people speak here in a way one is not used to hearing.
>
> (Guattari 2009a, 269)[9]

Similarly, Grifi's anthropology of disobedience 'opens up to forms of self-representation and unedited self-organisation and presents new ways of engaging in and expressing politics' (Scotini 2013). As Grifi (1975, my translation) explained: 'We stopped governing, selecting and orienting the people we wanted to film [...] Thus we created a place where everyone could create themselves'. In Grifi's films of the late 1970s, it is mostly women who come to 'create themselves' on screen, thereby becoming the political protagonists: *Anna* (1975) is followed by *Lia* (1977), *Dinni e la Normalina* (1978), and *Michele alla ricerca della felicità* (1978). As Luca Barratoni (2007, 16) points out,

> It is precisely the possibility to express another possible community and to forge the means for another consciousness and another sensibility that emerges [...] in Grifi's radical attempt to welcome the least privileged and most distant other and make her – the female protagonist – the foundation of a new society.

It is in the context of a new feminist politics of sexual difference that this 'other' female protagonist entered both the political arena and the cinematic space as an 'unexpected subject',[10] bringing with her the body, the unconscious, subjectivity, sexuality, affects, desires, fantasies, and fears. The discrepancy between the propagated equality of women and the factual persistence of their oppression and exclusion from politics forced the formation of a separationist women's movement based on the experience of sexual difference. Through

> A completely unforeseen gesture, women separated themselves from men [...] It was then – with a sundering that dislocated bodies in public space (men on the one side and women on the other) – that a female "common world" came to be.
>
> (Dominijanni 2009, 13)

This gesture of difference marked a *taglio* ('cut') from modern politics that constituted 'a real exodus from traditional politics, an exodus that divided the public sphere and brought to life a female agora based exclusively on the free relationships among women' (Dominijanni 2012, 159, my translation). With *Lia* and *Dinni e la Normalina*, Grifi captures how the female protagonist appears, unexpectedly, as an 'embodied and sexed singularity, born of tensions between reason and drives' (Dominijanni 2012, 159, my translation). She emerges against the figure of the twentieth-century male political subject, shattering the anthropology of modern politics – namely, the who, what, and how of politics.

## *Lia* (1977): 'Rivoglio la pancia mia'

In November 1977, students and workers gathered at the Fabbrica della Comunicazione in Milan to protest against an anti-psychiatric conference organised by Semiotica e Psicoanalisi, a psychoanalytic group around the 'star-psychoanalyst'[11] Armando Verdiglione, who attempted to anchor Lacanian thought in Italy.[12] In the protesters' eyes, Verdiglione and his conferences were the epitome of right-wing authoritarian cultural politics and a bourgeois 'falsa antipsichiatria' (Rossi 2017, 148) alienated from the proletarian struggle against psychiatry and the lived experiences of those institutionalized. (Rossi 2017, 145; Fiore 2008, 154). The 1977 conference, which included speakers such as Jean Oury, Fernand Deligny, and Gisela Pankow, was held with the theme of violence (see Verdiglione 1978). Given the eruption of political violence in 1977 – 'the year of violence' (Berardi 2009, 14) in which demonstrations and counter-assemblies, street fights and occupations, terrorist attacks, and state repression dominated the scene – the conference somewhat marked the psychoanalytical response to an escalating political situation. Whereas at the psychoanalytic conference psychiatric violence was primarily discussed at the level of language and the symbolic order (see Verdiglione 1980), at the counter-assembly the issue of violence extended beyond the psychiatric context to intersect with questions of class and gender, as well as the demonstrators' desire for new and embodied forms of politics on the Left (Licciardello 2017, 106).

Among those gathered at the counter-assembly was Alberto Grifi, who with his portable video camera captured the moment in a single 26-minute shot. While Grifi's experimental cinematographic practice of the 1960s was characterised by complex montage techniques – as, for example, in the cinematic fragmentation of scenes from Hollywood films in *Verifica incerta* (1964) – he moved away from this in *Lia*, instead using a continuous shot, a technique known as plan sequence. Grifi regarded montage as the cinematic equivalent of the Fordist assembly line and saw a structural resemblance between the filmmaker who organises and controls the order of images and the factory owner who holds power over his workforce and the division of labour. He thus employed the plan sequence as a disobedient cinematic technique in which montage operated through its negation.[13] As a body among other bodies, in unsteady movements and shaky camera pans, his camera closely follows the young psychology student Lia through the crowd and makes her, just like Anna, 'the point of absolute gravity' (Kushner 2012, 255). Lia speaks of violence and fear, of powerlessness and repression, and expresses her discontent with the discursive form of the counter-assembly. By taking hold of other people's hands, or grabbing their attention by yelling and screaming, she calls for collective, embodied protest. Her intervention is met with irritation and anger by one person in particular. He is a representative of the *Collettivo di lavoro contro i manicomi,* a workers' collective against institutional psychiatry. He criticises anti-psychiatry for its disregard of class issues and instead advocates for concrete political actions against psychiatric violence. One such action involves building a democratic front between psychiatrists and nurses. Annoyed by his sternly presented demands, read out loud with a microphone, Lia, seeking a more spontaneous form of political expression, interrupts his speech, imitates him, hugs him aggressively, and snatches his notes. (Figure 6.2).

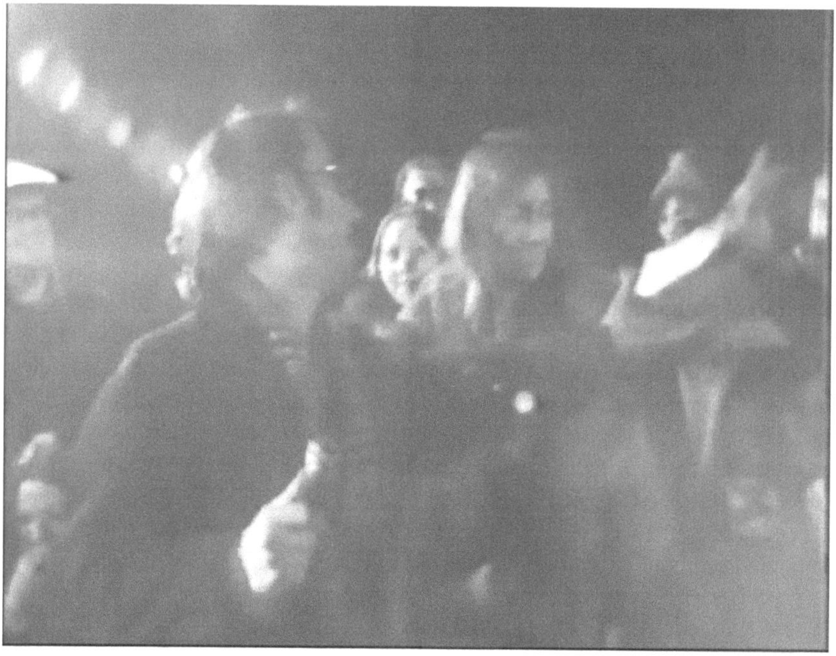

*Figure 6.2* Still from Alberto Grifi, *Lia*, 1977. Courtesy Associazione culturale Alberto Grifi, 00:16:01.

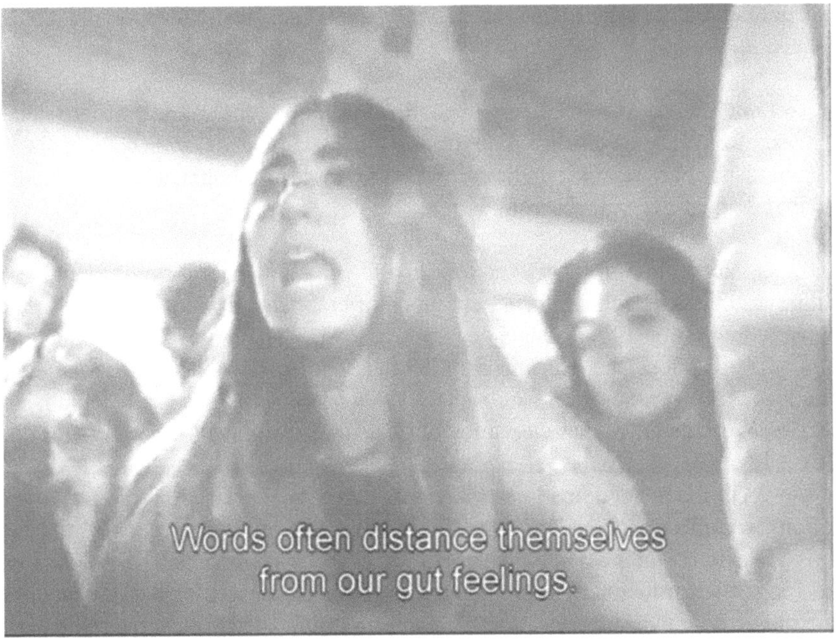


*Figure 6.3* Still from Alberto Grifi, *Lia*, 1977. Courtesy Associazione culturale Alberto Grifi. 00:08:36.

It is a telling exchange that hints at the political tensions between the workers' and the women's movement while also exposing their mutual anger and frustration with bourgeois anti-psychiatry. The representative of the workers' collective articulates the specificity of psychiatric violence, rooted in capitalist class relations, whereas Lia addresses a broader and subjective form of violence experienced at the level of affect and the body. Lia challenges his political discourse by mobilising her body, particularly her belly, against language and the rationality of the mind (Figure 6.3). She screams:

> Words often distance themselves from the belly, I reclaim my belly, I want to feel it! I want to feel it, along with all the other bellies that are here, I really can't bear my head anymore, I don't want it anymore, I want to feel the bellies![14]

Her exclamation 'rivoglio la pancia mia' ('I reclaim my belly') not only expresses a desire for embodied politics but also reflects the claims to bodily self-determination that were central to the feminist struggles of the 1970s, not least in the abortion campaign, which carried slogans such as 'l'utero è mio e lo gestisco io' ('the uterus is mine and I am in control of it'). In turning to the belly (*la pancia*), Lia attends to that part of the body traditionally most withdrawn from women's autonomy and often devalued as a site of knowledge. The philosopher Luisa Muraro (1994, 78) has pointed out that the Italian word *la pancia* is associated with a devaluation of female thinking:

> In Italian, to denote absolutely dequalified thinking, one says: "pensiero del cazzo" or if it is a woman's thought: she thinks with her belly. Language distinguishes between man and woman also in terms of thought, as a difference that de-qualifies thought from within.

In Lia's intervention, *la pancia* no longer refers to an inferior form of thought but rather functions as vehicle for a new mode of embodied political expression that subverts the rationality of language. She transforms her gut feeling into an act of embodied disobedience. Her intervention thus marks an 'an act of discourse that challenges both grammar and the alphabet, that becomes situated and "femalized", that recovers its voice or its gestures by becoming corporeal' (Scotini and Perna 2019, 12).

As such, Lia's embodied intervention, as noted by Rossi (2017, 148, my translation), signifies 'a pivotal moment in the discourse of anti-psychiatry' that not only reveals the movement's antagonistic positions on psychiatric violence but also logs the formation of feminist modes of political expression that accounted for subjectivity and the body (see Licciardello 2017, 105f.). The non-response of the Marxist activist to Lia's feminist intervention captures the traditional Left's inability to respond to a new feminist notion of politics and reflects what the Italian philosopher Ida Dominijanni (2012) has referred to as 'a crisis of politics from the perspective of a politics of sexual difference'. Grifi's recording of the counter-assembly illustrates how, amid this crisis, female difference emerges in contrast to the twentieth-century male political subject, rendering the latter's political performance in a parody of himself.

## Militant madness against the video-police

In Grifi's agitprop sci-fi film *Dinni e la Normalina, ovvero la videopolizia psichiatrica contro i sedicenti gruppi di follia militante*, which was commissioned and ultimately censored by the Italian public broadcasting company RAI, the female protagonist Dinni appears at the intersection of medical and media violence. The film is divided into two parts. The first is set in a dystopian state in which a despotic regime and its psychiatric video-police use a pharmaceutical product called 'Normalina', an alkaloid extracted from the faeces of diligent prototype workers of 'clinical normality', along with mass amounts of TV propaganda, to suppress and neutralise any form of political dissent and to restore political normality (Figure 6.4). In a televised study, a medical professor in a white coat explains the functions of Normalina and the role of the psychiatric video-police in hunting down members of militant madness, rebels who had escaped the control of Normalina – among them, the unemployed and underemployed, proletarian youth, thieves, women, drug addicts, and mad people – until the arrest of Dinni, a member of the group, is announced. This part is set in a television studio and ironically adopts the aesthetics

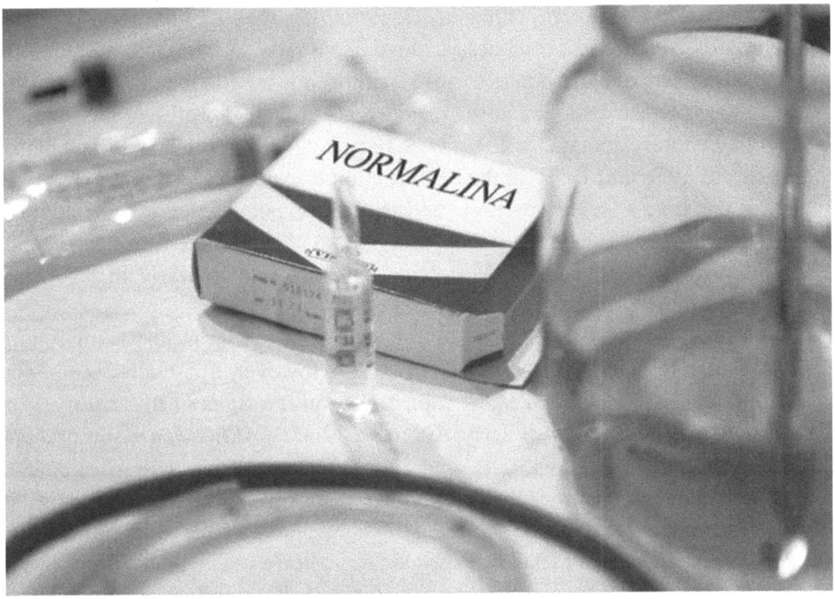


*Figure 6.4* A close-up of the packaging of Normalina, the pharmaceutical product used by the psychiatric video-police to normalize deviant citizens. From Alberto Grifi, *Dinni e la Normalina, ovvero la videopolizia psichiatrica contro i sedicenti nuclei di follia militante*, 1978. Courtesy Associazione culturale Alberto Grifi.

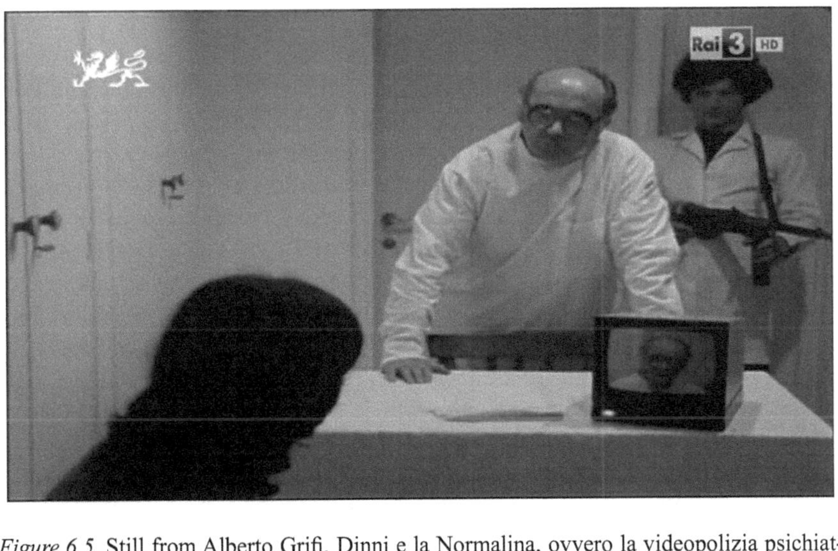

*Figure 6.5* Still from Alberto Grifi, Dinni e la Normalina, ovvero la videopolizia psichiatrica contro i sedicenti nuclei di follia militante, 1978. Courtesy Associazione culturale Alberto Grifi.

of mass media and state propaganda. Depicting images of monitors, cameras, clapperboards, and domestic scenes, it illustrates how elderly people and families internalise the propaganda news, thereby reinforcing the mediated fiction of this future scenario. The pseudo-scientific lecture by the medical professor incorporates Grifi's documentary footage of the protests against Verdiglione's anti-psychiatric congresses of 1976 and 1977. In the film's fictional scenario, this footage has been seized by the state's 'schizo-archive' and is utilised as evidence against activists of militant madness, including Dinni, described as 'one of the most determined antagonists of Verdiglione and all bourgeois and anti-proletarian psychiatry' (Fiore 2008, 153, my translation) (Figure 6.5).

The second part of the film reveals that the first part was just a nightmare. Dinni's awakening shifts to the reality of 1978. However, this reality seems just as dystopic as the unreality of her dream, and soon the signs of this reality – the streets of Rome, an edition of Jerry Rubin's *DO IT! FALLO!,* an issue of *Lotta Continua* – begin to merge with the scenario of the dream. Her landlord, a butcher in a white coat who resembles the medical professor of the video-police, identifies Dinni as one of the members of the Red Brigade wanted for the kidnapping of the former Prime Minister and leader of the Democrazia Cristiana, Aldo Moro, one of the main protagonists of the *compromesso storico*, whose abduction and eventual murder in 1978 marks both the high and end point of Italy's long 1970s.[15] *Dinni e la Normalina* ends with the butcher's call to the police.

Although Grifi himself described *Dinni e la Normalina* as a joke, a political parody amplified by the film's low-budget aesthetics, there lingers a sense of unease arising from the parallels between the fictional dystopia and the historical reality of 1978, a period characterised by escalating state repression and police violence.

By portraying both the pharmaceutical Normalina and television as state-administered drugs – characterising them as the new 'opium of the people' – Grifi illustrates in an exaggerated and ironic manner how medical and media power collaborate in restoring political normality and eliminating political dissent. Both psychiatry and state television are figured as biopolitical propaganda machines that create a falsifying reality and manipulate dissident bodies and behaviours.

The film's critique of mass media echoes the Situationists' analysis of the role of the proletarian in the entertainment society, in which he is no longer just a worker but also a consumer of illusions and a producer of surplus value. *Dinni e la Normalina* also seems to draw on some of the ideas on psychoanalysis and cinema articulated by Félix Guattari in his essay 'The Poor Man's Couch' (1975), in which he suggests, somewhat ironically, that both psychoanalysis and cinema confect

> A certain type of drug that, though technologically more sophisticated than the ordinary joint or pipe, nonetheless functions by transforming the mode of subjectivity of those who use it: one captures the energy of desire in order to turn it against itself to anaesthetise it, to cut it off from the external world in such a way that it ceases to threaten the organisation and values of the dominant social system.
>
> (Guattari 2009b, 259)

According to Guattari (2009b, 264), 'Commercial cinema is nothing else but a simple, inexpensive drug' utilised to establish 'a normalization of the social imaginary'. In *Dinni e la Normalina*, the state exercises control over both the dissident body and the means of communication to normalise and discipline the social imaginary, revealing 'that the power of psychiatry and the techniques of normalisation have invaded all the levels of our life, waking and sleeping' (Seem and Parkin, cited in Sedgwick 2015, 269). In his anthropology of disobedience, Grifi counters these techniques of normalisation with forms of militant madness, engaging them as political tools to resist and combat the escalating biopolitical repression by the state and the media. Both the 'real' activists at the anti-psychiatric counter-assembly in *Lia* and the fictitious groups of militant madness in *Dinni e la Normalina* call for a collective reappropriation of madness as a political tool against repression and an expression of political dissidence. Lia, for example, explains that she has been to asylums and worked with 'the mad' to then declare her own madness: 'Io sono matta' ('I am crazy!'). She recounts her experiences at the conference *Donne e Follia*, which took place at the San Salvi psychiatric hospital in Florence only a few days before the counter-conference and was attended by about 4000 women who discussed the relation between the female and the mad experience to establish a sense of solidarity between women and psychiatric patients: 'I went to *Donne e Follia* in Florence. I was there with mad women who were equal and identical to me'. In an article published shortly after the conference, another participant reflected: 'There is a shared element between the everyday madness of being a woman and the madness for which they lock you up in an asylum' (Tagliaferri 1977, my translation). This shared sense of madness is echoed by Dinni, who claims that 'madness is the property of the people, and it is the people's ability to collectively regain possession of it in order to oppose violence and repression'.

Giovanni Jervis, probably much like Lia's Marxist rival, could see in this reappropriation of madness only an escapist idealisation that avoided addressing the principal contradictions of mental illness rooted in class antagonism. As Jervis (1978, 17, my translation) explains, 'In militant circles, those of the counterculture and feminists, the contradictions of the movement seek their answers in the ideologies of exclusion, of madness, being out and psychic destruction, referring to a mythical idea of anti-psychiatry'.[16] In anti-psychiatric discourse, madness in general and the madness of the female subject in particular are often understood as political weapons against psychiatric destruction and social conformity. Just as psychoanalysis found its story of origin in the case study of Anna O., anti-psychiatry has Mary Barnes, the ex-nurse who had been diagnosed with incurable schizophrenia and sent to be treated at Kingsley Hall. There she effectively went through hell, something of a symbolic death, through which she eventually found herself born anew, this time as a talented artist. Barnes would go on to become a symbolic figure for the anti-psychiatry movement, representing the emancipatory potential of female madness (see Roudinesci and Plon 2004 45).

Grifi takes up the anti-psychiatric discourse that constructs female madness as a form of 'dissent to prevailing forms of normality, mediocrity and bourgeois "common sense"' (Jervis 1978, 141, my translation) and presents the figure of the mad woman as a model for revolutionary subjectivity. However, unlike R.D. Laing, Grifi does not exploit the suffering of his female protagonists – they do not suffer from real states of psychological distress but rather invoke madness as a form of political articulation that opposes the rationality of modern politics and resists the power and manipulation exercised by psychiatry, the state, and the media. Lia and Dinni revolt against these institutions, against the disciplining and normalisation of political expression, against the biopolitical destruction of the body, and sometimes against film itself. In Grifi's anthropology of disobedience, madness no longer appears as a pathological condition but instead is figured as a form of political dissent, an articulation of difference, and a last outcry amidst the end of a radical political moment.

## 1978: The end of an era

In 1977, Alberto Grifi found two black-and-white silent films in a small market in Milan that had presumably been commissioned by the scientific department of the Italian pharmaceutical company Roche S.A. in the late 1930s. The first and shorter film demonstrates the surgical technique of transorbital leukotomy of the frontal lobe of the brain. The second film documents the treatment of schizophrenic patients with a novel intravenously injected drug that induces a vascular storm. While the film aims to prove the benefits of this new method, the images show the patients, most of them women, suffering from terrible convulsions. Finally, as proof of their recovery, the patients raise their hands in a fascist salute. Grifi declared this *objet trouvé* to be a ready-made film and called it *Il preteso corpo* (1977) (Rossi 2017, 147). In doing so, Grifi transformed the film's signs and purpose, turning it into an indictment of the coercive and fascist violence exercised in psychiatric institutions, captured in its negative (Licciardello 2017, 109f.).

With *Lia* and *Dinni e la Normalina*, Grifi transcends the confines of the clinic and shifts the focus towards the madness and violence enacted and resisted outside medical institutions: on the streets, on the screen, and through the unexpected subject of the woman. While *Lia* and *Dinni* reveal the inner political conflicts and the increasing state repression that brought the movement of 1977 to an end, they also show the formation of unexpected political alliances and how the visual cultures of radical psychiatry connected the issue of psychiatric violence to questions of sexual difference, class issues and the (counter-)power of the image.

Grifi's anthropology of disobedience demonstrates how the 'mad body' is manipulated, disciplined, and normalised by biopolitical power exercised by both medical and media apparati, while suggesting that madness, and in particular the political madness of the woman, is not only a site of oppression but also one of struggle and resistance. Madness appears as a political affect, but it also signals the end of Italy's long 1970s. This end is foreshadowed by the Left's inability to respond effectively to the political inventions of the feminist movement and the collaboration of medical and media power in restoring normalcy, which would later fully manifest with the ascent of Berlusconi's biopolitical 'media empire'.[17]

The year 1978 marked the end of Italy's creeping May, leaving behind a failed revolutionary subject and shared 'wounds of separation and loss' (Dominijanni 2009, 137). Looking back at the intersections between the visual cultures of radical psychiatry and the feminist politics of sexual difference may not mend these wounds, but such reflection could potentially offer new perspectives for the reconstruction of political alliances. Grifi's anthropology of disobedience holds a sense of urgency, particularly now, at a time when the Left's concept of counter-information appears to have been fully absorbed by right-wing conspiracy theorists, and the feminist achievements of the 1970s, above all the decriminalisation of abortion, are once again being jeopardised by neo-fascist forces.

## Notes

1 Following this line of thought, Foster and Funke (2018) have noted that extending beyond the confines of the clinic holds particular significance for feminist research within the medical humanities, as it enables the consideration of sites and spaces that may have gone unnoticed but are integral to the lived experiences of women.
2 The term *videoteppista*, which roughly translates to 'video hooligan', describes the use of video as a new tool of political disobedience during the counter-informational video-activism in Italy in the 1970s. While today 'counter-information' is largely associated with the circulation of fake news and conspiracy theories by the political Right, cinematographic counter-information was used in 1970s Italy as a form of counter-power by the Left. Grifi's agitprop dystopian sci-fi *Dinni e la Normalina, ovvero la videopolizia psichiatrica contro i sedicenti nuclei di follia militante*, in which 'the psychiatric video police' manipulates information to denounce and persecute political dissidents, prefigures how the idea and practice of counter-information was to be co-opted by the state media apparatus of the Right.
3 I am borrowing this phrase from Vincent Bonin's essay 'In Abeyance: It Is Perhaps Now Time to Leave, Once More, the Clinic…' (2016), in which he reflects on cinematic and psychoanalytic performance as analytical acts and political interventions into the *dispositif* of the clinic.
4 For a detailed discussion of the social ethnography of R.D. Laing, see the chapter by Janina Klement in this volume.
5 In the absence of an English translation of Jervis's essay I used an early German translation.
6 According to Foot (2015, 251), the closure of asylums marked not an end but a beginning in the revolution of mental health care. Thousands of patients were discharged from psychiatric institutions and admitted to other facilities such as community housings, nursing or family homes. For a detailed analysis and critique of the law, see, e.g., Burns and Foot (2020).
7 The term *maggio strisciante* refers to the creeping movement of the Italian protest culture of the long 1970s which, unlike May 1968, did not culminate in a political climax but extended over a decade and 'crept ahead slowly in minor instances, flare-ups, and forms that were not de facto recognized as big, revolutionary, or obviously political' (Calder Williams 2013, 13).
8 Cesare Zavattini was an Italian screenwriter and the central theorist of neorealism. In his manifesto 'Some Ideas on the Cinema' (1966), he argued that the necessity of an imagined 'story' is 'simply a technique of superimposing dead formulas over living social facts' and called on filmmakers to 'excavate reality, to give it a power, a communication, a series of reflexes, which until recently we had never thought it had'. With the notion of *pedinamento*, Zavattini (2021, 148) described his vision of a cinematic form

of ethnography in which 'filmmakers leave their own home and make them shadow people'.

9 Other examples of what Guattari (2009a, 171) refers to as a cinema of combat or 'a minor cinema for minorities' include *Ce gamin-là* (Fernand Deligny and Renaud Victor, 1975), *Coup pour coup* (Marin Karmitz, 1972), *La ville bidon* (Jacques Baratier, 1971), *Histoire de Paul* (René Féret, 1975) and *Asylum* (Peter Robinson, 1972). One might also think of *Apollon: una fabbrica occupata* (Ugo Gregoretti, 1969), which tells the story of factory occupation from the perspective of the workers themselves, or *L'aggettivo donna* (1971) by the Collettivo Femminista Cinema-Roma, which aimed to instigate a feminist cinematic self-consciousness.

10 Carla Lonzi introduced the term il soggetto imprevisto to describe the sudden, unforeseen, and the yet-to-be-realized presence of the woman in history and politics. See, e.g., Scotini and Perna (2019).

11 In a 1986 article in the German magazine *Der Spiegel,* Armando Verdiglione is described, not without irony and contempt, as a self-proclaimed 'star-psychoanalyst' and 'Lacan's Italian prophet in Milan' (*Der Spiegel* 1986, my translation).

12 In the 1970s, Semitioica e Psicoanalisi organized several international congresses on anti-psychiatry that drew on psychoanalytic, linguistic and Marxist theories and included contributions by well-known 'luminari dell'antipsichiatria' (Rossi 2017, 148), such as Gilles Deleuze and Félix Guattari, but also philosophers of the New Right like André Glucksmann and Bernard-Henri Lévy. In large counter-assemblies, students and proletarian youth protested against Verdiglione's 'conference circus' (*Der Spiegel* 1986, my translation) and the co-opting of radical psychiatry by bourgeois, psychoanalytic forces. Grifi documented some of the protests in his films *Lia* (1977), *Gli autoriduttori al convegno di antipsichiatria di Milano* (1977) and *Dinni e la Normalina* (1978).

13 The film critic Amos Vogel (1974, 139f.) described the plan sequence as an assault on conventional montage that 'has contributed towards propelling cinema away from the petty-bourgeois sentimentalities of Hollywood into our real universe of unrest, uncertainty, anguish […] The assault on the old montage is therefore an attempt to strengthen immediacy, to capture the viewer by mystery and intimation, to increase his identification by forcing him into stronger mental response, thus jolting him from the comfortable safety of his own universe.'

14 All quotes from the films *Lia* and *Dinni e la Normalina* have been translated from Italian by the author.

15 The kidnapping and murder of Aldo Moro marks the beginning of the infamous *riflusso*, which put an end to the mass movements of the 1970s and instigated the conservatism of the 1980s (see, e.g., Uva 2015).

16 David Cooper responded to Jervis' thesis of the myth of anti-psychiatry with a short essay in which he discusses anti-psychiatry's role within the social revolution, understanding it as 'a part of that social revolution which must precede, accompany and follow the political revolution against class domination' (Cooper 1978, 73, my translation).

17 For a discussion on the relationship between biopolitics, neoliberalism, and mass media under Berlusconi, see Dominijanni (2014).

## References

Barattoni, Luca. 2007. *The Endless Pursuit of Truth: Subalternity and Marginalization in Post Neorealist Italian Film*. PhD dissertation, University of North Carolina at Chapel Hill. Accessed April 30, 2024. https://cdr.lib.unc.edu/concern/dissertations/3x816n368.

Basaglia, Franco. 2005. *L'utopia della realtà*, edited by Franca Basaglia Ongaro. Turino: Giulio Einaudi.

Bellocchio, Marco, Silvano Agosti, Stefano Rulli, and Sandro Petraglia. 1975. *Matti da slegare* (Fit to Be Untied).

Berardi, Franco. 2009. *Precarious Rhapsody: Semiocapitalism and the pathologies of the post-alpha generation*. London: Minor Compositions.

Bonin, Vincent. 2016. "In Abeyance. It Is Perhaps Now Time to Leave, Once More, the Clinic…" In *Putting Rehearsals to the Test: Practices of Rehearsal in Fine Arts, Film, Theater, Theory, and Politics*, edited by Sabeth Buchmann, Ilse Lafer, and Constanze Ruhm, 196–210. Berlin: Sternberg Press.

Burns, Tom, and John Foot. 2020. *Basaglia's International Legacy: From Asylum to Community*. Oxford and New York: Oxford University Press.

Calder Williams, Evan. 2013. *The Fog of Class War: Cinema, Circulation, and Refusal in Italy's Creeping '70s*. PhD dissertation, University of California, Santa Cruz.

Cooper, David. 1978. "Antipsychiatrie, Entmythologisiert." In *Giovanni Jervis, and Franco Rella: Der Mythos der Antipsychiatrie*, 72–78. Berlin: Merve-Verlag.

Crossley, Nick. 1998. "R. D. Laing and the British Anti-Psychiatry Movement: A Socio-Historical Analysis." *Social Science & Medicine* 47(7): 877–989.

Crossley, Nick. 2002. "Mental Health, Resistance and Social Movements: The Collective-Confrontational Dimension." *Health Education Journal* 61(2): 138–152.

Der Spiegel. 1986. "Dunkler Sinn." *Der Spiegel*. Accessed April 30, 2024. https://www.spiegel.de/panorama/dunkler-sinn-a-322570d3-0002-0001-0000-000013519550?context=issue

Dominijanni, Ida. 2009. "Wounds of the Common." *Diacritics* 39(4): 135–145.

Dominijanni, Ida. 2012. "Das Schielen der Venus. Die Krise der Politik aus der Sicht der Differenzpolitik." In *Inventionen 2*, edited by Isabell Lorey, Roberto Nigro, and Gerald Raunig, 158–173. Zürich: Diaphanes.

Dominijanni, Ida. 2014. "Das Gespenst der Sexualität – Frauen, Biopolitik und Neoliberalismus im heutigen Italien." *Feministische Studien* 32(2): 216–226.

Fiore, Angelita. 2008. "Corpi sconnessi, ovvero l'assenza di organi: La manipolazione delle menti tra comunicazione e (anti)psichiatria." In *Alberto Grifi: Oltre le regole del cinema*, edited by Manuela Tempesta, 149–155. Atripalda, AV: Edizioni Laceno.

Foot, John. 2015. *The Man Who Closed the Asylums: Franco Basaglia and the Revolution in Mental Health Care*. London and Brooklyn: Verso.

Foster, Sherri L., and Jana Funke. 2018. "Feminist Encounters with the Medical Humanities." *Feminist Encounters: A Journal of Critical Studies in Culture and Politics* 2(2): 1–6.

Goddard, Michael. 2021. "The So-Called Groups of Militant Insanity against the Video Police: Anti-Psychiatry and Autonomia in 1970s Italian Audiovisual Media." Séminaire INHALab. Association ATHAMAS – Art et antipsychiatrie, INHA Paris. Accessed April 30, 2024. https://westminsterresearch.westminster.ac.uk/download/f732dc1a470c05cd31afde57682f413ca63a1e5da93bc51c6043e1b6a46ecbb8/138489/Paris%20anti%20psychaiatry%20and%20autonomia%20talk.pdf.

Grifi, Alberto. 1975. "Interview mit Alberto Grifi." Accessed April 30, 2024. https://www.arsenal-berlin.de/assets/Legacy/katalog_blaetter/1975_Anna_19.pdf.

Grifi, Alberto. 1977. *Lia*.

Grifi, Alberto. 1977. *Il preteso corpo*.

Grifi, Alberto. 1978. *Dinni e la Normalina, ovvero la videopolizia psichiatrica contro i sedicenti gruppi di follia militante*.

Grifi, Alberto. 2008. "Cinema di lotta e d'invenzione." *Alias: Supplemento settimanale de Il Manifesto* 3(490): 2–4.

Grifi, Alberto, and Gianfranco Baruchello. 1964. *Verifica incerta*.

Grifi, Alberto, and Massimo Sarchielli. 1975. *Anna.*
Guattari, Félix. 2009a. "Not So Mad." In *Chaosophy: Texts and Interviews, 1972–1977*, edited by Sylvère Lotringer, 268–271. Los Angeles, CA: Semiotext(e).
Guattari, Félix. 2009b. "The Poor Man's Couch." In *Chaosophy: Texts and Interviews, 1972–1977*, edited by Sylvère Lotringer, 257–267. Los Angeles, CA: Semiotext(e).
Jervis, Giovanni. 1978. *Der Mythos der Antipsychiatrie.* Berlin: Merve-Verlag.
Kushner, Rachel. 2012. "Woman in Revolt: Alberto Grifi and Massimo Sarchielli's *Anna.*" *Artforum* 51(3): 254–259.
Licciardello, Annamaria. 2017. *Il cinema laboratorio di Alberto Grifi.* Alessandria: Edizioni Falsopiano.
Muraro, Luisa.1994. "Die denkende Differenz der Geschlechter. Eine italienische Einführung." *Feministische Studien* 12(2): 71–80.
Ongara Basaglia, Franca. 1987. "Preface." In *Psychiatry Inside Out: Selected Writings of Franco Basaglia,* edited by Nancy Scheper-Hughes and Anne M. Lovell, xi–xxv. New York: Columbia University Press.
Postel, Jacques, and David F. Allen. 1994. "History and Anti-Psychiatry in France." In *Discovering the History of Psychiatry*, edited by Mark S. Micale and Roy Porter, 384–414. New York: Oxford University Press.
Proctor, Hannah. 2016. "Lost Minds: Sedgwick, Laing and the Politics of Mental Illness." *Radical Philosophy* 197: 36–48.
Rossi, Stefania. 2017. *L'evoluzione biologica di una lacrima: Il cinema di Alberto Grifi.* Roma: Timía.
Roudinesco, Elisabeth, and Michel Plon. 2004. *Wörterbuch der Psychoanalyse: Namen, Länder, Werke, Begriffe.* Wien: Springer Wien.
Scheper-Hughes, Nancy, and Anne M. Lovell. 1987. "The Utopia of Reality: Franco Basaglia and the Practice of a Democratic Psychiatry." In *Psychiatry Inside Out: Selected Writings of Franco Basaglia*, edited by Nancy Scheper-Hughes and Anne M. Lovell, 1–50. New York: Columbia University Press.
Scotini, Marco. 2013. "Disobedient Images. Autonomia and the Politics of Representation." *Open! Platform for Art, Culture & the Public Domain.* Accessed April 30, 2024. https://www.onlineopen.org/disobedient-images.
Scotini, Marco, and Raffaela Perna. 2019. The Unexpected Subject – 1978 Art and Feminism in Italy. Milano: Flash Art.
Sedgwick, Peter R. 2015. *Psycho Politics: Laing, Foucault, Goffman, Szasz and the Future of Mass Psychiatry.* London: Unkant Publishers.
Tagliaferri, Marida. 1977. "Convegno di Firenze: dalla follia alla liberazione." *Effe. Archivio storico di effe mensile femminista autogestivo.* Accessed April 30, 2024. https://efferivistafemminista.it/2014/11/dalla-follia-alla-liberazione/.
Tolve, Antonello. 2008. "Hapax. Etica ed estetica nella grammatica cinematografica di Alberto Grifi." In *Alberto Grifi: Oltre le regole del cinema,* edited by Manuela Tempesta, 144–148. Atripalda, AV: Edizioni Laceno.
Trivelli, Elena. 2015. "Exploring a 'Remembering Crisis': 'Affective Attuning' and 'Assemblaged Archive' as Theoretical Frameworks and Research Methodologies." In *Affective Methodologies: Developing Cultural Research Strategies for the Study of Affect*, edited by Britta Timm Knudsen and Carsten Stage, 119–139. London: Palgrave Macmillan.
Uva, Christian. 2015. *L'immagine politica: forme del contropotere tra cinema, video efotografia nell'Italia degli anni Settanta.* Milano and Udine: Mimesis Edizioni.

Verdiglione, Armando. 1978. "Introduzione." In *Violenze e psicanalisi. Documenti del convegno internazionle di pscanalisi*. Milano, 24–26 Novembre 1977, edited by Armando Verdiglione, 7–11. Milano: Feltrinelli Editore.

Verdiglione. Armando. 1980. "La Questione." Accessed April 30, 2024. https://www.armandoverdiglione.com/testiW/1973/laquestione.htm.

Vogel, Amos. 1974. *Film as a Subversive Art*. New York: Random House.

Whitehead, Anne, and Angela Woods. 2016. "Introduction." In *The Edinburgh Companion to the Critical Medical Humanities*, edited by Anne Whitehead, Angela Woods, with Sarah Atkinson, Jane Macnaughton, and Jennifer Richards, 1–31. Edinburgh: Edinburgh University Press.

Zanza, Davide. 2004. "Memoria, verità. Le mani sul cinema. Un ritratto di Alberto Grifi e del suo macchinario lavanastri." *Alias: Supplemento Settimanale de Il Manifesto* 40(322)*:* 2–4.

Zavattini, Cesare. 1966. "Some Ideas on the Cinema." In *Film. A Montage of Theories*, edited by Richard Dyer MacCann, 216–228. New York: Dutton.

Zavattini, Cesare. 2021. "Shadowing." In *Selected Writings*, volume 2, edited and translated by David Brancaleone, 148–151. London: Bloomsbury Publishing.

# 7 The denied poetics of global psychiatry and Frantz Fanon's poetisation of science

*Lisa Schmidt-Herzog*

> *As it strives toward totality, literary work moreover forms the ethnography of its own subject matter. We see a poem by Brathwaite as the equivalent of a novel by Carpentier and an essay by Fanon. We go even farther in not distinguishing between genres when we deny that their divisions are necessary for us or when we create different divisions.*
>
> Édouard Glissant

## Introduction

In the humanities and social sciences, Fanon has been widely acknowledged, mostly for his books *Black Skin, White Masks* (1952) and *The Wretched of the Earth* (1961). However, not much notice has been taken of his thought within neurology and psychiatry, his main fields of expertise, even though he also published texts on a broad range of empirical work. These have been compiled as part of his collected writings only in 2015 (Khalfa and Young 2015b). The editors of his collected writings suggest that this might be the case due to 'their technical nature; Fanon's sustained interest in now discredited therapies like electroshocks or insulin coma therapy (methods that he used and on which he wrote scientific articles); or his experimentation with first-generation neuroleptics' (Khalfa and Young 2015, 167). In fact, electroshock therapy is still a common practice today, but even if it was not, this would not explain the total absence of *historicising* perspectives on his writings within the medical-psychiatric discourse, since works and figures do not just sink into oblivion simply because time and scientific progress have been moving forward (which they always do). Otherwise, a figure like German psychiatrist Emil Kraepelin, whose work on different cultures was dedicated to preventing racial 'degeneration', would not be presented as the predecessor of today's transcultural psychiatry section within the World Psychiatric Association (World Psychiatric Association 2023).

What else then would explain today's epistemic gap between the dominant medical-psy discourse and Fanon's work? It is true that his technical writings are largely attuned to the formal criteria of 'hard science', while the two books unfold dramaturgies that have been acknowledged and studied for their specific poetics (see, e.g., Keller 2007). However, when this supposed division is made into an

DOI: 10.4324/9781032660165-12

absolute, the epistemic value of the one realm is conceived of as incommensurable with the other – usually to the detriment of that which is considered as poetic. If such language is then not only rendered the Other of proper *scientific* knowledge but the Other of proper knowledge *in general*, the power to make assertions about reality is ultimately restricted to that way of speaking, which conforms to the rules of the dominant discourse.

If I argue here that a hiatus between scientific and poetic language is the result of a construction, then where are those marks that would indicate this constructedness and make it become visible? After all, in today's mainstream psychiatric literature there is no active stance being taken against Fanon or similar voices that are *implicitly* deemed as not belonging to the discourse. In fact, epistemic injustice as outlined by Miranda Fricker (2007) does not necessarily appear in the shape of a strongly articulated opposition against forms of knowledge that one wishes to suppress.[1] Rather, it is precisely this silent non-appearance that comes as a *performative* expression of neglection, which is so self-evident that it renders any *verbal* expression of a concrete criticism obsolete. However, just as racism cannot be explained away by someone saying that they had not intended to reproduce racist thought, the absence of knowledges and languages from a discourse must not (always) be thought of as intention – but still as meaningful. Thus, if there is no active condemnation of Fanon, then how to think of his non-appearance in the discourse on a structural level, which not only applies to his persona but to marginalised voices per se? The guiding proposition of the following analysis is that the epistemic injustice of being rendered the Other of (scientific and general) knowledge turns into a full-scale ontological violence when Otherness is being equated to neither belonging to reality nor being able to make legitimate assertions on it. That's why to Fanon, thinking of a possible 'cure' would always mean to create structures in which the individual speaks, acts and appears in the world – responsible for co-creating reality, rather than being excluded from it.

## The methodological turn of post-war medicine and psychiatry

Initially, the text that would later become known as *Black Skin, White Masks* was intended to be Fanon's medical dissertation at the University of Lyon in 1951. But it caused 'quite a scandal' and his supervisor Jean Dechaume suggested to him to not hand it in, because it did not fit the formal standards of a medical dissertation (Cherki 2000, 18). Responding to this, it was only two weeks later that Fanon presented a thesis on the neurological disorder Friedreich's ataxia (Fanon 1951) and the title was easily granted to him. But even if the eventual thesis was written in a much less polemic tone, it did contribute some radical work in challenging the belief of both a pure psychogenesis and a pure organogenesis of mental illness. These terms signify two very different ideas about the supposed origins of psychic suffering. While the organogetic approach goes back to the paradigm that every mental illness eventually can be traced back to a dysfunctional organ (Fanon 1952, XI; Khalfa and Young 2015, 175),[2] the psychogenetic viewpoint opts for conceiving of the suffering as a result of psychological alterations (for instance, due to traumatic events). Against this backdrop, it was Fanon's stance to consider – while not neglecting either of these two approaches – the *sociogenesis* of mental suffering. This meant to take physical, psychological, *and* social factors as crucial in contributing to the development of symptoms, without reducing them neither to empirical data nor to personal experience or social structure. However, Fanon renounced the idea that science could eventually detect *final origins* of mental illness and suffering and that the problem was to be solved by identifying one causal mechanism. Hence, the notion of 'sociogenesis' does not mean that the social was the one initiating pathogenetic factor to him. Rather, it indicates a shift in thought from focusing on supposed origins (which remain opaque) to paying attention to the given, that is, the present status of symptoms, which always only become manifest in a concrete social milieu.

Fanon's dissertation was set in a much more conventional clinical framework than his following books, but it paved a way that *Black Skin, White Masks* would take up and develop further. Published one year later by Éditions du Seuil,[3] the introduction leaves no room for misunderstanding that there is a clear change in tone, style, and approach

> It is good form to introduce a work in psychology with a statement of its methodological point of view. I shall be derelict. I leave methods to the botanists and the mathematicians. There is a point at which methods devour themselves.
>
> (Fanon 2021 [1952], 12)

Rejecting the idea of a proper methodology must have been received as a rather absurd endeavour amongst a scientific community at a time when psychiatrists around the globe were working fiercely on standardising their psychopathological descriptions, diagnoses, and classification systems. While advertising the idea of one *global health* after World War II, the WHO called for an expert group that was formed in 1959 to develop a methodology that would produce reliable and valid data on mental illness in different countries. Eventually, these considerations led to conducting the prominent first epidemiological study on schizophrenia (WHO 1975). In this sense, the emergence of today's psychiatry as a *global* endeavour was closely intertwined with the emergence of the first generation of transcultural psychiatry, because it provided the statistical data from which a worldwide comparability of incidences and prevalences was created.[4]

After the Holocaust and during the time of broad social movements, psychiatry found itself in a profound crisis, facing the demands of denazifying and decolonising the clinic, the social movements that protested the asylum policies in the 1960s, and the publication of prominent critical works, like those of Erving Goffman (1961) and Michel Foucault (1961). Reforms were more than necessary. One problem was the arbitrariness of diagnosis, which could differ between various psychiatrists because of the lack of an orienting fundament. The classical psychoanalytical approach to diagnosis as *Deutungskunst* (i.e., a skill that cannot simply be objectified) then meant that an individual doctor could diagnose far more at their own discretion than is the case today – an omnipotence that had become complicit with fascist ideology.

Countering this danger, mainstream psychiatry sought to implement a new ethics by standardising its methodological tools to make the discipline more 'objective'. Strikingly, the abolishment of any trace of a potentially violent and despotic subject in the sciences was introduced at the very moment in intellectual history when phenomenology and psychoanalysis reintroduced the notion of subjectivity into their discourses, underlining the importance of acknowledging it not only on an ethical level but also on an epistemological one. Camille Robcis (2021, 51) points out how Fanon continually stresses the 'importance of the social, of others and alterity in the formation of the self', a self that is able to live with others (i.e., being itself an other amongst others), acknowledging their reality. However, the same importance of the social, others, and alterity holds true for the formation of a world which consists of a plurality of external objects and existences that cannot simply be absorbed. Fanon's subject of this self-formation and worldbuilding *is* undeniably a subject, yet it does not subject the world to its own premises but rather integrates it by engaging with it.

Against the backdrop of the intellectual climate prevalent within the medical department in Lyon, Fanon makes it very explicit in his writings that he does not speak from the 'objective' perspective of a neutral, unaffected ghost. Rather, his own horizon is that of a racialised person under a gaze that makes him the Other

> Maman, look, a N***; I'm scared!
> Scared! Scared! Now they were beginning to be scared of me. I wanted to kill myself laughing, but laughter had become out of the question. [...]
> Look how handsome that N*** is.
> The handsome N*** says, Fuck you, madame.
>
> (Fanon 1952, 919)[5]

It is a common strategy to diminish the argument of someone who is personally affected by the discrimination they are fighting against. But here, Fanon's stance is that his involvement in the matter, which is interlaced with every act of his speaking, is not other than anybody else's involvement, since thought and speech are *always* profoundly shaped by a person's life and experiences. Precisely because this holds true for him just as much as it holds true for any patient or doctor (whatever skin colour they may have), concepts of pure organogenesis and pure psychogenesis fall short in their approaches to mental illness. These theories exclude the subject from their theory and therefore lack in establishing a meaningful connection between the mental state and the lived experience of an individual. Fanon not only sets the subject of experience at the centre of his theory, but he also discloses the author (i.e., himself) as being necessarily interwoven with the text. His grammatical mixture of third- and-first-person narration, for example, can be read as an expression of an ambivalent subjectivity that is aware of its own being-in-the-world, translating it into a specific being-in-the-text. While description and analysis in the third-person mode seem to render a speaker invisible, neutral, and 'objective', the rhetoric of the first-person mode usually serves for introspection. Certainly, a too-quick identification of the third person with the 'objective' and the first person with the 'subjective' appears problematic. Nevertheless, it has been argued that especially the discipline of anthropology has made use of these two poles and their corresponding grammatical persons. Philosopher Ernst Tugendhat, for example, claims that it is exactly this grammatical constellation that corresponds to anthropology's aim to understand the world *and* oneself (Tugendhat 2007). When Fanon outlined the subject position to such an extent, this inevitably ran contrary to the methodological turn in mainstream psychiatry and its attempt to diminish any subjectivity while strengthening scientific 'objectivity'.

## The reality of fiction

The objectivity that psy-disciplinary knowledge aims at relies on empirical testing of hypotheses, which are conveyed into studies and translated into statistical data. Validity and comparability are assured by means of replication (i.e., by guaranteeing that an experiment can be repeated at all times). However, psy disciplines themselves have reflected on the fact that the results of many scientific studies cannot be reproduced at all times, and the concomitant disillusionment with this basic pillar has led to a fundamental *replication crisis* (see Malich and Munafò 2022). Contrary to an epistemology of the *experiment*, it becomes apparent how Fanon's epistemology of *experience* took a markedly different approach to what would even be considered as knowledge. In that sense, he could elaborate on subject matters that did not even count as such within the psychiatric framework, such as anecdotes, movies, and fictional characters. This is not to say that no psychiatrist ever felt called to comment on literary or mythological figures. On the contrary, there is a vast reservoir of analytical work on such matters, Sigmund Freud's choice of Oedipus as *the* eponym for his theory being the best example. However, while such attempts took their cases from the annals of European cultural history, making use of Greek mythology to construct a fundament for their anthropological claims, it was a very different enterprise to take the ordinary, the trivial, and everyday language as an analytical point of departure, constantly risking allegations of intellectual banality (something that thinkers like Roland Barthes and Michel de Certeau had to grapple with, as well).

In the third chapter of *Black Skin, White Masks*, Fanon (2021, 45) recalls an urban legend of a *Black* man who is said to have slept with a *White* woman, exclaiming 'Long live Schœlcher!' at the height of orgasm. The allusion indicates that this sexual encounter was only made possible thanks to Victor Schœlcher, a French politician who had visited the South of the United States in 1829 and afterwards concentrated all his political work on the abolition of slavery. Twenty years later, he was the initiator of the *Décret d'abolition de l'esclavage du 27 avril 1848*, which, in fact, established the end of slavery in France and its colonies. Drawing on such a story – hearsay or maybe even a common joke, that is, something that under no circumstances could be counted as statistical data – clearly opposes psychiatric textbook knowledge. Fanon (1952, 45, emphasis added) anticipates arguments that would disqualify making use of such a common narrative when he writes: 'People will argue that this anecdote has not been *verified*. But the fact that it has taken shape and survived through the years, is an unmistakable indication that it addresses a tension, explicit or latent, but *real*'.

By emphasizing that what is stored in collective memories is part of *reality*, Fanon touches on a crucial point. Only by stressing the necessity of not conceiving reality as that which can be verified does it become apparent how common it has become in psy-disciplinary language to place in doubt the very existence of phenomena that cannot be translated into statistical data. 'If fiction and reality are to be linked, it must be in terms not of opposition but of communication, for the one is not the mere opposite of the other – fiction is a means of telling us something about reality' (Iser 1975, 7). What literature theorist Wolfgang Iser has pointed out regarding the ontological status of literary works does also hold true for Fanon's use of such to make arguments about societal conditions.

It is in this sense that Fanon makes the same argument for the epistemological value of the Schœlcher anecdote and for his use of René Marans' novel *Un homme pareil aux autres* (1947) for analytical purposes: the reality of the text, which plays such an important role in *Black Skin, White Masks*, cannot be verified in any statistical or empirical sense, even though it is autobiographically inspired. However, it must be considered as real, especially because its topic touches the core of French racism during the 1940s, which is a sociological fact that continues to be stored in collective memory. Marans' *Un homme pareil aux autres* serves as a paradigmatic piece for Fanon to analyse the unconscious suffering of the Black protagonist Jean Veneuse, which becomes most apparent when he and the White woman Andrée mutually fall in love, but it is impossible for him to believe that she returns his affection. Fanon appropriates the story – or the case – not to develop a clinical theory of neurosis that would take the psychic as an expression of the individual's life circumstances but rather to stress the general psychic milieu within a colonial situation, which both the colonised *and* the coloniser are being subjugated to.

Turning a fictional character into a quasi-case study must already be read as an original poetic act that subverts psychiatry's epistemological system with regard to its claim of reality. However, subversion also takes place on the level of Fanon's own language, which he allows to produce paradoxes. Especially when pointing out the psychic condition of Veneuse, Fanon repeatedly draws on the irritating notion that something is *and* is not the case. This is best demonstrated when he speaks of the character as a representative for the psychic suffering experienced through racial discrimination. On the one hand, he claims that 'Jean Veneuse is a magnificent example that will allow us to study in depth the attitude of the black man' (Fanon 1952, 46); on the other hand, he writes that 'it is our opinion that Jean Veneuse is not representative of the black-white-experience; rather, he represents a certain way for a neurotic, who happens to be black' (Fanon 1952, 61).

Keeping in mind that the argument running throughout all of Fanon's writing continually stresses the structural, social, and therefore political aspects of psychic suffering, this statement must provoke irritation at first glance. It appears as if he put into question that the character's suffering, his anxiety, and his self-devaluation showing in the face of a potential romantic relationship could be of any use for a structural analysis. In fact, it sounds like a repetition of the old argument that would individualise pathology, depicting it as an unlucky accident. It is in this sense that ethnopsychiatry as it was understood by the School of Algiers de-politicised pathology and pathologised political uprisings and resistance movements. Moreover, one could read the passage stating that Veneuse is a 'neurotic, who happens to be black' as an affirmation of an alleged non-influence of skin colour on the psychic, neglecting how colourism would emerge exactly from the statement that someone 'doesn't see colour' (see Bergo 2015). After all, to make the correlation between skin colour and psychic suffering appear accidental means devaluing the particular, the individual, and the subjective, rendering it as something that does not belong to the world, something that does not tell anything about the general intersection of racism and the psyche.

However, while it is true that any pathology is particular in the sense that it is a unique expression of a subject's lived experience that no other consciousness and no other body could ever feel in the same way, it is not true that this particularity indicates the inexistence or meaninglessness of the structural. This is the crucial point for Fanon when he states that Veneuse might be a neurotic no matter what. He constantly stresses that Black *and* White people are suffering from alienation under a colonial situation, which is why the seemingly paradoxical passage has to be understood in the sense that a man *like* Veneuse would be suffering from a colonial situation no matter what. This *likeness* interconnects strikingly with the title of Maran's novel itself: *Un homme pareil aux autres* – 'a man like any other'. It is only in this respect that the colour of his body does not matter, because colonialism makes *all* bodies suffer, even if their sufferings might appear very different in each case and even if the coloniser does not even realize (at first) that their body is in a constant state of suffering. They might not suffer from oppression, since they themselves are the oppressors, deeply alienated from oneself and from others. But to Fanon, this will to oppress is itself a suffering, not a sign of healthy strength. Mistaking the one for the other is not only a simple error. In fact, it belongs to the dominion of racism being a form of bad faith, which is repeatedly pointed out by Lewis R. Gordon throughout his work (see Gordon 1995). To put it clearly, the aforementioned passage would then have to be read with a different stress, and thus with a very different meaning: 'It is our opinion that Jean Veneuse is not representative of *the* black-white-experience; rather, he represents *a certain way* for a neurotic, who happens to be black'. Veneuse's neurosis exhibits *one* (particular, individual, subjective) possible psychic reaction to a *general* (structural, social, political) situation under colonialism.

While mainstream medicine and the psychiatry of the post-war era took a methodological turn against potentially harmful forms of subjectivity, Fanon put the subject at the core of his analysis. This was not only in sharp contrast to the dominant discourse, but it also provoked harsh critique, for instance, from feminist scholars (see Fuss 1994; Bergner 1995; Mercer 1996). However, their argument was not to condemn any lack of 'objectivity' in his thought but rather to claim that the specific subjectivity Fanon addressed was highly male-centric and that his analysis excluded any female subject position and their lived experience. With regard to the woman of colour, he would say: 'I know nothing of her' (Fanon 1952, 145). If this essay is concerned with violent exclusions from discourses, it becomes apparent how this is not only an issue of one dominant position repressing one minoritarian thought. Rather, there is heterogeneity within dominance and within minority, and the appearance of one voice always raises the question if it can speak for other voices as well or whether it makes them unheard.

In this sense, one would have to address the question of violence found also in Fanon's own thought, language, and political action. Only recently, philosopher Kwame Appiah (2022) compiled little-known accounts from Fanon's life, portraying him as an 'anti-Gandhi' who would not shy away from supporting an Angolan rebel group that massacred a Portuguese settler village. However, the emphasis here is not on asking about his take on violence as a 'cleansing force' during liberation struggles but rather on epistemic exclusions. If Fanon's subjectivity mutes other voices, the question arises whether the appearance of a speaking subject does not always carry violent potential, since its presence always creates the absence of an other – at least temporarily. Linguistic structuralism has pointed out that to speak about one thing necessarily implies not speaking about another, so that one would have to assume that there is always already violence in speaking. However, if one does not accept the idea that the only ethical approach to the world would then be to mute oneself, it must be asked what an ethical language, which speaks in the awareness of always being violent, might look like. Could there be a language of nonviolent violence? A language that takes a strong position without claiming to be universal? To speak while an Other does not would then not necessarily mean silencing or annihilating them but giving an example for others to speak from their specific lived experience as well.

Thus, Fanon's emphasis on one particular subjectivity does not per se recall the potentially violent omnipotence that mainstream medicine and psychiatry in the post-war era were trying to defeat. It would be a mistake to read the feminist claim for other *subjects* to appear in his analysis as a claim for more '*objectivity*'. Just as Fanon (1952, 12) claims that 'intelligence has never saved anyone', scientific objectivity has never prevented anyone from being excluded. However, if *no* discourse exists that does not exclude, the problem with the dominant medical and psy-disciplinary knowledge is not so much that a voice like Fanon's simply does not appear, but rather that non-appearance is framed as non-knowledge for reasons of being too subjective, while the language of these disciplines presents itself as perfectly objective, scientific, and neutral. If the poetisation of science means to give shape to a subject matter through language, while making this very act explicit as the horizon one speaks from, there is a liberating potential in this, opening up the possibility to recognise one's own violence and to develop an ethical language of non-violent violence. On the contrary, if a discourse shapes its subject matter through language and denies its own poetics, it makes claims to universalism and pretends that the language used was nothing more than strict representation, as if it could simply depict what *is* real.

## The politics of constructing reality

The construction of reality is a genuine dimension of power. If a dominant discourse categorically excludes languages and knowledge that are framed as too 'subjective', this discourse exhibits its very own political agenda while concealing it at the same time. There is a striking analogy in how this onto-epistemological power relation plays out on the structural level of discourse *and* on the concrete level of the medical setting. Fanon (1952) himself addresses the violent dimension of the clinic when he points out how French colonial doctors declared the suffering of their African patients as pseudo-pathology. These patients described somatic pains that could not be located in the organs, which is why doctors thought of it as something that did not exist. Fanon describes how the racist image of the malingering African patient is directly connected to the fact that their symptoms did not fit into what French medicine considered *real* diseases in the 1950s, since the common conviction was still that any disease would appear with an organic correlate.

When phenomena that cannot be translated into the language of psychiatry are suggested to not be real, this exhibits a specific understanding of the epistemic value of language as such. Language then either appears as a conveyer of objective truth or as a false statement. When colonial doctors reinterpreted the exhibited suffering as pseudo-pathology, they ignored the positive value of the patient's particular utterance (i.e., the complaint about an experienced – and therefore real – pain). What these patients were saying was not perceived as reliable information but rather as empty speech or blatant lies. It was only interesting insofar as it could be counted as a symptom – not for a *real* pathology but for a *non-existent* pseudo-pathology.

But just as Fanon argued for the epistemic value of the Schœlcher anecdote and of Maran's novel, and just as he pointed out their inherent reality that resists verification, he argued for the reality of those patients' symptoms that colonial psychiatry annihilated: 'A thing is said to be vague when it is lacking in consistency, in objective reality. The North African's pain, for which we can find no lesional basis, is judged to have no consistency, no reality' (Fanon 1952a, 6). Fanon himself described a pain that could not be found in the organs: the colonial situation. His lived experience was shaped around this situation and his language was witness of that. Hence, if it is exactly such language that is being framed as 'too subjective' (as opposed to mainstream medicine and psy disciplines' 'objectivity'), it is not only that the dominant discourse created a structure in which Fanon's poetisation appeared as lacking consistency. This structure also paved a fundament that rendered the very psychic effects of colonial racism as particular, individual, subjective, and therefore allegedly irreal, just like the symptoms of those patients described above.

## Conclusion

It is remarkable how this specific notion of what is real and what is not goes hand in hand with corresponding notions of what language is supposed to be and do.

Psychiatry's methodological turn in the post-war era must not only be read as a singular reaction to problems specific to this very discipline, allegedly separate from other epistemic systems. Instead, it can be situated in a much broader context of objectification of knowledge and language that constituted one strand within the so-called linguistic turn. The old philosophical argument about the value and truthfulness of rhetoric reappeared in the twentieth century as a debate on how to think of the interconnection of language as expression and language as a pure means of communication. If psychiatry chose the latter to uphold its own scientific ideal, the corresponding language had to prove itself to be the exact opposite of what was taken as the falsidical pseudo-language described above, and therefore appear as clear, reporting, and perfectly descriptive.

However, if Fanon emphasises the performative qualities of language – creating meaning not only on a level of clearly determinate communication but also on a level of effect – this is not to say that his work might slide into obscurity or be lacking a very empirical, materialist basis. In this sense, Michael Allan (2023, 50) argues that Fanon takes the Arabic term *istiqla* ('independence') as it appears on an Algerian radio station 'less as a word whose meaning is to be decrypted than as a call to action for those committed to the struggle'. Regarding his vast spectrum of analytical work, Fanon's thought is not to be considered *the Other* of science. He always called for science to reflect on its own premises, one of them being that *any* knowledge production is inherently shaped by the poetics of language. This is why Lewis Gordon (2018, 24) argues that Fanon's

> [A]esthetics is not, then, the dessert we have after our nutritional needs have been met but instead, as perhaps also dessert should be understood, part of the entire constellation of meeting such needs. It is as central to what it means to live a human life as the various other converging dimensions of human existence.

Science, being a mode of knowledge production, is conveyed through, formed by, and inevitably entangled with language, whose poetics becomes manifest in every act of expression.

That is why Fanon was strongly critical of the concept of Négritude as it was conceived by Aimé Cesaire, arguing that it essentialised African ways of living and thinking as being more rhythmic, passionate, and poetic than Western thought, and therefore othering itself. In *this* sense, Fanon's language is *not more* poetic than the language of mainstream medicine and psy disciplines, since every language carries a specific poetics. Fanon's intervention (especially in *Black Skin, White Masks*) *is* a poetisation of science in the sense that his strategy to make an argument is to employ a language that is explicitly not neutral, bearing witness to the lived experience of an actual subject. Hence, while it needs to be emphasised that Fanon's textual work demonstrates how aesthetics, and therefore poetic language, is a medium 'through which human beings in effect make themselves at home with reality' (Gordon 2018, 20), it must not be forgotten that this is a process that does not take place *outside* the realm of science. In fact, the construction of reality as world-making encompasses every act of speaking and writing – in the sciences, in the arts, and in the everyday speech act. Only in acknowledging this can the alleged hiatus between subjectivity, poetics, politics, and science be deconstructed, and only in this can there be a liberating potential in poetisation.

## Notes

1 See also Daniele Lorenzini's contribution to this volume.

2 By the end of the nineteenth century, this conviction was most prominently postulated by the German neurologist Wilhelm Griesinger. To him, the dysfunctional organ in question could only be the brain; hence, he claimed that every mental illness is an illness of the brain.

3 It was due to the mediation of the editor-in-chief at the journal Esprit that Fanon made contact with the publishing house. His biographer David Macey indicates that this was a stroke of good fortune, since the book would have been hard to publish also with publishing houses focused on literature, such as Gallimard, because it juxtaposes poetic allusions with the technicality of empirical data from the clinic (see Macey 2000, 153).

4 In an in-depth case study, Andrew Lakoff exemplifies how a hegemony of knowledge systems is produced when universalising techniques like the DSM form a nexus with global capitalism. It was in 1997 that the French genomics company Genset collaborated with an Argentinian hospital on a project that investigated the DNA of bipolar patients. The hospital was asked to provide the needed blood samples; however, Argentina has a strong psychoanalytic tradition, in which the diagnosis 'bipolar disorder' was unknown; thus, the question was how to mediate between these diverging notions of illness. Eventually, the hospital needed the money Genset was paying them, and doctors diagnosed bipolarity in cases they would have diagnosed differently before (Lakoff 2007).

5 The racial slur in the original was censored for the sake of the current publication.

## References

Allan, Michael. 2023. "The Language(s) of Self-Representation: Toward a Postcolonial Theory of Voice." *Critical Times: Interventions in Global Critical Theory* 6(1): 39–57.

Appiah, Kwame Anthony. 2022. "Liberation Psychology." *The New York Review of Books* LXIX(3): 43–46.

Bergner, Gwen. 1995. "Who Is that Masked Woman? or, The Role of Gender in Fanon's Black Skin, White Masks." *Publications of the Modern Language Association* 110(1): 75–88.

Bergo, Bettina, and Nicholls, Tracey. 2015. *I Don't See Color. Personal and Critical Perspectives on White Privilege.* Pennsylvania: Penn State University Press.

Cherki, Alice. 2006. *Fanon. A Portrait* (2000). Ithaca, NY, London: Cornell University Press.Fanon, Frantz. 1951. *Troubles mentaux et syndromes psychiatriques dans l'hérédo-dégénérescence spino-cérébelleuse. Un cas de malade de Friedrich avec délire de possession.* thèse méd., Lyon.

Fanon, Frantz. 1964. "The 'North African Syndrome'" (1952a). In *Toward the African Revolution.* edited by Haakon Chevalier, 3–16. New York: Grove Press.

Fanon, Frantz. 2021. *Black Skin, White Masks* (1952). London: Penguin Books.Foucault, Michel. 1965. *Madness and Civilization. A History of Insanity in the Age of Reason* (1961). London: Tavistock.

Fricker, Miranda. 2007. *Epistemic Injustice: Power and the Ethics of Knowing*. Oxford: Oxford University Press.

Fuss, Diana. 1994. "Interior Colonies: Frantz Fanon and the Politics of Identification." *Diacritics*, 24(2/3): 20–39.

Goffman, Erwing. 1961. *Asylums: Essays on the Social Situations of Mental Patients and other Inmates*. New York City: Anchor Books.

Gordon, Lewis R. 1995. *Bad Faith and Antiblack Racism*. Amherst: Humanity Books.

Gordon, Lewis R. 2018. "Black Aesthetics, Black Value." *Public Culture* 30(2): 19–34.

Iser, Wolfgang. 1975. "The Reality of Fiction. A Functionalist Approach to Literature." *New Literary History* 7(1): 7–38.

Keller, Richard C. 2007. "Violence, Resistance, and the Poetics of Suffering: Colonial Madness between Frantz Fanon and Kateb Yacine." In Keller, Richard C. *Colonial Madness. Psychiatry in French North Africa*, 161–190. Chicago, IL: Chicago University Press.

Khalfa, Jean, and Robert C. Young. 2015a. "The Organogenesis and Psychogenesis of Mental Illness." In *Alienation and Freedom, Frantz Fanon*, edited by Jean Khalfa and Robert C. Young, 175–183. London: Bloomsbury Publishing.

Khalfa, Jean, and Robert C. Young. (eds). 2015b. *Alienation and Freedom. Frantz Fanon*. London: Bloomsbury Publishing.

Lakoff, Andrew. 2007. *Pharmaceutical Reason. Knowledge and Value in Global Psychiatry.* Cambridge: Cambridge University Press

Macey, David. 2000. *Frantz Fanon*. London: Granta Books.

Malich, Lisa, and Marcus R. Munafò (eds). 2022. "Special Issue: Replication of Crises – Interdisciplinary Reflections on the Phenomenon of the Replication Crisis in Psychology." *Review of General Psychology* 26(2): 127–273.

Maran, René. 1947. *Un homme pareil aux autres*. Paris: Arc-en-ciels.

Mercer, Kobena. 1996. "Decolonisation and Disappointment: Reading Fanon's Sexual Politics." In *The Fact of Blackness: Frantz Fanon and Visual Culture*, edited by Alan Read, 114–131. Seattle: Bay Press.

Robcis, Camille. 2021. *Disalienation: Politics, Philosophy, and Radical Psychiatry in Postwar France*. Chicago, IL: University of Chicago Press.

Tugendhat, Ernst. 2007. *Anthropologie statt Metaphysik*. München: Beck.

World Health Organization. 1975. *Schizophrenia. A Multinational Study. A Summary of the Initial Evaluation Phase of the International Pilot Study of Schizophrenia*. Geneva: World Health Organization.

World Psychiatric Association. 2023. "About Transcultural Psychiatry Section." https://www.wpa-tps.org/about-wpa-tps/transcultural-psychiatry.

# Musing 3

## Fanon, epistemic injustice, and the colonial medical encounter

*Daniele Lorenzini*

As is well known, Miranda Fricker (2007, 1) defines epistemic injustice as 'a wrong done to someone specifically in their capacity as a knower' and focuses on two main kinds of (discriminatory) epistemic injustice: *testimonial injustice*, on the one hand, where 'prejudice causes a hearer to give a deflated level of credibility to a speaker's word' (e.g., a jury that does not believe a defendant's testimony because of their accent, sex, or skin colour), and *hermeneutical injustice*, on the other, where 'a gap in collective interpretive resources puts someone at an unfair disadvantage when it comes to making sense of their social experiences' and/or rendering them communicatively intelligible to others. This gap, according to Fricker, is caused by the hermeneutical marginalisation of the group to which the subject belongs.

The medical encounter is clearly a space in which these forms of epistemic injustice or violence can, and often do, take place (Carel and Kidd 2017). In this chapter, I focus on one of these forms: the problematic passage from *objectivity* to *objectification* within the medical encounter in the colonial context. To illustrate this point, I rely on Frantz Fanon's psychiatric writings.

Fanon, who was born in Martinique but trained as a psychiatrist in France, began his residency at Saint-Alban in 1951 under the mentorship of François Tosquelles. After completing his residency, he moved to Algeria (at the time still a French colony) and, from 1953 to 1956, he worked as *chef de service* in the Blida-Joinville psychiatric hospital. In his writings from these years, Fanon addresses and reflects upon his experience of treating Algerian patients, both in France and in Algeria, focusing in particular on how the words and behaviour of the 'North African' constantly raised suspicion among the medical staff as to the *reality* of their illness. Indeed, Fanon observes that, when asked to describe their pain and symptoms, the colonised subject rarely conforms to the established (Western) medical discourse: 'the North African presents himself cloaked in vagueness', he claims that 'it hurts everywhere', and he 'seems hostile to conforming to categories of time', as 'the past, for him, is a distressing time' (Fanon 2014, 41–42). Fanon describes several frustrating conversations, or *failed* encounters, between doctor and patient in this context characterised by colonial relations of power:

– Where does it hurt?
– In my belly (He points to his thorax and abdomen.)

DOI: 10.4324/9781032660165-13

– When?
– All the time.
– Even at night?
– Especially at night.
– So, it hurts more at night than during the day?
– No. All the time.
– But more at night than during the day?
– No. All the time.
– And where does it hurt the most?
– Here. (He points to his thorax and abdomen).

(Fanon 2014, 42)

Fanon (2014, 42–43) characterises his patient's experience in terms of them *becoming* their pain: 'He *is* his pain and refuses to understand any kind of language and it is but a short step to the conclusion: It is because I am Arab that they are not treating me like everyone else.' The medical staff too often feels frustrated: their patients' responses are vague, their explanations contradictory, and most of the time careful examinations and X-rays show nothing at all. Thus, Fanon (2014, 43) writes, 'the North African's pain, for which we can find no lesional basis, is found to have no consistency, no reality'; however – and this is the crucial point for Fanon – 'the North African *is* also the-kind-who-doesn't-like-work, such that everything he does is interpreted *a priori* on this basis', and the North African is thus seen as a faker, a liar, a phony.

It seems clear that, since it originates from prejudice, this conclusion constitutes a case of epistemic injustice, one in which the subject is wronged in their capacity as a knower – here, a knower of their own subjectivity, of their body and pain. From this perspective, the encounters between doctor and patient that Fanon describes seem to be straightforward cases of *testimonial* injustice, where prejudice causes the (French) medical staff to give to the patient's words a deflated level of credibility, or no credibility at all. Hence the invention of the so-called 'North African syndrome', an imaginary syndrome, a 'pseudo-pathology' that reduces the colonised patient to the stereotype: 'the North African is a faker and a liar who doesn't want to work', even though, as Fanon (2014, 44–45) immediately remarks, there is actually 'no doubt in anyone's mind that [the patient] is ill'.

Yet the situation that Fanon describes is more complex than that. What about the well-intentioned doctor who *does* fight against the potential influence of prejudice during the consultation but ends up unable to find any 'reasonable' medical explanation for her patient's pain? Is her feeling of frustration at her patient's 'comedy, or drama' (Fanon 2014, 43) unjustified in this case? Is her conclusion that, after all, the patient's words must not be trusted *irrational*? Fanon writes:

> Any patient who complains of headaches, ringing in the ears, and dizziness *must* also have high blood pressure. But if these same symptoms are present with no sign of high blood pressure or brain tumours or anything testing positive, the doctor *will have to* conclude that medical thinking is at

> fault; and since any thinking is thinking about something, he will find the *patient* at fault - an undocile, undisciplined patient unaware of *the rules of the game*. The rule, ever so strict, that states: every symptom presupposes a lesion.
>
> (Fanon 2014, 44, emphasis added)

One way to respond to the above-mentioned questions is to suggest that the well-intentioned doctor does not commit *testimonial* injustice, and that this is rather a case of *hermeneutical* injustice. Although Fanon does not use this expression, I believe this is exactly what he is getting at, namely, that the reasons that, in this context, lead a well-intentioned doctor to discount her patient's words are *structural*. In other words, the problem is not a specific subjective prejudice that affects the doctor's thinking, but the systemic effects of the colonial and racist order of things. Indeed, as Fanon has convincingly demonstrated in his works, it is the colonial order of things that literally makes the patient sick, and conversely the patient's – conscious or unconscious – refusal to play the coloniser's medical 'game of truth' (to use an expression borrowed from Michel Foucault) is not a sign of their being inconsequential, untrustworthy, or straightforwardly deceitful (Fanon 2014, 45). It is instead a form of – significant, albeit minimal – resistance or counter-conduct on their part.

The problem here is that the French doctor is unable to take into account the consequences of colonial domination on her patient because of what Lewis Gordon (2010, 8) calls 'epistemic colonisation': the medical categories that she relies on do not make space for such considerations, not considering them salient. Consequently, the medical encounter is a failure even when the doctor does her best to *personally* or *subjectively* counteract the influence of prejudice. Thus, Fanon's contribution helps us to problematise a merely ethical approach to epistemic injustice in terms of individual virtues.

In *The Wretched of the Earth*, Fanon (2004, 37) famously claims that 'for the colonised subject, objectivity is always directed against him'. This is the case because, in the colonial context, objectivity – or the rules of the (Western) medical game of truth – necessarily triggers effects of *objectification*, thus undermining any beneficial effect that the medical encounter is supposed to produce. Interestingly, Fanon describes this situation as one that 'traps' *both* the patient and the doctor, thus suggesting that the mere revision of the Western medical discourse is not enough to counteract this form of injustice. The only way out, according to him, is a transformation at the social and political level: the end of colonial domination and the creation of radically new ways of living together.

## References

Carel, Havi, and Ian James Kidd. 2017. "Epistemic Injustice in Medicine and Healthcare." In *The Routledge Handbook of Epistemic Injustice*, edited by Ian James Kidd, José Medina, and Gaile Pohlhaus, Jr., 336–346. New York: Routledge.

Fanon, Frantz. 2004. *The Wretched of the Earth* (1961). New York: Grove Press.
Fanon, Frantz. 2014. *Decolonizing Madness: The Psychiatric Writings of Frantz Fanon*, edited by N. Gibson. Basingstoke: Palgrave Macmillan.
Fricker, Miranda. 2007. *Epistemic Injustice: Power and the Ethics of Knowing*. Oxford: Oxford University Press.
Gordon, Lewis R. 2010. "Fanon on Decolonizing Knowledge." In *Fanon and the Decolonization of Philosophy*, edited by Elizabeth A. Hoppe and Tracey Nicholls, 3–18. Lanham, MD: Lexington Books.

# Part 3

# Agency in illness and ethics of suffering

# 8 Narrative autonomy to the test of illness

*Silvia Pierosara*

## An irreparable loss of autonomy?

This chapter develops the thesis (Boyd 2000) that illness, in addition to being physical pain, is experienced as a radical loss of autonomy. Such loss could be interpreted as the ethical–practical side of the loss of meaning, accompanied by a sharpening of the question concerning the existence of evil in the form of physical and psychological suffering. From an existential standpoint, this awareness of the impoverishment of our capacity to effectively act in the world cannot be denied. However, it also opens the possibility for a different exercise of autonomy, which assumes a narrative form. Indeed, the more we are pervaded by a sense of bewilderment, the more we feel the need to understand and reconstruct meaning. Narrative practices are generally considered capable of shaping the meaning of experience due to their synthetic capacity, which accommodates negativity within a teleological dynamic oriented towards the good (Charon et al. 2017).

These practices, due to their connection to meaning and teleology, have often been criticised, especially in relation to cases in which meaning seems to become an automatism, and evil – understood as pain and suffering – appears to be too easily justified or, conversely, removed. If it is necessary to accept the invitation not to take the meaning for granted, it is equally relevant to recognise a critical-reconstructive dimension to narrativity. This dimension configures meaning and sense without permanently imposing them, and it offers the possibility of overturning pre-constituted meanings to give word to the experience of illness, albeit in imperfect, unfinished forms. Refusing to narrate due to fearing that the search for meaning will turn into an automatism that takes it for granted would mean, to a certain extent, that the experience of pain and illness is surrendered to silence and being suppressed. That is, it involuntarily becomes analogous to the perfectionist imperatives of performance society (Deleuze 1998).

In an always reversible manner, narration synthesises actions, events, universal norms, and concrete situations, following change that it attempts to explain by inserting it into a historical plot, even when the narrative gesture is destined to repeat and reshape itself and runs, at least apparently, 'in circles'. Therefore, narrating in various forms, be this not entirely conscious, allows one to resort to various dimensions of experiencing illness: from pain to suffering (Ricœur 2013), and from

DOI: 10.4324/9781032660165-15

the inner word that wonders 'why? why me? why now?' to the outer world and the relationship with care networks that carry the burden of accentuated dependence.

I propose to read the interaction between person, pain, and suffering as the trace of a loss of personal and moral autonomy, which indirectly corresponds to the need to acquire narrative autonomy. The nature of suffering and its paralysis of action urgently require a work of configuration and reconfiguration by the patient, thus giving urgency to their commitment in terms of restructuring the experience. Consequently, the autonomy painfully experienced in illness can be declined as narrative autonomy, whose historical and relational weaving always provides an emblematic picture of interdependence based on the suffering condition. Paradoxically, the worsening of dependence does not diminish the dignity manifested in autonomy. Rather, it turns it into a task, an exercise to be preserved. This exercise inevitably summons others and this summoning is recognisable in the faces of those who, for different reasons and with different skills, assist the patient in the experience of illness.

While it is undeniable that illness is commonly associated with the loss of autonomy understood as competence, that is, the ability to choose and act for oneself, it is also necessary to expand on this term and move away from singular meanings. For example, it includes recognising that the desire for autonomy persists, even when the presence of others becomes more necessary than ever and when limitation and finitude manifest themselves in a nameable, diagnosable way. Autonomy does not correspond to capacity and efficacy. Instead, it denotes a yearning for freedom, which is expressed in the demand for respect for one's own dignity, which in turn can be experienced in the form of will and authorship in relation to reorganising the existence around illness. This demand and its consequences make clear what often remains implicit in assumptions about autonomy: it does not arise *despite* others and without limits but emerges from a suffering, unchosen condition of relationality that fosters responsibility. Therefore, it makes sense to speak of 'autonomy', because the experience of pain more than any other thing occurs without delegation, arising in the first person, and those affected must cope with it, perhaps not passively, even in the residual form of resisting and imagining otherwise. That is, we suffer the event-disease, not the question about its meaning and the precarious answers arising from it.

By placing the noun 'autonomy' next to the adjective 'narrative', we understand how patients, under certain conditions, can be differently autonomous due to their capability of inserting themselves within a web of meaning and relations arising from the unwanted event. At least initially, this event escapes comprehension and threatens personal integrity. Through the lens of pain, we understand how 'narrative autonomy' constantly operates on the edge of meaning, without guarantees, accepting the risk of a question that is continuously raised (Blanchot 1995). By losing some grip on life, through fragmentary narrative and through the narrating body, people rediscover their dignity from the wound, and through words they can resist their slide to non-sense. The greater the sense of bewilderment, the more frequent the recourse to narration: 'stories have to repair the damage that illness has done to the person's sense of where she is in her life, and where she may be going. Stories are a way of redrawing maps and finding new destinations' (Frank 1995, 53).

After this brief review of the ways in which narration and illness meet, also through an examination of the related literature, it is necessary to explore the possibilities and limitations of narrative autonomy. Specifically, this is to ask how narrative autonomy can be declined from the perspective of the suffering person; what categories it allows us to rethink; where the margins of this autonomy are concretely revealed; and what kinds of support and assistance it receives from people in the care network. Whether understood as a road from experience to reflection, or as reversing the route, it will then become clear that autonomy, rather than being an individual competence, acquires the features of a 'relational' task anchored to the historical condition of the human being.

## The encounter between narration and illness 'is told in many ways'

As a preliminary point, I will review some angles from which narration is commonly used while experiencing illness, although not always explicitly.

From a social standpoint, listening to narratives allows an understanding of illness not only as an individual process but also – and primarily – as a systemic one. The interconnections between agent and context; relations with others; the role in society; and symbolic, imaginary horizons of meanings transpire from the way a traumatic event is perceived and narrated. Consequently, narration provides an interconnection between patient and society, making its interpretative categories and *emplotment* strategies available to decipher sickness, its genesis, and its social meaning. Resorting to narration, in this sense, represents a trace of a holistic conception of sickness.

From an epistemological standpoint, the encounter between narration and illness has two possible perspectives: on the one hand, illness itself can be compared to an event with narrative structure, and it can therefore be diagnosed and understood through narration and its 'textuality'; on the other, narrative language itself can offer a structure that is analogous to the manifestation of illness.

Let us focus on the first perspective. Narration reinterprets the processes of causal inference in a non-rigidly deterministic sense, taking responsibility for the dialogue between explanation and comprehension, as claimed by exponents of narrative medicine and *medical humanities*. Narration, one might say, prevents 'the fall into objectivity' (Foucault 2001, 443) from being definitive or irrevocable. Moreover, narration entered medical history as disease came to be considered as a text requiring attention, with the capacity for representation and connection, as masterfully underlined by Michel Foucault (1973). In reconstructing the birth of clinical medicine, the philosopher underlines how the symptom becomes a sign

> Beneath a gaze that is sensitive to difference, simultaneity or succession, and frequency; the symptom therefore becomes a sign – a spontaneously differential operation, devoted to totality and to memory, and calculating as well; an act, therefore, that joins, in a single movement, the element and the connection of the elements among themselves.
>
> (94)

Following Foucault's interpretation, one could hypothesise that clinical medicine originated with narration, because it is approached as a practice and technique of sign interpretation, presupposing an analogy between illness and text that makes it a technique and practice of interpretation, as well as a gaze and language of truth. This passage shows how the interpretative attitude can be traced back to an objectifying practice

> In this regular alternation of speech and gaze, the disease gradually declares its truth, a truth that it offers to the eye and ear, whose theme, although possessing only one sense, can be restored, in its indubitable totality, only by two senses: that which sees and that which listens. This is why the questionnaire without the examination and the examination without the interrogation were doomed to an endless task: it belongs to neither to fill the gaps within the province of the other.
>
> (112)

Carlo Ginzburg, who admirably described the circumstantial paradigm (Ginzburg 1992), is among those who combined perspectives on medical semiotics and narration. The 'circumstantial' paradigm inscribed in clinical practice appears in narrative medicine on two levels: the physician not only reads illness as a text but also collects and connects clues in relation to the patient's narrative. If the circumstantial paradigm is inescapable in medicine, we should distance ourselves from an interpretative excess that might become as violent as negligence: sometimes silence happens without underlying reasons, and the assumption of a hidden meaning is the first step towards its imposition. Being aware of this possible drift allows the critical use of narration as an instrument to construct and deconstruct interconnections, while keeping at a remove the risk of objectification: if the narrator of the illness is recognised as a co-author and co-protagonist in the process of 'reading' and caring for oneself, the 'circumstantial' paradigm does not necessarily lead to a reification of the patient's body and discourse.

As for the second perspective, according to which narrative language itself can offer a structure that is analogous to the manifestation of illness, Bühler (1934) identifies three fundamental functions of the linguistic sign: it is a symptom, since it expresses the interiority of the user; it is a signal if we refer to the addressee; and it is a symbol in relation to the external world that it aims to indicate or represent. From this thesis, it is possible to trace a 'circumstantial' character in the very nature of language, compared to which narration performs a connective function by telling a story that, through symbols, links symptom and the inner state with the signal. If language is, by its very nature, a sign – that is, a symptom, signal, and symbol at the same time – then it can embrace the experience of illness, which is analogous in terms of its manifestation.

Anthropologically speaking, narration allows illness to be understood as a cultural event in which personal history is inscribed, assigning to it a different meaning depending on the context and values of the community of reference, both in a diachronic, intracultural sense and in a synchronic, intercultural sense.

Medical anthropology documents the astonishing variety of the cultural meanings of sickness in relation to context; however, medical anthropologists (e.g., Byron Good) identify narration as a transcultural process by which coming to terms with illness. Illness and disease themselves, argues Byron Good, have a narrative structure. In other words, the narrativity of sickness is evidenced in the historicity and temporality of human existence: 'Illness is grounded in human historicity, in the temporality of individuals and families and communities' (Byron Good 1994, 157).

From an ethical–anthropological standpoint, the experience of illness implies its narration by the patient: if, on one hand, the intensification of pain takes away the word and appears inexpressible, on the other it needs to be shared, told, and expressed through narration. From the view of the carer, the space for narration represents a 'third' space of common deliberation thanks to the imaginative capacity, which hosts horizons of deciphering, sharing, and 'circulation' of good practices. Narrative autonomy is thus recognisable in both the patient and physician as a meeting point, where meaning is found between at least two similar needs. Therefore, the ethical–anthropological assumption that enables thinking of narrative autonomy in care contexts consists of acknowledging the doctor–patient encounter as a relationship. This fact, which may appear banal or be overlooked, is actually at the root of any ethical consideration related to contexts of care. By extension, all deviations or pathologies of that encounter can easily appear to be an irrelevant interaction or the provision of a service, thus renouncing the most ambitious statute of relationship.

Gabriel Marcel underlines this with unequivocal simplicity when reconstructing the reasons behind the increasingly pervasive depersonalisation of medicine. According to him, there was a time when the relationship between physician and patient was the norm – and had a normative relevance; nowadays, the establishment of this kind of relationship has become the exception (Marcel 1953). To ensure that the encounter between doctor and patient retains the traits of a relationship, they both need to be aware that they cannot objectify each other: that they belong to being, and not that they have it at their disposal.

The normative scope of the relationship between doctor and patient, based on trust and unchosen intimacy, also implies an anthropology of the non-objectifiable, which cannot reduce stories to mere data or bodies to objects. Therefore, it can be argued that narrative medicine arises precisely from this ethical–anthropological awareness. It does not originate from the need to find an ethical corrective to an eminently technical–instrumental interaction, but rather from the recognition that the ethical and normative dimension is the enabling condition for the encounter between doctor and patient. Before technique, and along with it, comes vocation. Narrative medicine must rest on these foundations in order not to surrender to the double temptation of reducing narration to a mere technical competence, and to the opposite one of assigning an almost thaumaturgic virtue to it. There is no cure in narration with no relationship behind it. The doctor/patient relationship is at risk of double objectification: that of the doctor towards the patient-object and that of the patient, who might consider the doctor a provider of services in return for payment. Therefore, the world of care delivery establishes an exposed relationship, which is vulnerable (Russo 2006) to reification; against this, narration constitutes the 'third space' in which doctor and patient can consolidate a relationship of trust while resisting the double objectification.

From this angle, I will attempt to explore the consistency of narrative autonomy in caring contexts.

## Resisting non-sense: The narrative autonomy of the sufferer

As mentioned above, the experience of illness is commonly associated with a loss of autonomy, which makes the person partially or totally dependent on the care of others. This condition of radical vulnerability leaves the sufferer in the hands of others and at their mercy (Ferrarese 2018). According to this vision, vulnerability and autonomy are mutually exclusive. Such a view is based on a conflation of autonomy with independence, or with a set of skills reflecting individual effectiveness and performance within a hyper-competitive society, or with self-mastery or total control. It is undeniable that sickness exposes the individual to harm by others, even by those responsible for caring. However, patients do not lose their autonomy as narrators; as interpreters, they are able to cultivate hope in the future and manage their own vulnerability by coming to terms with it. The autonomy of a patient, paradoxically, is directly – and not inversely – proportional to the vulnerability experienced while suffering. This situation sharpens the demand for meaning, intensifying it in the experience-limit of pain. The demand for meaning must be answered by a self that keeps starting over without renouncing a view towards the future.

Patients are capable of narrating – not just describing – their symptoms, and of articulating and linking themselves into a story, along with those who share their biographical journey. The sick person is someone who asks – and by asking prefigures scenarios, follows possible developments, makes suppositions, and commits to act in concert with the carers, for example, following therapies, indications, and suggestions, and inserting these in a plot. Already during anamnesis, patients experience an intensification of their narrative autonomy as a capacity to synthesise, an attempt to reconcile irreconcilable events and actions, and an inconceivable asymmetry between what they want and what they have or are. When illness becomes more difficult, the task of configuration becomes greater. It is a fragile capacity, made up of silences and exposed to misunderstanding and misinterpretation, and it requires care.

Even when the disease is known, the patient can experience narrative autonomy as the ability to trace connections and counterfactual thinking directed towards the future, towards the possibility of salvation. Antonio Casado da Rocha (2014, 207) has outlined the contours of narrative autonomy in the context of the ethics of care: 'People are narratively autonomous if they can interact with others through a shared history that links past and future [...] Narrative autonomy requires a connection between patients' audience and environment, and their sense of time'. Therefore, narrative autonomy can be defined as 'the ability of patients to develop a shared story by linking past and future' (207). This capacity is not comparable with a competence that increases performance effectiveness. Rather, it is an undedicated trace of responsibility even under painful conditions. Narrative autonomy is not simply about interpreting but also about acting in the world, starting from the possibility for the patient to reorganise horizons of meanings.

Narrative recounting involves gestures charged with ethical and existential implications. There are several reasons for this. First, this recounting begins from a situation that has not been chosen. It arises from a self expropriated by sickness that translates into words an involuntary condition that irrevocably 'pertains' to it. That is, recounting happens from a condition that speaks for the self and starts from the self to project an elsewhere, to imagine something else, and to approach the world it narrates precisely while narrating it. The self becomes the narrated illness, but it also becomes other than illness. Second, narration and self-evaluation allow some escape from the condition of loneliness that entraps the patient. By recognising that others are suffering from the same pain, the narrator avoids a risk of absolutisation that victimises and further isolates. From this perspective, narrativity can have a universalising function, allowing the uniqueness of one's concrete experience to be recognised as similar to others'. Finally, narrating and recounting are much more precious when included in the plots of a silence to be respected without violation: we cannot presume to interpret or understand beyond ourselves. In this sense, narrative autonomy can also be a choice not to narrate, omit, or defend a self that uses words as a protection from indiscretion, objectification, and the blame that sometimes accompanies care practices.

In relation to how the person acts in the world in relation to sickness, narrative autonomy can be declined in relation to several meanings. The first relates to the corporeality of the narrated stories. The second connects to notions of self-care as a practice of freedom and responsibility. Renouncing it would mean, at most, being replaced by neutral apparatuses, thus substituting technique with relationship. The third involves recognising the sick person as capable of repayment.

Regarding the first meaning, the act of narrative autonomy intersects with suffering: to recognise oneself as autonomous, one must not deny the dimension of uncontrollable, defective corporeality. According to Frank (1995, 27), 'The body is not mute, but it is inarticulate; it does not use speech, yet begets it'. When confronted with such language, patients must be able to recognise themselves as capable of articulation and, at the same time, they must be able to recognise the corporeality of their narrative autonomy. This autonomy is not only an interpretative capacity, but also a gesture, an action originating from the body.

Regarding the second meaning, the person who suffers is also narratively autonomous because, if possible, that person must be able to exercise self-care without being entirely replaced by the doctor. Care is also a story written by at least two authors: it is a cooperative enterprise that is built together, preventing asymmetries of roles and knowledge from becoming barriers that produce domination. In his famous and controversial *Medical Nemesis*, Ivan Illich makes some remarkable considerations about this:

> Any kind of dependence turns into an obstacle to autonomous mutual care, coping, adapting and healing and, what is worse, into a device by which

people are stopped from transforming the conditions at work and at home which do make them sick.

(Illich 1975, 70)

When faced with suffering, the patient's autonomy is preserved when they are encouraged to take care of themselves and their own health, left to find the meaning of what is happening by framing it within a story that is being witnessed in the first person, without falling into the 'neo-liberal' temptation of blaming patients that do not respond, making them unrealistically responsible for their own illness (Sontag 1978). On the contrary, exasperating the dependence on an inaccessible system of knowledge, which provides services without giving time for justification, leads people to forget the possible social and contextual reasons that contribute to determining the illness itself.

Even in sickness it is possible to exercise a self-care that shifts from dominating biological states to a conscious co-existence with sickness. This is about not giving up taking care of oneself, compared to passively submitting to the mercy of others. Consequently, being autonomous with respect to health and illness means, on one hand, recognising ourselves as capable of facilitating the physiological processes that ensure the maintenance of health and, on the other, of 'making one's illness speak', within the historical horizon of a network of narratives by which we are identified and that make the experience of pain not certainly comprehensible but at least expressible – and therefore accessible to a question of meaning.

Following this definition of narrative autonomy between health and illness, Illich (1975, 168) once again offers some valuable points: 'health is a task, and as such not comparable to the physiological balance of beasts'. Even the physiological condition of health, which is natural and immediate in other living beings, among humans seems to be earned through 'having to be', through artifice or a task. The natural becomes ethical, designating a relationship that is not only interpersonal but also intrapersonal. Caring for oneself is a task of narrative autonomy because it unfolds over time; it comes from others in terms of practical wisdom, it has a history, and the patient becomes the protagonist of a task of self-interpretation that reverberates with action.

According to the third meaning, narrative autonomy is also the capacity to maintain a relationship of giving and receiving: we don't just give, we also receive (Ricœur 2000; Kemp 1987). The sufferer is therefore autonomous in giving, having the capacity to give back, not only to take. This is also narratively so because they contribute to setting up a plot, starting from their historicity. In fact, sickness seems to exacerbate the 'debtor' quality of relationships with others due to one aggravating factor: repayment, which in all its forms appears to be impeded by objectively insurmountable conditions. Having is always a 'having from' that intensifies during the illness. The ultimate impossibility of repayment experienced in sickness requires additional attention and care. The sufferer must always be able to think of themselves as capable of repayment, which does not mean repaying any debt but putting into circulation and relaunching a good that goes beyond the self.

Finally, narrative autonomy appears to be the eventual accentuation of a decentralisation of the constitutive self. It gives shape to the voice of the narrated illness and allows narrative autonomy to become self-care; finally, it allows to imagine repayment where being in debt would risk becoming the other side of oppression and definitive expropriation. The narrative autonomy recognisable in the person living in sickness is provisional. For this reason, the imperative of relationships, even in borderline cases and until death, is a trace of responsibility for others that opens the door to the future.

## Sharing and building narrative autonomy

Narrative autonomy can also be found in those receiving care. Experiencing illness is a relational event, which inevitably involves a network of people at different distances and proximities. As is well known, Ricœur calls this community 'the cell of good advice', namely, 'something that, compared to illness, can have the same role played by friendship in relationships established in a state of good health' (Ricœur 2000, 6; see also Alici 2015). At various levels, those taking care of the sufferer exercise a type of autonomy that can rightly be called narrative (Domingo Moratalla 2015).

On one hand, since it coincides with responsibility, narrative autonomy is found among people who are part of the care network. The task of caring can be ascribed to the author of a story that tends towards emancipating from pain, even when it is not possible in absolute terms. On the other, guarding the narrative autonomy of the patient becomes an eminent task for the carer.

People in the care network must exercise narrative autonomy while being responsible for the suffering of others they care for. From an ethical standpoint, accompanying the sufferer by creating a space of narrative sharing means operating at three levels: the level of caring, the level of transforming, and the level of consoling. At the caring level, the doctor operates narratively when they listen in order to give a diagnosis, connect signs and symptoms, decide on the future by organising it, and propose courses of action to configure the event within a biography. At the transforming level, in the relational space between doctor and patient, the hopes of healing are materialised, as well as stories about future projects, which must be continuously cultivated. In this sense, medical practice is the transformation of a desperate gaze into a gaze of acceptance and decentralisation, of hope in the future of others. At the consoling level, narration intervenes as a 'palliative', and the word 'powerless' becomes a balm for wounds when confronted with the inevitable, opening up imaginative worlds (Honneth 2010) that are not an escape before the end but ways to keep living up to dignity.

On the other hand, doctors also need to build autonomy; they must prevent the diagnosis from becoming a verdict of radical and definitive dependence, which deprives the self of its accessibility and leaves it to the narration of the other. Given the possibility of '*narrative surrender*' (Frank 1995, 6) by the patient, the doctor must work to ensure that they continue to recognise themselves as capable of self-narration, despite the transformation. For this to happen, it is necessary for the doctor or caregiver to renounce their exercise of power coming from their role to unilaterally establish the truth, in favour of a shared construction of the narrative.

Returning the experience of suffering to the humanity of the encounter without abandoning its meaning to pure technique means going beyond the dichotomy between art and science, and between skilful doctors and good doctors: a skilful doctor is also a good doctor (Tesio 2015), able to recognise that the patient has a voice to keep telling their story, in order to come to terms with their pain; such a doctor also avoids providing them with surrogate meanings, which sacrifice the depth of the question of 'why' to the clarity of 'how'. An expert and fair diagnosis will also be a 'good' diagnosis, that is, one that does not exclude the possibility of good. This also applies to all the caregivers, not only to the doctors.

Promoting and relaunching the hermeneutic circle between explanation and comprehension, making the sufferer capable of understanding what is happening, and sharing the necessary information and tools necessary to make them intelligible means contributing to building the patient's narrative autonomy in a process of care that is mutual reliance, an intersection of transformation stories. Therefore, accompanying and supporting the patient's narrative autonomy also means together recognising the transformation – not the definitive disappearance – of their capacities by discovering new ones, and creating and encouraging the identification of contexts in which patients can still experience their capabilities.

Sharing and constructing narrative autonomy mostly depends on the physician and their 'narrative humility'. This expression, which comes from a well-known article by Sayantani DasGupta (2008), summarises a series of attitudes that characterise medical practice as sensitive to narrative autonomy: first, the presence of a third space in which the sufferer is free to say or not to say, to let the illness or silence speak; secondly, the abandonment of the claim of interpretative omnipotence that reads in every empty space a horizon of imposed meanings with the excuse of an asymmetry of roles, in favour of a process of mutual knowledge that respects the opacity of the other; and finally, the willingness to question themselves, 'knowing that they don't know', in that they are not the masters of others' lives, let alone of the meaning transpiring from their stories. According to DasGupta,

> Narrative humility acknowledges that our patients' stories aren't objects that we can understand or master, but rather dynamic entities that we can approach or interact with, while simultaneously remaining open to their ambiguity and contradiction, and engaging in constant self-assessment and self-criticism regarding issues such as our role in the story, our expectations from the story, our responsibilities to that story, and our identifications with the story – how the story attracts or repels us because it reminds us of a number of personal stories.
>
> (2008, 1)

The narrative autonomy of the patient, therefore, must correspond to the narrative humility of the physician or caregiver: this is the condition to start the cooperative enterprise that is caring. In particular, this mutual support of autonomy and humility allows a shaping of the transformative possibility of narration as something that becomes different from illness and starts from it. In the same way, it allows a shaping of the consoling ability, which remains the only practicable path when every promise of meaning seems to be shattered in the smooth walls without footholds of a pain that leaves no escape. It is only through exercising and practising narrative humility that one can move away from the tendency to fill silence by reading it as presence within absence, and from being tempted to identify once and for all the person with the story that has been heard – thus testifying to the dynamic freedom contained in every story, as what is being told is a continuous becoming and at the same time a way to go beyond it, to let it go.

It is according to the promise for a cure contained in the story which links transforming and consoling that one might consider narrative autonomy as an expression of decentralisation, of a displacement that never becomes dissipation, of a becoming that crosses illness and is crossed, modified, and contaminated by it, without allowing dispersion to get the better of it, and without at the same time renouncing possible changes. Narrative autonomy is not only a way of experiencing the condition of suffering but also a way of healing, assuming a non-guilt-ridden responsibility for it. Only through the respect inscribed in narrative humility can the world of care establish a relationship that is exposed and vulnerable to the abuse of power but endowed with the necessary antidote to the risk of turning illness into a further opportunity for domination and objectification. By respecting the dynamism of a story that creates itself without pre-assigned meaning, without its form becoming definitive, in the same way it is possible to respect the narrative autonomy of the sufferer.

Where autonomy and humility intersect, transformation and consolation – segments of a story with at least two authors – stand side by side. If their normative core resides in the duty to not settle for surrogates of meaning, not fabricating oversimplified ones when meaning cannot be seen but is constructed together, their ethical core is to be found in the reciprocal capacity to decentralise for the benefit of the stories to come. Care does not exhaust the relationship between the two. It only makes full sense when it is awaiting the future and preparing for it, recognising itself as a social principle, the origin and source of conservation of society itself (Fraser 2016; Pulcini 2020). Narrative autonomy is a trace of historicity that inhabits us and by which we are inhabited; it is a form of human dignity which finds the highest expression in relationship and cooperation with others, even when life weakens and 'power' is replaced by 'suffering' (Alici 2017).

## References

Alici, Luca. 2017. *Patire e potere. Politica e questione antropologica.* Perugia: Morlacchi.

Alici, Luigino (ed.). 2015. *La "cellula del buon consiglio". Condividere la deliberazione pratica.* Rome: Aracne.

Blanchot, Maurice. 1995. *The Writing of the Disaster* (1980), trans. A. Smock. Lincoln and London: University of Nebraska Press.

Boyd, Kenneth M. 2000. "Disease, Illness, Sickness, Health, Healing and Wholeness: Exploring Some Elusive Concepts." *Journal of Medical Ethics: Medical Humanities,* 26: 9–17. https://mh.bmj.com/content/26/1/9.

Bühler, Karl. 1934. *Spracktheorie: Die Darstellungsfunktion der Sprache*. Jena: Fischer.
Byron Good, J. 1994. *Medicine, Rationality, and Experience. An Anthropological Perspective*. Cambridge: Cambridge University Press.
Casado da Rocha, Antonio. 2014. "Narrative Autonomy: Three Literary Models of Healthcare in the End of Life." *Cambridge Quarterly of Healthcare Ethics* 2: 200–208.
Charon, Rita, Sayantani DasGupta, Nellie Hermann, Craig Irvine, Eric R. Marcus, Colsn Edgar Rivera, Danielle Spencer, and Maura Spiegel. 2017. *The Principles and Practice of Narrative Medicine*. Oxford: Oxford University Press.
DasGupta, Sayantani. 2008. "Narrative Humility." *The Lancet* 371(9617): 980–981.
Deleuze, Gilles. 1998. *Essays Critical and Clinical* [1993], trans. D. W. Smith, M. A. Greco. London: Verso.
Domingo Moratalla, Augustín. 2015. "Ragione dialogica e discernimento morale." In *La "cellula del buon consiglio". Condividere la deliberazione pratica*, edited by Alici Luigino, 41–56. Rome: Aracne.
Ferrarese, Estelle. 2018. *Vulnerability and Critical Theory*. Leiden: Brill.
Foucault, Michel. 1973. *The Birth of the Clinic. An Archaelolgy of Medical Percepiton* (1963), trans. A.M. Sheridan Smith. London: Tavistock.
Foucault, Michel. 2001. *Madness and Civilization. A History of Insanity in the Age of Reason* Frank, Arthur W. 1995. *The Wounded Storyteller. Body, Illness, and Ethics*. Chicago, IL: University of Chicago Press.
Fraser, Nancy. 2016. "Contradictions of Capital and Care." 100 *New Left Review*. https://newleftreview.org/issues/ii100/articles/nancy-fraser-contradictions-of-capital-and-care.
Ginzburg, Carlo. 1992. "Clues. Roots of an Evidential Paradigm." In *Clues, Myths, and the Historical Method* (1986), trans. John and Anne C. Tedeschi, 87–113. Baltimore, MD: Johns Hopkins University Press.
Honneth, Axel. 2010. "Entmächtigungen der Realität. Säkulare Formen des Trostes." In *Das Ich im Wir. Studien zur Anerkennungstheorie*, 298–305. Frankfurt am Main: Suhrkamp.
Illich, Ivan. 1975. *Medical Nemesis. The Expropriation of Health*. London: Calder & Boyars.
Kemp, Peter. 1987. *Éthique et médicine*. Paris: Tierce.
Marcel, Gabriel. 1953. "Remarques sur la dépersonnalisation de la médecine." In *Qu'attendez-vous du médecin?* edited by Gabriel Marcel et al., 17–28. Paris: Plon.
Pulcini, Elena. 2020. *Tra cura e giustizia. Le passioni come risorsa sociale*. Turin: Bollati Boringhieri.
Ricœur, Paul. 2000. *Etica e vivere bene. Conversazione con Paul Ricœur*. In AA.VV. *Il male*, 1–14. Milan: Raffaello Cortina.
Ricœur, Paul. 2013. "La souffrance n'est pas la douleur." In *Souffrance et douleur. Autour de Paul Ricœur*, edited by Nathalie Zaccäi-Reyners and Claire Marin, 13–34. Paris: PUF.
Russo, Maria Teresa. 2006. *La ferita di Chirone. Itinerari di antropologia medica in medicina*. Milan: Vita & Pensiero.
Sontag, Susan. 1978. *Illness as Metaphor*. New York: Farrar, Straus & Giroux
Tesio, Luigi. 2015. *I bravi e i buoni. Perché la medicina clinica può essere una scienza*. Roma: Il pensiero scientifico.

# 9 Plumbing the perpetual loss of paradise

## Susan Taubes and sacred suffering

*Rachel Pafe*

In early 1930s Paris, French philosopher-mystic Simone Weil met feminist philosopher Simone de Beauvoir and famously exclaimed, 'It's easy to see you've never been hungry', thereby seeming to accuse the other thinker of a privileged life of thought about – rather than experience of – struggle and suffering. I will depart with a similar anecdote about Susan Taubes, an American-Hungarian thinker, to problematise the tension between writing about the suffering of others and taking it on personally. I will particularly unpack how such a tension is challenged by Taubes' critique of Weil's need to find an absolute solution to suffering. Taubes was drawn to Weil's powerful critique of the violence of modernity and her recognition that there was no divine solution to such violence, yet she accuses Weil of still needing a total solution to suffering. Taubes asserts that when Weil realised that political action cannot solve violence, she turned to a theology that promotes the individual acceptance of suffering as the only chance for salvation. I assert that Taubes' reflections on suffering and violence stemming from a critique of Weil are particularly relevant for problematising binary and linear notions of the medical encounter. That is, suffering is not considered as a mere lack, loss, or impediment to be overcome, but rather explored in murkier territory as conversely containing ethical lessons and resources.

While Taubes argues that loss and suffering are sources of immanent communal ethics based on imperfect and ongoing protests against violence, her proposal for concretely enacting such an ethics is vague. I argue that the questions that arise from the gap between Taubes' ethics and their lack of material political positioning highlights the unresolved tension between Taubes, Weil, and beyond, and through this it is possible to explore what forms an ethics to address suffering would take in the realm of the community, namely, communal political life. This is rooted in the balance between an ethics based on the critique of the quantification of particular forms of suffering yet able to provide enough structure to its worldly realisation to prevent its potential abuse. I explore this last arena by speculating on how such questions resonate with an oft-overlooked short text by Taubes, 'The White Mask Falls' (1963), a review of Jean Genet's play *The Blacks: A Clown Show.*

Susan Taubes was born to secular Jewish parents in Budapest, Hungary on 12 January 1928. She moved with her father to the United States in 1939, and in the late forties and early fifties, Taubes studied philosophy at Bryn Mawr College

DOI: 10.4324/9781032660165-16

in Pennsylvania and the Sorbonne in Paris. In 1956, she earned a PhD at Harvard (Radcliffe) with her dissertation *The Absent God: A Study of Simone Weil*, the half-erased subtitle – *On the Religious Use of Tyranny* – is still faintly visible. This still-unpublished dissertation is Taubes' major work on Weil, which I will soon discuss at greater length. After its completion, Taubes lectured at Columbia University and Barnard College, and worked as curator at Columbia's Bush Collection of Religion and Culture. During this time, she actively participated in the New York literary scene and began to focus on more experimental writing, which likewise drew upon the issues of violence and alienation that underpin her dissertation. In many ways, this is embodied in her final, recently republished novel, *Divorcing*, which contains poetic visions of Taubes' ethical vision. Shortly after *Divorcing* was published in 1969, Taubes took her own life.

In turning now to Taubes' ethical vision, I will first recall an anecdote about her. I do so fully aware that her legacy is still mainly tied to anecdotes of her relationship with her husband, rabbi and philosopher Jacob Taubes, but I aim to use it as a jumping off point to highlight how suffering is problematised in Taubes' thought. Shortly after marrying Jacob Taubes in 1949, Susan Taubes visited him in Israel with the idea that perhaps the couple would live there more permanently. As Christina Pareigis (2011) recounts in her afterword to the 1950–1951 volume of letters between the Taubeses, Susan Taubes was quite wholeheartedly rejected by the circle of European Jewish thinkers who stood behind the founding of Hebrew University and its attempt to rethink post-war Jewish thought, including Martin Buber, Hugo Bergman, and Gershom Scholem. The arrival of Taubes among this community who had fled the horrors of a war and genocide largely experienced first-hand, Pareigis writes, proved triggering. This community, who had largely lost their fortunes and often health in the war, found her expensive North American clothes, jewellery, and glamour offensive. They excluded her from the social encounters of the quite small circle, effectively rebuking her for parading her material wealth and robust health in the face of their lingering suffering.

I find this episode fascinating for several reasons, the first in that it draws a parallel to Weil's encounter with de Beauvoir. Weil was accusing de Beauvoir of a privileged life of thought. Taubes, on the other hand, was rejected before even introducing her ideas, excluded for the abundance of her material and physical presence. Shortly thereafter, Taubes returned to New York.

At the base of both episodes is also a more primary yet abstract accusation that each thinker had somehow not suffered enough to be taken seriously. This rests on a slippery slope of comparison of loss and suffering during a time when many were traumatised from the horrors of the war and the events leading up to it. Weil, who grew up in an upper-middle-class Jewish family, struggled to find the best way to combat suffering. Her quest echoes a longer history of Western European intellectuals endowed with the means and leisure to write on this topic. How to address the disquieting feeling that one is witnessing the violence and pain of others from a comfortable, privileged environment and, perhaps even more violently, using it as one's subject matter? This question forms a starting point for understanding the contrast between how Weil and Taubes respectively approached suffering.

Taubes repudiates what she describes as Weil's aim to suffer the plight of those experiencing violence around her, followed by a radical disassociation from such violence upon realisation it is not curable. Taubes takes this accusation of not suffering enough and turns it on its head. She argues that addressing such suffering does not lie in taking it on but rather a radical affirmation that, indeed, we have *not* suffered enough, and that this is the source of both her critique and ethical riches. Yet, as I will shortly discuss, her thought arrives at its own limits regarding how to concretely address such ethical riches in the realm of political action.

Taubes' 1956 dissertation on Weil is divided into three parts: a discussion of Weil's political writings, an analysis of her 'theological turn', and the proposal of her own ethical vision. It positions Weil's earlier years of political (syndicalist) activism as connected to her attempts to not only shed her material wealth but actively take on the suffering of others. It references Weil's infamous episode of joining workers in harsh factory conditions and only eating the meagre rations allotted to those in perilous conditions (Petrement 1976). But Taubes asserts that Weil became disillusioned with the Marxist struggle when she discovered that political revolution would never permanently solve the problems of violence. Taubes (1956, 140) writes that, disillusioned with political struggles, Weil pursued an absolute solution to 'the silence of God [...] by radicalizing a secular dilemma to the point where it demands a theological solution'. Taubes interprets Weil's theology of an absent, impotent God who wills human suffering as a conclusive attempt to find an absolute explanation for suffering by linking violence and oppression to supernatural causes.

Taubes describes Weil's theology as characterised by the assertion that the only solution to violence is for individuals to accept extreme suffering as God's will. I argue that Taubes understands this as a refusal to recognise that suffering has no total explanation or solution and therefore must be perpetually and collectively combatted. This idea of permanent and unchanging sin contrasts with Weil's earlier encounter with de Beauvoir. In that context, suffering was taken on in the name of the powerful individual contributing to a larger political cause. In this latter one, the earth is so cruel that individual acceptance of suffering and a return to the God who wills it is the only way to save oneself. Suffering is no longer about shared political struggle but rather the only means of spiritual salvation.

In this context, Taubes both draws upon and bitterly critiques Weil. On the one hand, Weil importantly recognises that there is no divine solution to the extreme violence of modernity. Yet, Taubes' critique rests on Weil's attribution of injustice to God's will as the essential condition of the world. Taubes argues that Weil refuses to accept that God has been indefinitely lost and that nothing, not even the supernatural, can totally solve suffering. This need for a solution results in a vision of suffering that perpetuates – rather than challenges – structures of violence, because the only explanation Weil can find is that God wills such suffering. Taubes (1956, 185) writes that, while Weil's 'identification with the defeated gives her mysticism a somewhat "leftist" flavor', it actually 'does not challenge the status quo but perpetuates it in the form of destiny'.

In this schema, Weil's unwavering demand to find a solution to suffering, both in the need to experience it in political activism and in then submitting to it in theology, results in its perpetuation. Taubes declares that, in contrast, when God is viewed as irrecoverably lost, responses to such suffering fall into human, decidedly imperfect hands. Suffering should not be embraced as violence that must be personally felt to empathise with others or save one's soul, but rather as a demand for communal responsibility to combat violence.

## On Taubes' ethical critique of Weil

In now turning to Taubes' ethical vision, I will first discuss how it is rooted in a critique of Weil's idea of a world in which an impotent God wills permanent violence. While Weil turns to the notion of an individual's *decreation*, or destruction of the personal self, as the only solution to such worldly suffering, Taubes emphasises the community as a space for multiple and ongoing solutions to suffering. In this section, I will first unpack how Weil defines the term 'decreation' and then discuss how Taubes' failure to provide a detailed definition of what community means for her ethical vision often renders it problematic. I conversely explore how the shaping of the aforementioned paradoxical medical encounter, based on reappropriating the riches of suffering, is rooted in it as a necessarily frustrating, incomplete, and non-linear encounter.

Taubes posits that God is not impotent but completely lost, and that this loss and its echoes in the history of human suffering and the protest against it imbue spiritual nourishment in immanent, material communities and their ongoing struggles for justice and responsibility for one another. Taubes (1956, 302) asserts that for Weil, man's suffering is God's will and we 'should love him as the author of evil'. For Weil, there is no correspondence between earthly sin and punishment, but human existence as such is a sin. In this context, Taubes argues that Weil's designation of an otherworldly God as the only possible site of good denies the chance for immanent human collectivity, struggle, and justice. While Taubes is likewise of the opinion that ownership of the good has often been abused by the powerful, an ideal good is still a means to accept that human justice and virtue are responsibilities to challenge violence and oppression in social reality.

The practical core of Taubes' critique of Weil is rooted in countering the assertion that reality cannot be challenged. Weil's notoriously vague concept of decreation is set out in a chapter of the same name in *Gravity and Grace*:

> Decreation: to make something created pass into the uncreated. Destruction: to make something created pass into nothingness [...] Creation is an act of love and it is perpetual. At each moment our existence is God's love for us. But God can only love himself. His love for us is love for himself through us. Thus, he who gives us our being loves in us the acceptance of not being. Our existence is made up only of his waiting for our acceptance not to exist. He is perpetually begging from us that existence which he gives. He gives it to us in order to beg it from us.
>
> (Weil 2003, 32)

In this passage, Weil seems to propose that while human existence is based on God's love, there is an inherent problem in the limits of God's love, which does not leave the realm of the divine: namely, it cannot enter the human world and self. To bridge this gap, Weil suggests that God demands that humans freely accept destruction of their physical selves. Thus, the 'decreation' of the human body is the only way of reciprocating God's love. Responding to this, Taubes argues that in Weil's theological vision, to receive salvation one must not only reject the human community but ultimately the self. In this vision, the only response to suffering is to personally experience it to such a degree that one does not survive. Sharply opposing this 'solution', Taubes suggests that suffering should rather be understood as a source of inspiration. She writes

> It is the specific mark of human suffering that it points beyond the sheer immediacy of pain to an ideal norm which applies to man as such within a historical reality. The chain of the oppressed of all the ages burdens man not merely by its physical weight, but as a wrong [...] [Weil's thought] reaches its most scandalous expression in the view that the suffering of the innocent is a special sign of the love of God. Thereby religion not only sanctions the present sufferings of the injured but paralyzes the nerves of a historical human community based on a mutual responsibility between the generations.
> (Taubes 1956, 312)

Taubes reproaches Weil's vision of individual suffering, asserting that this passive acceptance of violence as the state of the world that must end in the destruction of the self sanctions violence and provides no challenge to structures of oppression. Taubes (1956, 312) argues that the solution to such violence is not to accept and take on violence against oneself but rather to turn to suffering as a concept that reveals an ideal which inspires humans to take collective action within historical reality and erect a 'historical human community based on mutual responsibility between the generations'. The medical encounter inferred in these reflections thus becomes more nuanced; namely, suffering in this context is most potent as a historical concept tied to struggle against violence rather than a desirable condition. Taubes asserts that Weil's overemphasis on the elimination of suffering results in its proliferation rather than eradication; more broadly, it is implied that such a position critiques a binary medical encounter focused on limited ideas of a cure as a clearly marked and linear solution.

## On Taubes' ethics

The last section of Taubes' dissertation proposes a patchwork ethical vision that draws on Jewish, Protestant, and Hindu thought in combination with Greek mythology. At its core is the idea of loss inspiring an ideal of responsibility and critiques rooted in memories of human suffering and protests against it stretching back to the creation of humankind. Suffering for a particular cause is not a prerequisite for action or thought; instead, it is counterproductive when quantified and solidified. Rather, one must perpetually engage in a ritual exercise rooted in a critical re-reading of sacred symbols of suffering throughout history. But as I alluded to earlier, this ritual is never concretely fleshed out, leading to gaps as to what such a community would look like and how it would act and move in the world. Thus, the question is one of maintaining a balance between an ethics that is rooted in the critique of the quantification of particular forms of suffering yet able to provide enough structure to its worldly realisation, in order to prevent its potential abuse.

Her ethical vision first takes the form of the ritual recovery of sacred symbols of 'man's perpetual loss of paradise' (Taubes 1956, 367). She suggests that this could be accomplished by a 'hermeneutics of man', essentially an exercise of close reading that strips particular symbols from their religious and institutional contexts and focuses on how they value forms of human rebellion against oppression and violence. As I will unpack later, Taubes couples this hermeneutical act with a ritual one, the details of which remain vague. Her understanding of the sacred in this context is similar to that of Émile Durkheim, who in *Elementary Forms of Religious Life* (1915) proposes the sacred not as connected to God but as something that has the power to ritually unite communities. For Taubes, this sense of the sacred traverses history in the memory of human suffering and the struggle against it. It is rooted in the idea of embracing the loss of God as a chance to collapse categories of the sacred and secular.

Taubes argues that Weil's theology hints at this task, but just as its strength lies in the lack of consolation in a world in which God does not intervene, so does it conversely lack human solutions because agency is ultimately placed in an impotent God. As Taubes (1956, 385) asserts, 'We would like to develop the notion of atheistic purification more radically than Simone Weil'. If only, Taubes bemoans, Weil was able to admit that God does not exist and will not intervene, a whole new arena of historical possibility built on the power of human intervention could open up.

Taubes (1956, 367) underlines,

> The expulsion from paradise perpetuated in the Promethean revolt represents the beginning of the birth of the redeemer in man; this is so because the Promethean rebel figures as a compassionate healer, helper, and liberator. But he himself is bound in chains.

Such ideals of healing, helping, and liberation are inextricably bound with the loss of paradise and ensuing oppression and suffering. Communities need both loss to hold themselves together and the struggle to embrace it as a call to recognise the suffering of others. Taubes' notion of sacred symbols is a way to support ideals of responsibility and justice amidst this paradox. She draws on a constellation of symbols to support this claim: Dionysus, Orpheus, Job, Vedic myths, and Christ serve as 'mythical content, which does not compromise man's memory of paradise and hope for redemption, which affirms a form of human community where there will be peace, love, and understanding between man and man' (Taubes 1956, 371). These symbols are sources of hope for an ideal community that resonate in the instability of immanent communal life. The historical symbols of humans both suffering due to their worldly chains and fighting against them provide a means for communities to foment love and revolt against the oppression around them. This sheds light on a nuanced site of suffering that can modify the notion of the medical encounter as not only linear and finite but also as an experience between an individual and medical professionals. In this schema, a community deals with suffering together, stretching back through the generations of the past and looking to the future to come.

As mentioned earlier, Taubes proposes the retrieval of historical symbols of suffering from their various ties to institutions, politics, religion, and God through an act of close reading and a critical interpretation of various religious and spiritual texts. This is supported by the argument that

> The diverse symbolic representations of man's confrontation with divine power are no longer mere signs or stepping stones in the unfolding of a subsequentially constructed divine plan, but recover their own specific gravity and archetypal character, and as pure myth can become new points of departure.
>
> (Taubes 1956, 359–360)

This act crumbles the division between human and God, immanence and transcendence. It is a means of reclaiming the good as a communal ideal that does not depend on God. Loss is a means to find alternative sources of spiritual nourishment that take suffering seriously without quantifying or ultimately trying to solve it. This entails a journey in which loss serves as a radical examination of the structures that once provided surety in life, ones that purported to stave off suffering but ultimately promoted it. It means ridding oneself of both belief in God and the human historical abuses that created suffering in the name of a divine plan. It is an ongoing and unpredictable process that must be repeated situationally, relocating the sacred in ongoing human struggle. Such a history of the oppressed would be constantly remade through ritual practices that oscillate between immanence and transcendence:

> Repetition implies the ambiguity, the danger of impurity or perdition cannot be surmounted once and for all, but only instance by instance by confronting it again and again in every given situation. Repetition suggests moreover, that the function of religious forms is not simply to overcome anxiety, to attain purity peace or salvation in the sense defined by the conventional frame, but to return to the primordial "danger," to participate in the unconstrained, chaotic potency of the sacred.
>
> (Taubes 1956, 390)

On the one hand, this passage describes an endless ritual of accessing pure symbols that denies a fixed idea of religion, the divine, and history. It seems to suggest a history of humans seizing the sacred for themselves without reliance on divine intervention. While this sacred denies the surety of salvation, it provides a means to gather power for the imperfect struggle of combatting oppression, violence, and suffering in the world. Yet, the ritual practice implied by this passage is vague. What does Taubes mean by her insistence on 'purifying' mythological-religious symbols to deny 'purity'? While she seems to clarify this discrepancy by describing the latter as purity 'defined by the conventional frame', how is this vision regulated to not end up in unjust hands?

## The contours of community

Taubes never puts forth a concrete political vision. On the one hand, this fits within her broader critique of the pitfalls of institutional religions and political systems, which she does get into with much detail through her critiques of the inefficacy of post-war Marxist thought and traditional Judaism. While the verve of Taubes' reclamation of suffering is persuasive, problems arise in how she attempts to go about such a task, which is built on the call to 'purify' religious and spiritual elements from their transcendent elements to recover their force for the organisation of immanent political communities. A few elements jump out as inherently problematic, the most glaring being the idea of pure access to original myths of suffering. How can one ever find such an uncontaminated myth and who would regulate that it is used by the right forces? I will first unpack such issues in Taubes' ethics and then speculate on how they perhaps find grounding in a short review she wrote about Jean Genet's play *The Blacks* (1963) as a subversive enactment of community through the medium of theatre.

As discussed earlier, Taubes was particularly interested in symbols across various religious and mythological traditions that manage to preserve the memory of 'man's perpetual loss of paradise'. Such symbols present the struggle against oppression and violence as tied to a broader history that stretches back to the creation of humankind. The crux of turning to such symbols is that, while they focus on something that has been lost again and again throughout the ages, they contain 'a mythical content, which does not compromise man's memory of paradise and hope' (Taubes 1956, 371). It is here that Taubes denotes that such purified symbols of loss should be understood as affirming hope for an ideal future community, from which an imperfect immanent community can draw spiritual nourishment.

Yet, the dimensions of a communal practice founded on accessing such mythological symbols remain ambiguous. Does not the search for a form of purity, or pure myth and symbols in connection to formations of community, simply imply a repetition of the religious-political constellations Taubes critiques? How does one ensure that such a vision would not fall into the wrong hands? Taubes fails to answer this fundamental question of *what kind of community*.

While Taubes never formulates this as a concrete declaration in any of her philosophical writings, one short and often overlooked essay, 'The White Mask Falls' (1963), touches on many such themes. While I do not read this essay as a definitive answer to the aforementioned questions, I argue that it provides an interesting glimpse of how they could be explored by turning to Taubes' broader, multidisciplinary body of writing. 'The White Mask Falls' is a review of the English-language performance of Jean Genet's *The Blacks: A Clown Show* (*Les Nègres*). While it does discuss the play as such, it mainly focuses on the power of theatre as a means of reflecting on the impossible gap between contemplating the suffering of others and how this leads to the building up, tearing down, and subversion of the idea of community.

Genet's *The Blacks* is a meta-play, a play within a play, that seeks to reflect racial prejudices and stereotyping. First performed in English in New York at St Mark's Playhouse in 1961, the plot loosely follows a 13-member, all-Black cast; 8 members perform the trial and resulting murder of a white woman, while 5 wear whiteface to play a jury and a presiding queen. Genet clearly underlines that the involvement of a white playwright and white audience is another layer of ritual theatricality in the play. He states:

> This play, written, I repeat, by a white man, is intended for a white audience, but if, which is unlikely, it is ever performed before a black audience, then a white person, male or female, should be invited every evening. The organizer of the show should welcome him formally, dress him in ceremonial costume and lead him to his seat, preferably in the first row of the orchestra. The actors will play for him. A spotlight should be focused upon this symbolic white throughout the performance.
>
> (Genet 1994, 8)

These elaborate layers of ritual theatricality are meant to evoke the complexities of racial prejudices, white patriarchy, and the impossibility of communication under the oppression of structures of domination in which the audience is complicit. Taubes is likewise interested in the potential of such a form of theatricality described in the above passage. She writes

> What makes *The Blacks* an entirely unique, entrancing, and disturbing theatrical venture is that the very ground of theatrical experience—the community of understanding and sympathy between the people in the audience and the humanity represented on the stage—seems to be pulled out from under our feet.
>
> (Taubes 1963, 85)

In this context, Taubes is interested in how the typical understanding of community as comprised of mutual sympathy and understanding is, as she puts it later in the article, exposed as a 'sham'. The underlying motive behind such an exposure is moral, Taubes asserts (1963, 85). She argues that while one might think of Bertolt Brecht for epic – or dialectical – theatre that draws audience members into participation, resulting in speculation and political action, Genet is more subtle in his enactments of what became known as 'theatre of the absurd'. The 'naturalistic theatre' exemplified by Brecht draws in the audience to act out 'representations of humanity' as 'we project ourselves in what seems to be our reflection in some hidden and mysterious process of identification and union'. In contrast, 'Genet's theater lays bare the mechanism of projection and vicarious satisfaction that underlies theatrical make-believe' (Taubes 1963, 87). Taubes asserts that Genet does not seek to draw the audience into an ultimately artificial political resolution, but instead leaves them stewing in the realisation of the constructed nature of their own violence and prejudices, without providing any clear resolution.

In bringing up this passage, I am interested in how such a 'sham' community made up of the recognition of violence and oppression ties back to the aforementioned discussion of Taubes' ethics of suffering. As touched upon earlier, Taubes' ethics emphasise the need for repetitive ritual without resolution that draw on the history of man's symbolic and mythical intergenerational and historical suffering. What does Taubes' understanding of Genet's approach to community in *The Blacks* mean in this context? Could her idea of the repetitive enactment of a sham community serve as one means to add details to some of the sketchier parts of her ethical oeuvre? Namely, can her interpretation of *The Blacks* be seen as one example of the ritual re-enactment of collective remembrance of historical symbols of suffering?

Taubes (1963, 90) points to the connection between the space of the play and real life, writing, 'To see the meaning behind this "architecture of emptiness and words" we must refer once more to the relationship between the theatre and real action'. *The Blacks*, Taubes argues, plays with the division between the constructed world of action within the play and the real world outside; this happens when an announcement interrupts the play, declaring it has served as a diversion for the real events happening outside, a secret offstage trial. In this context:

> Genet's final exposure of the theater as diversion does not seem to destroy the 'truth' of the theater; on the contrary, for a moment we almost believe that we have wakened out of our trance when in truth (and this is the truth of the theatre) we are hopelessly enchanted—nor will the real threat prevent us from clapping at the end because we are in a theatre.
>
> (Taubes 1963, 91)

Taubes thus positions the power of Genet's play as the careful drawing of an audience into a ritual that they think they are unmasking. It is the tension between almost believing that one has broken free from the trance that holds one within their respective societal place but then instead remaining in the same place as before, despite this glimpse of possibility. This momentary look does nothing to prevent 'the real threat' of danger in the world outside the play or the audience's enthusiasm amidst this real danger. As discussed earlier, Taubes is interested in drawing on the memory of mythical forms of man's unending struggle against the chains of the world, exemplified by the figure of Prometheus, as a kind of spiritual nourishment that would serve to fuel the similarly unending struggle for immanent communal justice. In this setting, the repetition of such a ritual is essential, as it denotes the ambiguous nature of the task and underscores that it is based on the continuous confrontation of danger in each arising contextual situation.

*The Blacks* seems to function as one example of such a microcosm of danger in which one glimpses historical suffering only to be plunged back into reality with the necessity of repeating the task anew, *ad infinitum*. It does not answer the question of Taubes' proposed process of purification of myths except with a resounding answer that supposedly stable concepts such as community, spectatorship, audience, inside, and outside must be continuously frustrated. It likewise illustrates that Taubes' political alliances fall more within the infamous struggle within existential thought exemplified by the fight between Sartre and one of Taubes' favourite thinkers, Camus. Does the embrace of man's freedom in the face of absurdity lead to the necessity for political action or the denouncement of the absurdity of all institutional political structures? These questions remain unanswered in Taubes' thought, but she seems to side with the latter. Yet she also seems to point to a potential form of communal justice rooted in the recognition of both suffering and absurdity.

Indeed, Taubes goes on to argue that the ritual of audience and community in *The Blacks* is important because it reveals the participants' fears of a broader overthrow of the societal structures of violence and domination in which they are complicit:

> We came, after all, because we are ashamed, and the play in which we witness our condemnation and overthrow, not only makes visible our secret fears of the vengeance of the oppressed, but in some measure makes it acceptable, because in the theatre at least, only the *white mask* falls.
>
> (Taubes 1963, 92)

The emphasis on the mixture of shame and fear that arises from this ritual ties back powerfully to the anecdote of Weil and de Beauvoir referenced at the beginning of this essay, as well as the later one concerning Taubes. Taubes ultimately underlines that thinking about suffering is an inextricably fraught task. Through her critique of Weil, she argues that the attempt to find an absolute solution to such a question ultimately leads down the paths of orthodoxy, self-denial, and destruction. Thinkers must constantly struggle with loss and suffering rather than attempting to quantify them as measuring sticks for authentic thought and action. Approaching suffering as a site of multiplicity, contradiction, and protest opens it up as an ideal inspired by perpetual loss throughout history and the immanent, communal, and material struggle against it. Imagining a medical encounter entangled with such fraught ethics means viewing it as a site in which notions of violence, care, and cure are inextricably intertwined in a dance of mutual frustration and nourishment.

For Taubes, it is an ongoing task that must be repeated situationally and collectively, yet the tensions in her own thought reveal the pitfalls of her own search for what forms this would take in the realm of communal political life. While I attempted to bridge this gap by speculating on how it could be potentially fleshed out, perhaps this is wishful thinking on my part, a desire for engagement with suffering to reap some material rewards, however small. In that sense I can somewhat empathise with the frustration of Weil's ghost as Taubes faced her, grinning, repeatedly whispering, 'no, it will never be enough'.

## References

Genet, Jean. 1994. *The Blacks: A Clown Show*. Genet the Blacks. Trans. Bernard Frechtman. NewYork: Grove Press.

Pareigis, Christina. 2011. "The Connecting Paths of Nomads, Wanderers, Exiles. Stationen einer Korrespondenz. Nachwort." In Susan Taubes, *Die Korrespondenz mit Jacob Taubes 1950–1951*, edited by C. Pareigis, 259–288. Munich: William Fink Verlag.

Petrement, Simone. 1976. *Simone Weil: A Life*, trans. Raymond Rosenthal. New York: Pantheon Books.

Taubes, Susan. 1956. *The Absent God: A Study of Simone Weil.* Unpublished dissertation, Harvard University.

Taubes, Susan. 1963. "The White Mask Falls." *The Tulane Drama Review* 7(3): 6–16. https://www.jstor.org/stable/1125086.

Weil, Simone. 2003. *Gravity and Grace*, trans. Emma Crawford and Mario von der Ruhr. London: Routledge.

# 10 Almodóvar's anatomies

*Hannah Parlett*

The world of medicine has been a vital and persistent source of influence in the work of Spanish film director Pedro Almodóvar. The hospital, as both architecture and institution, has provided an instrumental setting for a number of his most important films, including *All About My Mother* (1999) and *Talk to Her* (2002), both of which garnered major international acclaim and won Academy Awards. Centred on clinical practices and medical procedures such as organ transplantation and palliative care, these films are closely attuned to the physical needs and biological rhythms of the body, as well as the various acts of nurture required to preserve human life. The following essay argues that Almodóvar's significant interest in medicine must be read as part of his broader philosophical engagement with the daily work of 'care', both in a professional, clinical sense (demonstrated by the various nurses and doctors that make up the characters of his films) and as a more universal mode of domestic labour. The ethical considerations raised by medicine in Almodóvar's work, glimpsed through patient experiences of vulnerability and exposure, are closely aligned with the psychoanalytic questions summoned by the director's well-known interest in maternity and reproduction. Numerous scholars have examined how Almodóvar's engagement with maternity has sought to subvert conservative patriarchal scripts surrounding reproduction. Emma Wilson (2020) writes, 'maternity is rescued from the preserves of Catholicism and Franco's regime, with its vision of motherhood as a means of keeping women in the home and of rebuilding Spain and realised as erotic, savage, selfless, unnatural, perverse, and beautiful'. The affective experience of being a clinical patient, of being largely dependent on another subject to receive care and protection, mirrors the foundational relationship between mother and child that Almodóvar has repeatedly explored throughout his long career in films such as *Volver* (2006) and, most recently, *Parallel Mothers* (2021). The intense feelings of vulnerability that constitute early life as a child return to us during the modern medical encounter as depicted by Almodóvar, an experience similarly characterised by risk and the threat of damage. For Almodóvar, both medicine and maternity emerge as important existential sites on screen to explore a fundamental ambivalence at the heart of human subjectivity – that enduring conflict between love and hate, pleasure and pain, and care and violence.

DOI: 10.4324/9781032660165-17

## Between care and violence: The hospital bed

In Almodóvar's films, the hospital bed is imagined as a space where this ethical question becomes particularly charged. The imbalance of power that takes shape between patient and physician in his medical films speaks to broader anxieties about relationality and the nature of our contact with the exterior world. To reach out to the other for care or cure is to essentially open oneself to the simultaneous possibilities of tender intimacy or invasive injury. This primordial dilemma, the dilemma of dependency, was the subject of Melanie Klein's famous psychoanalytic investigations into the internal life of young babies who rely on the care of others to survive. Klein (1946) famously argued that the earliest days of human subjectivity are characterised by intense trauma and anxiety about subsistence, as well as overwhelming fear of the external object who cares for it (in Klein's original case study, this was the mother). Within the grip of hunger and paranoia, the infant directs destructive fantasies of splitting towards the external object, a mental state known as the 'paranoid-schizoid position'. The carer, carrying out various acts of feeding and cleaning, is experienced by the baby as a distinctly ominous figure, simultaneously capable of both nurturing and, more violently, wounding. This is the conflict between 'good mother' and 'bad mother', a psychic splitting driven by the oppositional feelings of pleasure and pain. For Klein, this early experience of dependency in infancy establishes an essential ambivalence within the human subject that continues to a greater or lesser extent in adulthood. As Mignon Nixon has outlined, the theoretical foundation of Klein's theory is rooted in these tactile acts of physical care

> Entirely dependent on hands that, in feeding, in cleaning, and otherwise tending, also graze or breach its boundaries, the infant fears what it also craves. Survival depends on enduring an invasive touch. Penetration, if too rough, is traumatic. Holding, if too tight, is suffocating. But even contact that is not injurious—even touch that is solicitous—underlines the infant's predicament. To be cared for as an infant [...] establishes an indissoluble link between Eros and Thanatos, a lifelong attraction to "experiences which are simultaneously life-giving and death-threatening.
>
> (Nixon 2005, 180)

Whilst Klein's findings most obviously describe the primal scene between mother and child, her seminal account of binary splitting and ambivalence offers a useful framework in which to read Almodóvar's representation of clinical medicine. This idea that care solicits both comfort and terror proves particularly compelling for an analysis of Almodóvar's complex characters. Klein's analysis of human dependency speaks more broadly to a universal condition of existence that continues far beyond infancy. This visceral sense of exposure is felt most palpably during the moments of life that Almodóvar depicts in his hospital films, including moments of physical pain, suffering, and corporeal weakness. As Judith Butler (2014) has argued in relation to Klein's central thesis, 'dependency fundamentally defines us: it is something I never quite outgrow, no matter how old and how individuated I may seem'. Like the young infant who nervously waits to be tended, the hospital patients in Almodóvar's films face a similar predicament. Almodóvar's cinematic worlds present a similar set of paradoxical possibilities, situated precariously between the twin affective poles of care and violence.

For example, in *All About My Mother*, Almodóvar imagines the hospital bed as a site of life-saving scientific intervention. At the beginning of the film, he tracks the daily work of Manuela, an Argentine nurse who oversees donor organ transplants in Ramón y Cajal Hospital in Madrid. In his depiction of this critical procedure, Almodóvar exposes the precarious and liminal borders between life and death. This apprehension of human life as fragile and in need of protection imbues Manuela's work as a nurse with philosophical and symbolic significance. This corporeal vulnerability becomes painfully acute with the tragic and unexpected death of Manuela's son and the subsequent donation of his biological heart to another man. In his autobiographical essay *L'Intrus*, the philosopher Jean Luc Nancy (2010) describes how the medical practice of transplant surgery interrupts the fantasy of the self as individual and independent. For Nancy, the organ transplant is an extreme, corporeal example of an original human state of dispersal and exposure to others. For Laura McMahon (2008, 464), Nancy's figure of intrusion denotes not only

> A question of otherness issuing from the outside—whether this be the transplantation of a new heart, the arrival of an immigrant, or the welcoming of a stranger—but also to signal a form of opening, exteriority, and exposure which is always already inside—"une intimité plus profonde que toute intériorité [...] exposition infinite".

It is this sense of openness to the other, deftly symbolised by the narrative of the heart transplant, that Almodóvar's film carries in its affective register and its important representation of tolerance, and community. Later on in the film, in Barcelona, Almodóvar returns us to another clinical setting when Manuela visits her pregnant friend Rosa (Penelope Cruz) before she is about to give birth. The hospital's *mise-en-scène* marks both the character's geographical journey (the move from Madrid to Barcelona) and her symbolic shift throughout the film. Hospital rooms bookend Manuela's trajectory between two states of maternity: one biological and filial, another adopted and embraced. In this scene between Manuela and Rosa, the hospital bed emerges as a space for affective connection, emotional support, and shared knowledge between two maternal figures. These tender, therapeutic images of medical healing are embedded within Almodóvar's larger cinematic meditation on matrilineal care, kinship, and chosen families. Marsha Kinder (2004) has argued that *All About My Mother* reworks and modernises the historical ideology of Spain as Motherland:

> Moving masterfully among a trinity of female roles (as actress, nurse, and mother), Manuela carries the story of the Motherland back from the pueblos of Latin America to Spain's metropolitan centres of Madrid and Barcelona,

where she embodies Almodóvar's new super-maternal stereotype for a globalized Spain.

This benevolent scene is replaced by something altogether more sinister and invasive in Almodóvar's next film, *Talk to Her.* Like Klein's ambivalent ego, Almodóvar's cinematic universe swings in a different direction and considers the potential violence latent within the scene of the hospital bed. In this film, we encounter Benigno (Javier Cámara), a male nurse who is responsible for the daily medical care of a comatose patient, Alicia (Leonor Watling). It is within this private clinic that Benigno meets Marco (Darío Grandinetti), the boyfriend of another comatose patient. The men bond over their shared situation and attend to each woman's bedside with gifts, gestures, and delicate care. It soon becomes clear that Benigno's intimate knowledge of Alicia's body, collected through various acts of cleaning and dressing, is a predatory form of violation. The patient's unconscious passivity, a result of her vegetative state, is brutally exploited by the subject responsible for her clinical treatment. Emma Wilson (2012, 91) has illustrated how *Talk to Her* offers 'lavish and disturbing images of silent and stilled femininity, of women effectively gagged and bound in their comatose state'. Medical surveillance within the hospital quickly resembles violence, rather than any attempt to 'cure'. Benigno's close access to Alicia's body within the hospital bed enables a non-reciprocal erotic obsession to develop, and it eventually facilitates the patriarchal, sexual mastery of the sick female body. Benigno's crimes disrupt the gentle image offered by his Spanish name, literally meaning 'benign', kind, and benevolent. His penetrative intrusion results in Alicia's pregnancy, a biological and tangible index of the violence that has taken place. This involuntary gestation is itself a form of corporeal invasion, encroaching upon the unwilling subject. *Talk to Her* offers an unsettling vision of nursing as a practice, one that transgresses its conventional associations with empathy, nurture, and protection. Instead, Almodóvar signals the ways in which medicine itself might be felt as its own form of injury.

Almodóvar extends this radical vision of medicine in *The Skin I Live In* (2011), a film that looks at surgical practice as a mode of corporeal disintegration and fragmentation. The film borrows from a number of classic horror tropes, including the familiar 'mad scientist' prototype via the figure of Robert Ledgard, a troubled plastic surgeon portrayed by Antonio Banderas. Through the strictly forbidden process of transgenesis, Ledgard develops an artificial skin and transforms the body of his daughter's rapist Vincente (Jan Cornet) into Vera (Elena Anaya) on the operating table. Ledgard justifies his research into transgenesis to a colleague at a medical symposium as follows: 'We intervene in everything around us. Meat, clothes, vegetables, fruit, everything! Why not use scientific advances to improve our species? You know how many diseases we could cure with transgenesis? Or the genetic malformations that could be avoided?' He does not disclose, however, the carceral circumstances of his experiments. This violent medical intervention is driven by revenge and mourning, as Ledgard's plastic surgery carefully manipulates his victim's flesh to resemble both his late wife and daughter. As many critics have remarked, the film is heavily influenced by Georges Franju's film *Eyes*

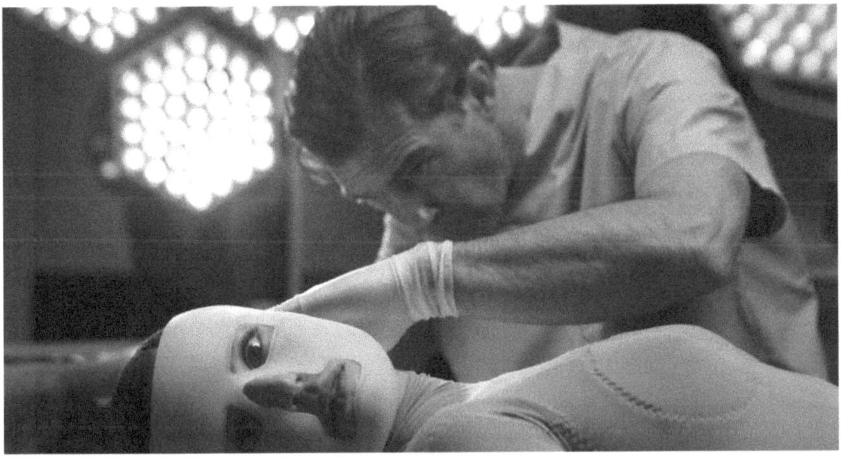

*Figure 10.1* A still from *The Skin I Live In* (*La piel que habito*, dir. Pedro Almodóvar), Pathé 2011.

*Without a Face* (1960). This earlier French film also features a grief-stricken doctor who performs a series of skin grafts on his victim as a desperate response to paternal loss. Both films 'involve talented surgeons carrying out medical procedures to transform their respective victims into replacements for their disfigured or dead daughters' (Eggert 2022). Medicine is visualised as the domain of the 'patriarch' quite literally, governed by paternalism and the law of the father.

The aesthetic economy of cutting, slicing, and sewing in Almodóvar's film draws on the double-edged logic of the 'stitch' as a form of both repair and destruction (Figure 10.1).

The therapeutic 'suture' is a way for Ledgard to mend bodies, and make psychic amends, following trauma. His specialised medical expertise, usually reserved for healing burn victims with corrective surgery, is repurposed for personal reasons. Vital for Almodóvar's film is the symbolism of the needle and thread, deployed to visualise the surgical disintegration and reconstruction of human anatomy, as well as to evoke the sartorial world of fabric. Dressmaking is an important thematic point of reference in *The Skin I Live In*, as we first encounter the future prisoner/patient at work in his mother's atelier, and later watch him tear the floral dresses given to him into a million pieces. It is within this register that Almodóvar also invokes the artistic legacy of Louise Bourgeois, with numerous citations and copies of her work reappearing in the film's mise-en-scene. Vincente/Vera watches documentaries about the artist's sculptural practice in Ledgard's underground cell and learns how to recreate the fabric sculptures from Bourgeois' late career, uncanny figures which boldly annihilate and reimagine the human form. For Tarja Laine (2014),

> Vera's works of art, made from her clothing, share significant parallels with Bourgeois's fabric sculptures and express both her experience of living in

> an "alien skin" and the gender identity that she is "dressed in" [...] Like Bourgeois' sculptures, Vera's skin looks as though it has been assembled from pieces of fabric, her body a patchwork in which different sections are simultaneously united and divided by scars.

With this close attention to the human form as something that can be moulded and reshaped, Almodóvar makes visible the 'plasticity' of both plastic surgery and the plastic arts. The film's various scenes of morphological transformation rehearse the original definition given to Ledgard's profession – the art of modelling malleable flesh.

*The Skin I Live In* also introduces us to Almodóvar's recurrent interest in anatomical art, and its unique and uncanny visualisation of human corporeal structures. The teaser poster for the film, designed by Almodóvar's long-standing collaborator Juan Gatti, features an *ecorché* figure, depicting a body without skin to starkly reveal the red muscles and internal organs beneath. This image, which also appears on the walls of Ledgard's grand home office, recalls the medical gaze of early modern Europe and its fascination with the dissection of corpses as a route to anatomical knowledge. Like these earlier illustrations, Gatti's poster for Almodóvar's film straddles the porous borders between science and art, resembling an instructional diagram just as it functions as a highly aesthetised mediation on mortality.

## The body as geometry

This brief survey of Almodóvar's cinema via the lens of medicine offers insight into how his films have reflected on the hospital bed as a site of ambivalence. On the one hand, this clinical encounter represents important possibilities for healing, connection, and rebirth. On the other, this is a moment marked by defencelessness and violence. Fundamentally, the hospital bed indexes an opening, the exposure of one body to another. Returning us continuously in his work to the scene of the clinic, Almodóvar highlights our ontology as relational beings, vulnerable and dependent on each other. For the feminist philosopher Adriana Cavarero (2016, 105), 'emphasising vulnerability is not a matter of correcting individualistic ontology by inserting the category of relation into it. It is rather to think relation itself as originary and constitutive, as an essential dimension of the human'. Cavarero develops a feminist ethics based on our mutual exposure to damage and argues that the corporeal posture of 'bending' formalises this alternative model of subjectivity. She critiques the vertical axis of 'rectitude' that has characterised much of masculinist, Western philosophy and instead calls for a horizontal structure grounded in 'inclination'. She argues

> In its radical version, which liquidates any residue of individualistic ontology, the relational model does not in fact allow for any symmetry at all but only for a continuous interweaving of multiple and singular dependence. At its most extreme, it is exemplified by scenarios in which the protagonists are altogether unbalanced.
>
> (Cavarero 2016, 13)

Cavarero is interested in the geometric shape of bodies that bend over and how this gestural economy maps an alternative ethics rooted in alterity. Asymmetry, or imbalance, represents an ethical situation, because one subject has power over another and the ability to respond to the exposure of the vulnerable with either care or a wound. For Cavarero, this paradigm of the human as relational is most neatly expressed in paintings of mother and baby from art history, especially Leonardo Da Vinci's *The Virgin and Child with St. Anne* (1503–1519). The scene of natality, with the mother bending down to tend to the infant, gives visual shape to the most extreme form of inclination towards the other. She continues:

> we are in the presence of the scene in which the vulnerable par excellence, the infant, not only unilaterally consigns itself to the other but also, and more importantly, provides for an originary bending, for a certain anomalous slope, for a posture. It is as if the fundamental concept of ethics were now seen, despite ages of sermons on moral uprightness, from the perspective of the vulnerable, or more to the point, inclination.
>
> (Cavarero 2016, 14)

Like Cavarero, Almodóvar also maps these ethical questions around care and medicine aesthetically, via the gestural and geometric composition of his hospital images. The bodies of those responsible for providing medical care in his films bend over the bodies of patients, a horizontal curve which maps an imbalance of power. This asymmetry visually traces an ethical question because, as Cavarero (2016, 14) has shown, 'the alternative between care and wound, as well as that between love and violence, is entirely inscribed in inclination as a predisposition to respond'. In *All About My Mother*, the uneven slope between the bodies of Penelope Cruz and Cecilia Roth seated on either side of the hospital bed denotes altruism and care. Manuela physically leans out in response to the needs of the other, providing comfort to the patient and promising to take on the reproductive labour of raising Rosa's unborn child. In *Volver*, Almodóvar returns to an almost identical image of the two women in the clinic. This geometric shape reappears when Raimunda visits her sick cousin Irene in a cancer ward in Madrid. The body of Penelope Cruz (previously a patient in Almodóvar's universe) bends over Blanca Portillo in the hospital bed, creating a gestural incline that sketches support and a warm embrace of the vulnerable. It is this unquestioned willingness to give up one's own sense of balance that makes the incline a fundamentally ethical posture for Cavarero:

> The one leaning out to the other in an act of care is herself unbalanced, tipped off her autarchic centre of gravity, not fully in control and exposed even as she leans out to respond to the constitutive exposure of another.
>
> (Huzar 2021, 27)

The horizontal composition of Almodóvar's images across these two films gives formal shape to an ethics of female community, friendship, and unconditional solidarity. Like Cavarero's case studies of mother and child from Renaissance art history, these moments of bending and leaning outline a feminist ethics of reciprocity within the hospital space.

However, as Cavarero (2016, 14) reminds us, care is 'not an automatic or obvious response of inclination; it is instead the ordinary and indeed desirable side of a violence [...] This relation is without reciprocity, it is structurally asymmetrical'. In *Talk to Her* and *The Skin I Live In*, the asymmetry of inclination instead denotes violence. The uneven slope depicted in these more troubling images of patient and physician outlines a lack of symmetry as a lack of reciprocity and consensual exchange. The medical encounter, as depicted here, emerges as the dialectical opposite of care and visualises an injurious response to the other characterised by an invasive medical gaze. The stark opposition between Benigno's vertical, active posture and Alicia's comatose, flat body is a geometric index of their differential agency, a structural imbalance that can (and will) be exploited. The angle of this line is sharper, harsher, and more pronounced than the curved slope between the women in the images described above. Similarly, the tactile contact between Ledgard and Vera is figured by Almodóvar as an intrusive touch, a medical encounter that is unwanted but cannot be resisted by the patient beneath. Almodóvar deploys the postural economy of his onscreen bodies to outline the dialectical shifts between care and violence that oscillate in his medical films. The human body, as formal structure, becomes a vital medium to think through the political, the ethical, and the social. Cavarero's model of relational ethics, based on maternal inclination as a paradigm, offers a useful lens through which to read Almodóvar's use of gesture on screen. Cavarero's work based on the maternal as an ethical model is also a helpful point of reference for thinking about Almodóvar's work more generally, given that both figures have continuously returned to the figure of the mother to ask larger, philosophical questions around community, life, and death. The work of the philosopher and the filmmaker intersect in their shared attention to the human body itself as an ethical medium. Both thinkers are interested in the body as form and the value of gesture as a site of philosophical investigation.

However, Almodóvar's cinematic images go one step further than the static, Renaissance paintings Cavarero references. The stillness of these historical postures is rejected and set into motion via the animation of the moving image, as Almodóvar's profilmic bodies exhibit the dynamism of human movement. For Giorgio Agamben, the specificity of cinema lies within this unique capacity to release static images into gesture and make visible the radical potentiality of human action. In an influential essay entitled *Notes on Gesture*, Agamben (2000, 50) argues: 'gesture is the exhibition of a mediality: it is the process of making a means visible as such. It allows the emergence of the being-in-a-medium of human beings and thus it opens the ethical dimension for them'. For Agamben, cinema radically resists the biopolitical appropriation of corporeal movement that the modern medical gaze had established in the late nineteenth century. He argues that protocinematic studies of human motion and gait undertaken by historical figures such as Gilles de Tourette and Edward Muybridge represent an attempt to predict, master, and discipline the organic rhythms of the body for capitalist ends. As Deborah Levitt (2012, 198–199) has put it,

> As these postures are broken down and analysed, exposed, and taken over by an eye of this kind, the undertakings of the individual and the moving images of expression and communication are exposed, decomposed, and re-established. These alienated artifacts become, in Agamben's terms, "indecipherable", and the Western world ends up being caught in a crisis of human gesture, in a crisis of the meaning and the interpretation of the human itself.

The liberation of image into gesture promised by cinema, however, reacquaints us with the human as medium and restores the progressive possibility of change via the body. For Agamben, the display of human gesture on screen marks cinema's flight from the field of aesthetics into the sphere of ethics and politics because the release of the still image into cinema exhibits 'the pure mediality of the human body in motion, unhinging biopolitical relations and grasping the potentiality of bare life' (Agamben 2000, 50). Without any predetermined behaviour or telos, the body re-emerges as a vehicle and/or medium for change. The film scholar Karl Schoonover (2014, 105) has extended Agamben's theory of gesture to argue that

> Cinema's registration of physicality is uniquely suited to disputing modernity's attempts to reify human life in the body, to regulate its vitality in measurable units, and thus to reduce its potential force for change by assuming to know the shape of history ahead of time.

Cinematic gesture, including the scenes of bending and contact that Almodóvar stages, enables this ethical potentiality to come into view, displaying the human body's status as medium with agency. It is this close attention to the human body as form, and cinema's unique capacity to represent this structure, that I will consider next.

## 'Anatomía'

As a coda to this discussion of Almodóvar, I turn now to a moment in the director's career when his interest in medicine reached a new aesthetic height. This particular example in Almodóvar's recent catalogue is the director's most explicit and distinctive engagement with medical knowledge, biology, and the body. In Pain and Glory (2019), Salvador Mallo (Antonio Banderas) reflects on his declining health and acute experience of embodied pain. The character is an aging film director living in Madrid who suffers from countless physical ailments and desperately seeks a form of pain relief, experimenting with both heroin and prescription drugs. The film's anxieties about corporeal expiry and finitude have been read by numerous critics as autobiographical, given the clear parallels between Salvador and Almodóvar. It is therefore possible to read *Pain and Glory* as a self-reflexive film, or at least a deeply personal attempt to grapple with the visceral and alienating experience of illness. In an interview with *The Guardian* in 2016, Almodóvar shared his own struggles with the debilitating effects of migraines and tinnitus, both health conditions that also plague Salvador in *Pain and Glory*: 'I have a lot of migraines; I don't hear with one ear and I'm photophobic. I don't go to award ceremonies because TV lights mean having a migraine the whole evening' (Romney 2016). Understood in these terms, filmmaking becomes its own form of pain relief for Almodóvar, being a therapeutic outlet to work through the ineffable feelings that accompany chronic suffering. Salvador also comes to understand the creative process in this way, as the experience of making art based on his life emerges as an unexpected form of cure. As spectators, we learn that *Pain and Glory*'s frequent and evocative flashbacks to the character's childhood in Paterna are in fact a product of this diegetic creation, a metatextual residue of Salvador's artistic healing. This postmodern and deconstructive approach to narrative invites us to read Almodóvar's film as a response to his own lived experiences of being a medical patient. The material and temporal body behind the camera (Almodóvar) becomes an essential point of interstitial contact between the profilmic body of Salvador (textually represented by Banderas) and the spectatorial body in front of the screen. This spectatorial body, itself an ephemeral and fragile object, brings its own host of medical histories and corporeal experiences to the cinematic encounter. With the film's close attention to the tangible and visceral rhythms of biological life, Almodóvar solicits this embodied knowledge and activates our sensory memories of physical pain.

In one early scene, Salvador describes all of the different medical problems afflicting his body and explains the anatomical origins of his chronic pain. As he recites this extensive list (insomnia, otitis, acid reflux, chronic pharyngitis, ulcers, intrinsic asthma, tinnitus, constant muscle aches, an unidentified lump in his throat), the film suddenly departs from live-action images and enters an entirely new formal register with a vivid animated sequence entitled 'Anatomía'. As Salvador narrates his biological decline, bright anatomical sketches provide an aesthetic means to map the locations of these various afflictions within the body. In an interview about the production of the film (Duralde 2019), Almodóvar explains the background of this striking sequence, which is the director's first use of animation in his long career

> I chose it to get the point across in the least amount of time. I'm introducing a character with multiple pains and afflictions, and that's no fun to direct or to discuss. Pains aren't very cinematic, unless they're tied up with action, but to show headaches or backaches, there aren't a lot of ways to shoot that in an interesting way. So I made a list of all the character's aches, and I gave it to Alberto [Iglesias] to set it to music, and once I had the music, I gave it to [graphic designer] Juan Gatti to animate it. At first, it was a whim; it amused me to go from the characters to animated drawings. I was amused by the narrative risk. But on the other hand, as I usually do, I appreciated how practical it was—the viewer learns what they need to very quickly, and it's visually interesting.

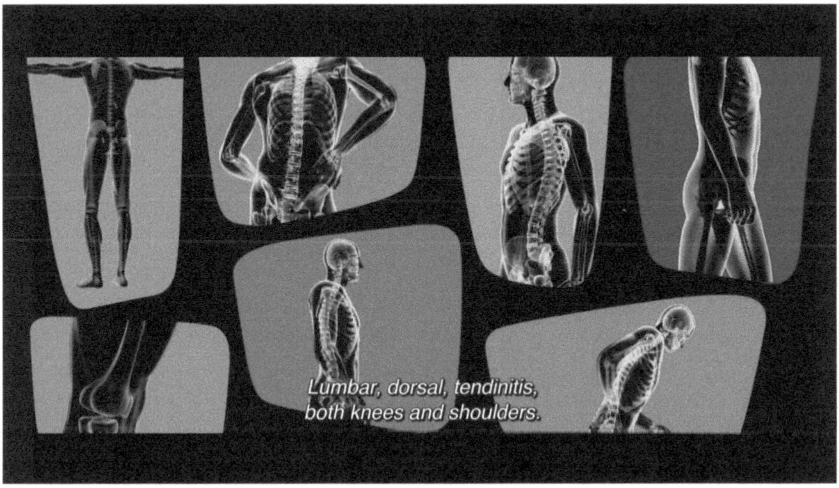


*Figure 10.2* 'Anatomía': A still from *Pain and Glory* (*Dolor y gloria*, dir. Pedro Almodóvar), Sony Pictures 2019.

As Almodóvar explains, the anatomical sketch has an important pedagogical and practical function here. The diagram transmits essential biological knowledge to viewers of the film, just as it has historically been a vital touchstone of medical education. Numerous curators and critics, such as Joanna Ebenstein and Martin Kemp, have recently turned to the longer history of anatomical art, tracing its development in dialogue with centuries of scientific attempts to better understand and preserve the human body. Almodóvar's anatomical illustration, dubbed a 'narrative risk' by the director, also carries philosophical implications. The sudden shift from live action to animation enacts a radical abstraction of the human form, flattening the haptic depth of Banderas' body to the sharp geometry of notation (Figure 10.2). Deployed to track the interior mechanisms of the body, the medical gaze necessitates the reduction of flesh to pure line. The stark formal shift from photography to computer-generated images indexes the disparity between our daily, phenomenological experience of the human body and its alternative representation by clinical medicine. There is a fundamental violence at the heart of this morphological transformation, estranging the human body to reimagine it as series of neat and sharp lines. In his reflections on Diderot's *Encyclopaedia*, Roland Barthes commented on the uncanny abstraction performed by the anatomical diagram as a mode of scientific demonstration

> We can say that there is not one plate of the *Encyclopaedia* which fails to vibrate well beyond its demonstrative intent [...] Consider the astonishing image of man reduced to his network of veins; here anatomical boldness unites with the great poetic and philosophic interrogation: *What is it?* What name to give it? How to give a name? A thousand names rise up, dislodging each other: a tree, a bear, a monster, a hair, a shirt, a fabric.
>
> (Barthes 2000, 229)

For Barthes, this particular form of medical iconography goes beyond pedagogy and situates the body at the very limits of the human. The clinician's curiosity about the interior operations of the body necessitates a total rearrangement of corporeal geography. This cartographic endeavour signals a form of rupture, as Barthes notes how this strange structure resists easy classification or categorisation: *What is it?* In a similar vein, the arrival of the anatomical sketch in Almodóvar's film figures interruption, as the experience of chronic illness throws both subject and body into taxonomic crisis. Salvador tells us that his medical diagnosis (granted visual expression via animated anatomical drawings) has led to an existential and psychic impasse. As aesthetic form, the anatomical sketch is deployed to signal the attack on Salvador's sense of embodiment and self-identity threatened by medical analysis.

In her book *Life-Destroying Diagrams* (2022), the film scholar Eugenie Brinkema has argued that the question of violence on screen is essentially a question of aesthetic form. She illustrates how corporeal destruction and degradation in contemporary horror cinema are rooted within a discourse of the body that explicates its potentially infinite capacity to be 'deformed' and reconfigured. In a bold analysis of Tom Six's infamous film, *The Human Centipede*, Brinkema suggests that it is the diagram of this abject structure (an anatomical inversion that brutally stiches bodies together) that communicates the sheer horror of this act. For Brinkema, the doctor's black-and-white sketch of this formal structure on pen and paper goes much further in visually denoting violence than the blood-stained image of the victims after this surgery has taken place. She writes:

> The entirety of the question of violence in *The Human Centipede* turns on the violence of an unmodifiable position, a rivetedness to a certain notation: the formality of a written bondedness violent in excess of any order stained with blood, vomit, pus, piss, shit, agony, weeping, terror. The diagram is what poses the formality of the problem of escape from the sequence that it is.
> (Brinkema 2016, 87)

Though Brinkema's analysis here focuses on an extreme and controversial example of modern body horror, her reading of the diagram is instructional. Salvador has not been the victim of a cruel surgical experiment, but he nonetheless feels trapped by his unmodifiable ontological form as a human body and cannot escape the biological burden this basic anatomy entails. Significantly, it is the abstract formality of geometric line on screen that traces this structural condition. The diagram formalises this ontological truth: there can be no escape from the body. Each animated diagram screened by Almodóvar maps the infinite possibilities for violence that are integral to the 'human' as form, from the fragility of human bones to the toxicity of malfunctioning lungs.

As these sketches take shape, Salvador explains how corporeal pain and intrusion are essential and constitutive features of the human as medium. His knowledge of this anatomical structure is tied to its innate capacity for disorder and decline, as he remarks: 'I started to know my body through pain and illness'. It is through the experience of chronic discomfort that Salvador becomes aware of his form, a consciousness shaped by the clinical gaze of modern science. As a discursive mode, medicine constructs the human body via its various pathologies and operates at an epistemological level by mapping the various locations of these possibilities. In an article about Almodóvar's film for the British medical journal *The Lancet*, the geriatrician Desmond O'Neill (2019) argues that Salvador's list of pains is a cinematic rendering of a famous medical dictum: 'health is the silence of the organs'. It is only via the experience of corporeal suffering, and the medical diagnosis of this affliction, that we become attentive to the material body as a life form with its own rhythms and vulnerabilities. This pain is not an external interruption or assault (like the violence inflicted in *The Skin I Live In* or *Talk to Her*) but a threat that resides within the body itself, embedded in the pure anatomy and ontology of the human. As Nancy illustrated in his autobiographical reflections on the heart transplant, the body itself is constituted by a fundamental strangeness and intrusion that becomes particularly acute during medical interventions. Despite our best efforts, we cannot avoid our basic exposure, being fragile, mortal, and temporal. If Salvador had previously existed in a state of blissful 'unawareness', he has quickly come to learn that the human form is plagued by limits and threats.

For Almodóvar, it is only the anatomical sketch that can make this fundamental condition clear on screen and it is only via the specificity of animation that he can give visual form to this diagrammatic economy. Freed from the anatomical constraints of the real, animation allows Almodóvar to visualise various corporeal shapes. These abstract figures morph and contort with the rhythm of Salvador's narration, consistently changing form to illustrate a different medical phenomenon. This metamorphosis rejects a stable structure, facilitating the continuous visual deformation of the human. This bold formal capacity to assume any possible shape might be read as an example of Sergei Eisenstein's 'plasmaticness'. In his famous reflections on Disney films from the 1930s and 1940s, the Russian film theorist Eisenstein was struck by the dynamic force and protean force of animation and figures like Mickey Mouse. As Pasi Väliaho (2017) has demonstrated, Eisenstein was drawn to the shape-shifting transformations staged by Disney characters and became interested in the particularities of animation as aesthetic form. Eistenstein (1986, 21) writes:

> For here we have a being represented in drawing, a being of definite form, a being which has attained a definite appearance, and which behaves like the primal protoplasm, not yet possessing a "stable" form, but capable of assuming any form and which, skipping along the rungs of the evolutionary ladder, attaches itself to any and all forms of animal existence.

Almodóvar, like Eisenstein (1986, 21) draws on the radical capacity of animation to reflect on human embodiment as a question of form and abstraction. As an aesthetic mode that allows for multiple mutations and transformations, animation allows Almodóvar to bring us as viewers into contact with the abstract violence performed by medicine and its estranging visual economies. Almodóvar's anatomical excursions on screen represent an important meeting point between the contemporary moving image (including both CGI and animation) and the longer history of the medical illustration, which reached the height of its popularity in Renaissance Europe. Anatomical sketches produced by artists and physicians such as Andreas Vesalius gradually replaced other pedagogical tools within medicine, substituting the need for the physical dissection of cadavers and corpses. The fascinating dialogue that Almodóvar sets up between contemporary screen culture and anatomical art is a project recently taken up by the filmmakers Lucien Castaing-Taylor and Véréna Paravel. Entitled *De Humani Corporis Fabrica* (2022), the documentary borrows its Latin name (which means 'the fabric of the human body') from Vesalius' seminal book of anatomical drawings originally published in 1543. The film uses the latest technological advances in medical imaging and photography to illustrate numerous surgeries and autopsies in contemporary Parisian hospitals. This includes ground-breaking footage from the inside of the human body, with tracking shots of the various organs, tissues, and fluids that make up our anatomy. Castaing-Taylor and Paravel reference Vesalius' major work in order to situate their own project as a contemporary artistic attempt to get us closer to what lies under the skin. Both artistic endeavours represent an attempt to grapple with the mystery of the human body, and the ineffable experience of being alive within one. In its representation of corporeal vulnerability and physical pain, *Pain and Glory* turns to animation (rather than documentary footage) to make sense of this strange experience.

This important example from *Pain and Glory* is illustrative of Almodóvar's broader cinematic project, which has repeatedly explored the ambivalence of psychic subjectivity. Our fundamental exposure represents opportunities for both care and violence, and medicine is a domain where this ethical question becomes particularly acute. In Almodóvar's films, the medical encounter indexes the dialectical opposition between the nurturing life drive and the more destructive death drive. The anatomical sketch is a compelling symbol of this tension. Its intellectual origins are rooted in historical attempts to cure bodies and preserve human life. However, scientific enquiry operates via the abstraction of the human body, and we often fail to recognise ourselves in the images medicine gives back to us. For Agamben, the analytic study of corporeal motion and gait resulted in a crisis of gesture and, by extension, a crisis of the 'human'. Almodóvar offers his distinctively cinematic iteration of this critique, looking at how medical imaging in its diagrammatic representation violently disrupts our perception of the body. This is violence conceived as a problem of form, between the enduring tension between the real and the abstract, or between flesh and line.

## References


Agamben, Giorgio. 2000. *Means Without End: Notes on Politics*, translated by Vincenzo Binetti and Cesare Casarino. Minneapolis: University of Minnesota Press.

Almodóvar, Pedro. 1999. *All About My Mother* (El Deseo).Almodóvar, Pedro. 2006. *Volver* (Warner Bros).

Almodóvar, Pedro. 2011. *The Skin I Live In* (El Deseo).

Almodóvar, Pedro. 2019. *Pain and Glory* (Sony Pictures)

Almodóvar, Pedro. 2021. *Parallel Mothers* (Sony Pictures).

Almodóvar, Pedro. 2022. *Talk to Her* (El Deseo).

Barthes, Roland. 2000. *A Roland Barthes Reader*. London: Vintage.

Brinkema, Eugenie. 2016. "Violence and the Diagram; Or, The Human Centipede." *Qui Parle*, 24(2): 75–108.

Brinkema, Eugenie. 2022. *Life-Destroying Diagrams*. Durham, NC: Duke University Press.

Butler, Judith. 2014. "On Cruelty." *London Review of Books*. https://www.lrb.co.uk/the-paper/v36/n14/judith-butler/on-cruelty.

Castaing-Taylor, Lucien, and Véréna Paravel. 2022. *De Humani Corporis Fabrica* (Norte Productions).

Cavarero, Adriana. 2016. *Inclinations: A Critique of Rectitude*. Stanford, CA: Stanford University Press.

Duralde, Alonso. 2019. "Pedro Almodóvar on the Real-Life Fears and Aches behind 'Pain and Glory'." *TheWrap*. https://www.thewrap.com/pedro-almodovar-pain-and-glory/.

Eggert, Brian. 2022. "The Skin I Live In (2011)." *Deep Focus Review*. https://deepfocusreview.com/definitives/the-skin-i-live-in/.

Eisenstein, Sergei. 1986. *Eisenstein on Disney*, edited by Jay Leyda. Kolkata: Seagull Books.

Huzar, Timonthy J. 2021. "Apprehending Care in the Flesh: Reading Cavarero with Spillers." *Diacritics* 49(3): 6–27. https://doi.org/10.1353/dia.2021.0027.

Kinder, Marsha. 2004. "Reinventing the Motherland: Almodóvar's Brain-Dead Trilogy." *Journal of Spanish Cultural Studies* 5(3): 245–260. doi:https://doi.org/10.1080/1463620040000282109.

Laine, Tarja. 2014. "Art as a Guaranty of Sanity: *The Skin I Live In*." *Alphaville: Journal of Film and Screen Media* 7: 4–38. https://doi.org/10.33178/alpha.7.02.

Levitt, Deborah. 2012. "Notes on Media and Biopolitics: 'Notes on Gesture'." In *The Work of Giorgio Agamben: law, literature, life*, edited by Justin Clemens, Nicholas Heron and Alex Murray 193–211. Edinburgh: Edinburgh University Press.

McMahon, Laura. 2008. "Figuring Intrusion: Nancy and Denis." *Contemporary French and Francophone Studies* 12(4): 463–470. https://doi.org/10.1080/17409290802447506.

Nancy, Jean-Luc. 2010. *L'intrus*. Paris: Galilée.

Nixon, Mignon. 2005. *Fantastic Reality: Louise Bourgeois and a Story of Modern Art*. Cambridge: MIT Press, 180.

O'Neill, Desmond. 2019. "The Pain and Glory of Ageing." *The Lancet* 394(10202): 909. https://doi.org/10.1016/s0140-6736(19)32089-6.

Romney, Jonathan. 2016. "Pedro Almodóvar: 'Nobody Sings. There's No Humour. I Just Wanted Restraint'." *The Observer*, 7 August. https://www.theguardian.com/film/2016/aug/07/pedro-almodovar-observer-interview.

Schoonover, Karl. 2014. "Histrionic Gestures and Historical Representation: Masina's Cabina, Bazin's Chaplin, and Fellini's Neorealism." *Cinema Journal* 53(2): 93–116. https://www.jstor.org/stable/43653570

Väliaho, Pasi. 2017. "Animation and the Powers of Plasticity." *Animation* 12(3): 259–271. https://doi.org/10.1177/1746847717740093.

Wilson, Emma. 2012. *Love, Mortality and the Moving Image*. Basingstoke: Palgrave Macmillan.

Wilson, Emma. 2020. "*All About My Mother:* Matriarchal Society." *The Criterion Collection*. https://www.criterion.com/current/posts/6795-all-about-my-mother-matriarchal-society.

# Musing 4

## On care and violence in medical humanities research collaborations

*Angela Woods*

In the following pages I would like to offer some reflections on a type of 'medical encounter' that too often goes unnoticed within medical humanities research, namely, encounters between researchers and collaborators in broader health and community settings. As I will show, these encounters, too, can be fraught with particular kinds of violence if we do not attend to them with care.

I come to these considerations in my capacity as the Co-Director of Hearing the Voice, a large interdisciplinary research project based at Durham University.[1] Over ten years, our interdisciplinary team of 38 researchers worked with nearly 150 other collaborators coming from fields as diverse as medieval history, cognitive psychology, anthropology, and theology, and including people who hear voices and who work across mental health services.

The experience of hearing voices was at the centre of the project. We sought to approach it first and foremost *as* an experience, not as a symptom or a pathology or as cognitive aberration. Recognising that voice-hearing can mean very different things across historical and cultural contexts, Hearing the Voice researchers looked in depth at voice-hearing in the Christian tradition (Cook 2018); in medieval and Early Modern Europe (Powell and Saunders 2021); in the contemporary ayahuasca clinics of Peru (Dupuis 2022); and in relation to writers' experience of hearing the voices of their characters (Foxwell et al. 2020). Central to our investigations were voice-hearing experiences that are intensely challenging and associated with severe mental distress, and voices that often lead people to psychiatric treatment and inpatient care. In seeking a deeper understanding that would challenge stigmatising stereotypes about voice-hearing, we collaborated closely with people who have experienced such distressing voices: partnering in research studies, helping to build networks of peer support, and co-producing a major online resource called Understanding Voices.[2]

A wide array of collaborations nourished a project of this size and complexity; here I focus on those related to an exhibition we co-curated called 'Hearing Voices: Suffering, Inspiration and the Everyday'.[3] This exhibition remains to our knowledge the world's largest such investigation of the experience of hearing voices,[4] and we were fortunate to have the resources to commission an artist to create a sound installation about these experiences. After a competitive process, this commission was awarded to Victoria Hume, whose work 'The Isle is Full of Noises' is

DOI: 10.4324/9781032660165-18

still available through the exhibition website. The installation is an animation that incorporates many different elements of testimony from voice-hearers across the North-East of England, who spoke about their experiences with her in a series of workshops. Victoria Patton (the project's exhibition lead) and I found this to be a compelling installation produced in a creative and respectful way. However, our enthusiasm for the piece was not unanimously shared by the exhibition's visitors. An email we received from another artist in the region testifies to a different viewing experience:

> ...Despite much excellence regionally, nationally and internationally hearing the voice currently appears tokenistic or even exclusionary of much of our diverse lived experiences... I'm sure Victoria Hume is a great sound artist yet I've learnt nothing about her personal experience of voice-hearing or mental distress in general. From my reading I understand she has been a long-term health manager (medical model?) now co-opting "our" experiences into her artwork. I am troubled by who really owns our voices and the potential to extend that abuse many of us experienced in our psychiatrisations.

Let me unpack this message, which contains much to reflect on. First, there is an accusation of being both tokenistic and in the same gesture exclusionary, an accusation of riding roughshod over the diversity of voice-hearing experiences. Yet perhaps the greatest violence being pointed to here is one that happens at a number of different registers, where someone who does not have, or does not disclose having, a set of experiences is being given the platform and resources to produce an artwork and engage audiences in the interpretation of those experiences. The commissioning of this artist is further seen in this context not as a violence that exists in a discrete or idiosyncratic moment but replicates a much wider set of power relations and of abuses of power that are associated with experiences of psychiatry and enforced psychiatric treatment.

Although Hearing the Voice has now ended, I have felt it important and productive critically to return to this moment. There is deep value in holding onto those things that trouble and conflict us as individuals working in collaborative research contexts, and in trying to trace the ways in which they have continued to influence our thinking and action. When we received that email, which was also shared publicly by the author, Victoria Patton and I talked for a long time about how best to respond. In the end, we decided to engage with the critical issues it raised by adding to the exhibition event programme an event entitled 'Who can speak about voices?' We invited the artist who sent the email to participate, along with a number of other speakers, and they delivered a performance piece that further challenged us in interesting ways. For us, that event was an attempt to open up questions of authority and expertise and incorporate some of the very vibrant scholarship and activism that takes place in mad studies, survivor-led research contexts, and in the context of participatory and co-produced research – thinking about how they relate to voice-hearing experiences, the production of artworks, and the staging of exhibitions.

That email and the discussions it generated highlight the importance of care as a concept when thinking about and shaping research collaborations. To care is 'to attend to', 'to bring our attention to', and 'to bring into focus' – in ways which might be curious and open-ended, requiring particular kinds of energy and affective investment across different forms of engagement.

But care also directs our attention to the question of investedness. What do we care about? What is the rationale for undertaking some activities and not others, working in this way and not that? Care focuses attention on the different goals that people bring to collaborations and the significance of the commitments they make personally, politically, ethically, and professionally. But here care can also imply 'tending' as a form of 'attending': creating spaces that can hold tension and conflict, and creating environments and processes from which people emerge with some sense of positive transformation. It is a simple question, but one that is rarely directly asked: 'What does it mean to care for each other in the context of the kind of interdisciplinary and cross-sector work that we do in medical humanities?' Holding onto care prompts us to recognise – and not just recognise but *embrace* – some of the ethical and political dimensions of collaborative work in the medical and health humanities, which can sometimes be a very difficult undertaking. Care is about many 'things' – many processes, many practices, many forms of behaviour – but, crucially, it is about a lot of emotional energy, including experiences where emotional labour is disregarded, or undervalued, or seen as the purview of certain bodies, certain genders, and certain people within the collaboration, but not others. The conclusion I have come to is that holding on to the concept of care is absolutely critical in thinking about the collaborative work that we, as scholars, do in the field of medical and health humanities, and beyond.

## Notes

1 The first phase of our project, which ran from 2012 to 2015, was funded by a Strategic Award from the Wellcome Trust (WT098455MA). In October 2015, we received a Wellcome Trust Collaborative Award in Humanities and Social Science (WT108720), which enabled us to continue our research on voice-hearing until 2022. https://hearingthevoice.org/.
2 See https://understandingvoices.com/.
3 'Hearing Voices: Suffering, Inspiration and the Everyday' was held at Palace Green Library, Durham, UK (5 November 2016–26 February 2017).
4 As well as touring to Hearing Voices Congresses in the USA, the Netherlands, and Canada, Hearing Voices was globally accessible via the online exhibition https://hearingvoicesdu.org/.

## References

Cook, Christopher C.H. 2018. *Hearing Voices, Demonic and Divine: Scientific and Theological Perspectives*. London: Routledge.

Dupuis, David. 2022. "Learning to Navigate Hallucinations: Comparing Voice Control Ability During Psychosis and in Ritual Use of Psychedelics." In *Voices in Psychosis:*

*Interdisciplinary Perspectives*, edited by Angela Woods, Ben Alderson-Day, and Charles Fernyhough, 194–202. Oxford: Oxford University Press.

Foxwell, John, Ben Alderson-Day, Charles Fernyhough, and Angela Woods. 2020 "'I've Learned I Need to Treat My Characters Like People': Varieties of Agency and Interaction in Writers' Experiences of their Characters' Voices." *Consciousness and Cognition* 79: 102901, 1–14.

Powell, Hilary, and Corinne Saunders. (eds). 2021. *Visions and Voice-Hearing in Medieval and Early Modern Contexts*. London: Palgrave Macmillan.

Woods, Angela, Ben Alderson-Day, and Charles Fernyhough (eds). 2022. *Voices in Psychosis: Interdisciplinary Perspectives*. Oxford: Oxford University Press.

# Part 4

# Anatomy of a transformation

# 11 T for trans

## An outraged investigation of non-binary medical transition in Germany

*Claude Kempen*

### Introduction: Coming up against 'health' insurance

In late 2019, I came out as non-binary. I started seeing a specialised therapist and began to think about surgical interventions and hormones. During this time, I learned that being a non-binary person in Germany meant being not recognised as trans by my insurance provider or by most other healthcare providers. While figuring out my very personal feelings about being trans and what that meant for me, I had to navigate the considerable institutional mazes of trans healthcare, insurance coverage, and seemingly endless medical appointments. Notably, in order to gain access to the healthcare I needed, I had to do all of this as if I was a binary trans man. I also had to become fluent in the ways and culture of German bureaucracy and its psychopathologising language. As I stumbled about, bumping into unfamiliar yet formidable obstacles, the essence of this struggle was finding out what trans meant in these different contexts, or what the implied meanings were around me. It seemed to have so many different definitions – 'trans' seems to carry within itself an experience of opposites and contradictions. I could feel the gap in how we as trans people perceived ourselves and how we were perceived and treated. I often struggled to keep my own definitions separate from those that my insurer, my surgeon(s), and my endocrinologist used or could comprehend.

In the following chapter,[1] I repeatedly ask the question 'What does trans mean?' in the (con)text at hand. Subsequently, I investigate the myriad definitions of trans and locate myself among them, asking 'Where am I in all of this?' Through this, I wish to demonstrate the discrepancy between my own lived experience of transness and the definitions I came up against within the medicolegal realm during my transition. Regarding trans is/as gap, understanding gap as a break in continuity, the gap I am alluding to lies between what trans means to the institutions I am encountering (e.g., insurers, surgeons, doctors) and what it means or could mean to me.

Following an autoethnographic method which I introduce in the next segment, I focus on one of the steps I took during my transition, namely, taking testosterone; that requires fleshing out the steps to accessing hormone replacement therapy (HRT). To analyse access to transition in Germany, there is no getting around its dominant health evaluation guideline on 'transsexualism', or so-called

DOI: 10.4324/9781032660165-20

*Begutachtungsanleitung* (BGA for short). When taking a close look at the BGA and my personal experience, it quickly becomes apparent that the German healthcare system imposes an extremely rigid regime that is both hard on binary trans people and impossible to navigate as a non-binary person. Only when one knows what to say, how to act, who to call, and who to pass as is there a chance to access healthcare and financial support. It is an experience packed with codes and definitions that require a certain amount of self-taught medicolegal knowledge.

## A praxiographic autoethnography

I am still in the midst of my transition. The ink on my legal documents is hardly dry. This simultaneity is unsettling at times, but I believe it holds value for the writer as well as the reader. It was Dafina-Lazarus Stewart who put this in perspective for me. She argues that good texts can emerge from 'living through/with moments of breakdown' (Stewart 2017, 286). Subsequently, I turned to other trans authors who have navigated life events and writing processes concurrently. In *Testo Junkie*, for example, Paul B. Preciado (2013) reflects both upon his testosterone intake and the intersections of sexuality, pornography, and pharmaceuticals. He calls his book 'a somato-political fiction, a theory of the self, or self-theory' (Preciado 2013, 11). These terms were later picked up by Maggie Nelson in the form of 'autotheory', first within her book *The* Argonauts (2016) and then in an interview with Micha McCrary, where she describes the genre as 'autobiographical writing that exceeds the boundaries of the "personal"' (cited in Wiegman 2020, 2). Gloria Anzaldúa's 'autohistoria' (1987) also comes to mind, but I have left her out in the present analysis to prioritise trans auto-theorists.

It is this 'encounter between first person narration and theory' (Wiegman 2020, 1) that I intend to focus on here. As previously stated, I turned to trans writers and academics, such as Sonny Nordmarken (2014), Eli Clare (2001, 2003), and Bobby Noble (2009b, 2009a, 2007), whose writing had an almost therapeutic effect on me and who made me realise that autoethnography was a valid way of producing academic texts. They have helped me feel affiliated with the autoethnographic genre, generally defined as 'an approach to research and writing that seeks to describe and systematically analyze (*graphy*) personal experience (*auto*) in order to understand cultural experience (*ethno*)' (Ellis, Adams, and Bochner 2010, 1). For me, this led to my wishing to describe and analyse my experience of transitioning in Germany, to grasp the cultural meanings of trans and to theorise it as a gap. It is a theory of self as well as culture.

The need for an autoethnographic take on this topic becomes evident when searching for literature on transitioning in Germany. Most texts are written by cis people about trans people, and many take the form of policy papers (see Amelung 2017; Nieder and Strauß 2015; Nieder and Strauß 2019). I hope to add a more personal perspective to this body of text, thereby acknowledging the importance of having an 'embodied stake in the matter at hand' (Stryker and Whittle 2006, 315) and of writing autoethnographically within the field of trans studies.[2] My answer to anyone critiquing my own work or that of others on the basis of it being unscientific, too personal, or inadequately 'objective' would be to point out this importance. I would also invite them to question their own approach to reading as an act of extractivism,[3] mining for more than what is being freely given.

Texts by George Scialabba (*How to be Depressed,* 2018) and Jordy Rosenberg (*Confessions of the Fox*, 2019) encouraged me to embrace a variety of sources in terms of their genre, using medical guidelines and autoethnographic and theoretical reflections. This textual multiplicity links nicely to the theoretical backdrop of this investigation as I draw on Annemarie Mol's *The Body Multiple: Ontology in Medical Practice* (2002). Therein, Mol analyses medical practices around atherosclerosis[4] and finds that this illness is 'multiple'. By this she means that the way that the illness might be described in a textbook differs from conversations had during a doctor's appointment. What is said about the illness in one context might even be at odds with what is said in another context. This insight is congruent with biosocial research undertaken by Columbia University (2019), stating that 'biological processes, rather than being fixed, immutable mechanisms that consign people to particular life outcomes, are instead fluid, dynamic responses to features of the social and physical environments humans inhabit'. Rebecca Jordan-Young and Katrina Karkazis (2019, 26) have also fruitfully drawn on Mol in their book *Testosterone: An Unauthorized Biography*, retrieving testosterone from its archaic attributions and demonstrating its biological and social multiplicity.

Mol (2002, 51) argues that 'as long as the practicalities of enacting a disease are kept unbracketed and out in the open, the varieties of "atherosclerosis" multiply'. Mol (2002, 31, 119–121) characterises analysis of this multiplicity as 'praxiography', which pays attention to how 'doing disease [is] part of the story' and acknowledges 'that no entity can innocently stay the same throughout the story, unaltered between various sites'. In his paper, '(Re)making sex: A Praxiography of the Gender Clinic', J.R. Latham (2017, 177–179) writes about his experiences as a trans man in Australia and draws on his medical records to identify '*how* sex is *enacted multiply* across a range of situations'. According to him, a 'Molian praxiographer [...] examines how phenomena materialise (multiply) in practice and how these enactments are related' (Latham 2017, 180). Mol and Latham have both set the cornerstones or my 'trans as gap' analysis. The gaping definitions of 'trans' that I encountered and on which I will elaborate were ever-changing, unstable, implied, or outright contradictory. 'Trans' was being done and spoken into existence, both by me with my own ideas, expectations, and dreams and by the healthcare system or providers who were expecting me to act a certain way, want certain things, and deliver a certain narrative.

## Everything is condition(al): Gatekeeping and binaries

Whoever thought of the packaging and product design for the testosterone gel I used knew exactly what they were doing. It would be difficult to come up with anything more phallic and dude-like. The bottle is black, white, and lime green, about 15 centimeters long, and fits lengthwise very comfortably in a cupped palm. It is sheathed by a plastic and rubber applicator almost as long as the bottle. The applicator also serves as a lid to seal the pump bottle. To get to the 'T', you first need to open the bottle by taking the applicator sheath off. This action makes a satisfying 'pop' sound. Once the lid is off, you pump the transparent gel out of the now-uncovered top of the bottle directly onto your skin and rub it in with the flat, white head of the applicator. I often opened and closed the applicator lid many times before and after using the gel because of how satisfying the sounds were. I fell for the design and I always used the bottle with a smirk on my face. I really liked the smell of the gel, too, although it is hard to describe: a whiff of alcohol and freshness that later mixed with my own new, musky smell.

When I took my first pump of T gel in October 2019, I was very lonely. I had single-handedly done my research about the particular recommendations and guidelines for transitioning on a low-dose of T. My partner was not supportive, and it looked like transitioning was going to mean the end of our relationship. During the summer of 2019, the urge to transition had grown but the process was painfully slow. I had talked to my doctor about taking T and she had been rather skeptical, being seemingly worried about my endocrine health. She told me to get the homeopathic version of T, which one can find in France, where I was headed for a trip. This form of T was supposed to prepare me for the hormones later. But while I was reading the mindblowing book *Stone Butch Blues* by Leslie Feinberg (2003 [1993]), sitting on a beach in the south of France with my then-partner and sucking on useless sugar pills, I felt awfully stuck, misunderstood, and alone. After the trip, another month passed before I started T with my doctor. She had had no experience of prescribing hormone intake for trans people at that point and (giving credit where credit is due) she looked into it for me. We began with one pump a week, which was as good as none at all. By the end of the year, I switched to one pump a day. In 2020, I decided I had waited long enough and took the full dose of testosterone every day for a few months. By this time, I had stopped informing my doctor about my intake of T, in order to avoid listening to her worries. Hoping to get more informed and affirmative support, I reached out to an endocrinologist, but more on that later.

One bottle of the gel I was taking costs around 60€. Full dosage requires about one bottle a month, costing 720€ a year. Despite having been given a prescription by my doctor, I had to pay up front at the pharmacy and apply to my private insurance provider for reimbursement. For that application, I needed to meet the expectations of my health insurance provider, which begin with a diagnosis: 'transsexualism'.

## Diagnosis and bureaucracy

> In the latter cases [of non-binary people] it is not a matter of transsexualism in the sense of this BGA.[5]

In 2020, the 'Medical Advisory Service of the Umbrella Organisation of Social Health Insurances' (Medizinischer Dienst des Spitzenverbandes Bund der Krankenkassen, or MDS) and their colleagues from the public health system (GKV Spitzenverband) updated their 2009 evaluation guidelines for public trans healthcare intending to further standardise the assessment of 'transsexuality'. The guidelines refer to and are based on the 'German Standards' (*Deutsche Standards*), which were developed in 1997 by a commission of so-called experts convened by the German Society for Sexual Research (DGfS).[6] Furthermore, the BGA references the International Classification of Diseases (ICD-10) of 1990, and more specifically its Chapter F64.0 on 'Transsexualism'. Health insurance providers in Germany have been obliged to cover the costs of gender reassignment treatment if it is considered clinically relevant as medical treatment for alleviating a condition. Despite the quite recent update of the BGA in August 2020, the standards of care for trans people in Germany are extremely outdated and rigid. Neither of the referential texts (namely, the ICD-10 and the standards of 1997) correspond to the current state of knowledge around trans issues. Although an attempt has been made in recent years to replace the 'German Standards' of 1997 (see Nieder and Strauß 2019), to this day the BGA and its references are still prioritised.

I am simultaneously dependent on and erased by the BGA. Non-binary people cannot be diagnosed as trans and therefore cannot access the gender-reassignment measures as the person they are. I accessed trans healthcare as a binary trans man – in other words, as someone who desires to live like a man and who suffers from his physical body being 'female'. Telling this story allowed me to meet the BGA's 'decisive criteria for the socio-medical appraisal of requested gender reassignment measures in case of transsexualism' (GKV Spitzenverband, Medizinischer Dienst der Krankenkassen, and Medizinischer Dienst des Spitzenverbandes Bund der Krankenkassen 2020, 30). Though I am not a man, Aren Aizura's *Mobile Subjects* notes that those who can provide "a coherent personal story" (2018, pp. 63–64) are more likely to convince medical practitioners and insurers of their "condition"—a criterion I fulfilled, leading to my diagnosis. An acceptable diagnosis according to the BGA includes a 'valid diagnosis of transsexualism according to the ICD-10 ('Transsexualism', F64.0), pathological suffering, and suffering that could not be sufficiently alleviated by psychiatric and psychotherapeutic means' (GKV Spitzenverband, Medizinischer Dienst der Krankenkassen, and Medizinischer Dienst des Spitzenverbandes Bund der Krankenkassen 2020, 30). Although I am not a man, according to Aren Aizura's *Mobile Subjects* (2018, 63–64), I was 'able to provide a coherent personal story' that convinced medical practitioners and my insurer of my 'condition', and so I received the required diagnosis. This was mostly due to how insistent I was about my physical dysphoria,[7] how that pushed me into telling lies, and how quick I was at learning the language of the insurers. In practice, this involved entirely omitting any mention of my actual identity as a non-binary person – exactly the thing which would have marked me as 'not trans' to those who had the final word on the matter – while at the same time describing my dysphoria very vividly and in great detail. This part of my lying was a lying by omission and perhaps by choice of emphasis. Other kinds of lying were also required of me, however.

'Transsexualism', according to the BGA, 'includes the desire to live and be recognised as a member of the other sex' and wanting 'hormonal and surgical treatment in order to make one's own body as similar as possible to the preferred sex' (GKV Spitzenverband, Medizinischer Dienst der Krankenkassen, and Medizinischer

Dienst des Spitzenverbandes Bund der Krankenkassen 2020, 13). Although 'the other sex' could include any other, as in more than two, the BGA explicitly 'refers to the division into male and female that is common in our society' and rules out recognising non-binary people as trans. Wishing to medically transition and being recognised as the 'preferred sex' is also part of the BGA's definition of 'transsexual' and hence part of defining who gets access to insurance. Furthermore, the guidelines stipulate that 'transsexualism' must have persisted for at least two years, and other mental disorders, 'intersexuality', genetic or chromosomatic 'anomalies' must be excluded prior to diagnosis (GKV Spitzenverband et al. 2020, 14). For the necessary socio-medical assessment, the following points are crucial for a comprehensive diagnosis: anamnesis with recording of psychosexual development, social anamnesis, biographical and medical anamnesis, assessment of the psychological findings (if necessary), a specialist's psychiatric or psychosomatic examination, and a physical examination with urological, gynaecological, and endocrinological findings (GKV Spitzenverband et al. 2020, 15).

Most of these points are clarified in a letter of recommendation by a therapist, the so-called *Indikationsschreiben*. The BGA establishes therapy as mandatory for a diagnosis and, therefore, coverage of the costs of transition. In order to access hormones, surgeries, or any other measures, one has to see a therapist at least 12 times in six months for 50 minutes per session (GKV Spitzenverband et al. 2020, 25). This requirement is not only very time-consuming, it also sounds and feels an awful lot like forced therapy. In *(Im)possible patients? Negotiating discourses of trans health in the UK*, Ruth Pearce (2016, 159) finds that many trans people compare the process of procuring a diagnosis to taking 'a test that might be "passed" or "failed"'. She argues that trans is viewed as a condition that 'requires identification from a qualified expert [...] with reference to a set of quite static criteria, usually rooted within binary conceptions of gender' (Pearce 2016, 7). This is especially cruel if the so-called expert or therapist, to whom one must prove one's transness as a matter of survival, is not supportive or affirming of trans people. Here it seems pertinent to repeat the phrase I used to introduce this chapter: I am simultaeously dependent on and erased by the medical practices imposed by the BGA. I need to procure a diagnosis to access dysphoria-diminishing measures that make my life more liveable, but the pathways towards that necessarily leads to not only inadequate and inaccurate diagnoses but also a reinforcing and reproduction of false and rigid labels and understandings of trans. Pearce (2016, 24) correctly notes that 'the power of medical diagnosis can work to both make trans lives possible, and limit the liveable scope of these possibilities'. Ironically, the prerequisite for transitioning – a word which in so many ways evokes movement in a desired direction – is having to stand still and submit to scrutiny.

## Endocri(m)e

> The diagnosis F64.0 (female-to-male transsexualism) was psychotherapeutically confirmed at the time of admission to therapy. The diagnosis can therefore be considered confirmed.[8]

After a long and exhausting search, I found a supportive therapist. During our sessions, he speaks to me about being non-binary, uses my pronouns correctly, and respects being non-binary as a valid way to be trans. He has taught me so much and I am grateful to have found him. Nevertheless, when he writes a letter of referral for me, he must completely switch his tone and write about me as 'he' and as a 'man'. He is extremely literate in the ways of the bureacratic institutions I mentioned above, so he knows what to say and how to formulate a 'proper' diagnosis according to the ICD-10 and the BGA. This is how I successfully 'pass the test' and receive my diagnosis. If I had had to pretend that I was a binary trans man in front of him, I would not be where I am today. But as a trans person who encounters not only insurance providers but multiple healthcare providers, this test needs to be passed over and over again.

When I went to my endocrinologist for the first time, for example, I quickly picked up on the fact that my encounters with her would be one test after another, and that I was very likely to fail them if something gave me away as non-binary. She was so afraid of people wanting to stop hormones, regretting taking them at all, or wanting to detransition that she constantly expected outright enthusiasm from my side: 'I want this – so much! – I simply cannot wait to be a man!' I saw her every two months. The nurses would take blood and the endocrinologist would check my T levels, which were never high enough for her. She would urge me to go higher because my current levels were only intermediate, neither 'man' nor 'woman'. I was so happy when she said that, but I needed to hide it. She looked me up and down, scanning my upper lip for stubble, my shoulders for width, my voice for depth, and my body for fat redistribution. At that point she got suspicious. She asked: 'Are you taking the three pumps as we discussed?' My brain just went blank. In truth, I was often unsure about taking T at all, and sometimes I only used one pump even though two were the average dose. I had started to feel quite uncomfortable with the smell and the hair growth it induced, and the substance made me feel uncomfortably sticky, both in my veins and on my skin. If the definition of trans meant wanting a medical transition, wanting to 'become the preferred sex', then it was clear that not wanting these things (at least not in the binary sense) was going to exclude me altogether from both the diagnosis and the transition process it entailed. It is exactly as Sandy Stone (2006, 231) has put it in the 'Posttranssexual Manifesto': 'There are several possible answers, but only one is clinically correct'. I answered the endocrinologist's question by saying yes, I was taking three pumps, but that my levels were super low to begin with. I was so close to failing that test – a test which should not have been necessary in any case.

A few sessions later, I was more assertive. I told her that I was feeling good with an intermediate level. I did not argue that I was non-binary, because it could have meant the end of our medical relationship, but I stressed that my level of comfort with the hormone should be more important than the superficial and physical outcome. Thankfully, she let it go.

At the time of this writing, I have been off testosterone for about eight months and have not seen her since. I later heard from trans people around me that the chain of medical care centres where I saw her has now withdrawn information on trans issues from their websites and is not seeing trans people anymore, arguing that hormones were given out to trans people too quickly and that this caused a high detransition rate. Considering that I (and others) had to be in therapy for months in order to even start hormones, this is a ridiculous claim. But it resonates with the exchanges I had with my endocrinologist. Since I did not go back and I am off the hormones, for her I am probably some kind of detransitioned failure to whom she should never have given hormones at all.

## T for trans

The insufficient care with which I was provided in terms of endocrinology led me to make several big decisions about their use completely on my own. That was a mistake, but it was also not my fault. When I came off T, something happened in my body and I had a terrible pain flare-up, the worst one in my years-long history with chronic pain and fibromyalgia. This should not have happened, and it would have been more easily avoided had I been able to freely speak of my needs to people with expert knowledge. I was clear about which effects of the hormone I was happy to experience and which I was not, and although I realised one cannot completely control these things, I also understood that my needs were almost certainly not compatible with long-term testosterone intake. It was always obvious to me that I would drop it some day. But speaking about it to someone sympathetic, who knew the effects and dangers around T and could supervise me through that, was not a possibility. I relied on community advice and group meetings, but it seemed nobody had experienced such pain in relation to coming off T. My point here is important. Rigid and binary gender practices around transition cause harm to non-binary people. In this vein, my story is just one of many.

If drawing on praxiography means to realise 'how phenomena materialise (multiply) in practice and how these enactments are related' (Latham 2017, 180), I would argue that the BGA materialised as letters and reports, as medical practice, and as limited at times ill-informed steps in my transition. In this materialisation, 'Words participate, too. Paperwork. Rooms, buildings. The insurance system' (Mol 2002, 25–26). Simultaneously, an explicit or implied definition of 'trans' materialises or is communicated to us by the medical institution. What does trans mean, therefore, thus far? I will attempt a glossary.

- Trans is binary
- Trans is FtM, MtF[9]
- Trans is wanting medical transition
- Trans is always having to be sure
- Trans is needing supervision
- Trans needs proof
- Trans is a mental, a medical condition
- Trans is a diagnosis that is precarious and conditional, based on the steps one takes
- Trans must be highly and performatively articulate

- Trans must always be able to communicate expertly in the language of the oppressive system one is currently negotiating

Latham (2019, 26) asks how one can 'traverse a medical system based on these self-evident and self-referential assumptions when none of them makes sense to you'. I had to make sense of them in a way that was completely detached from my lived reality. What the BGA and the practical consequences of this document define as trans is miles away from me. Exactly as Annemarie Mol argues, what a disease (in this case, trans) means in one place 'is actually at odds with what it is in other settings' (as summarised by Jordan-Young & Karkazis (2019, 26). What has trans meant to me up until this point?

- I am non-binary
- I am considering certain physical changes to alleviate my dysphoria
- I am trans no matter the medical steps I do or do not take
- I am finding things out as I go, and this needs time
- I need support to find what is right for me, not to prove myself
- I am always already trans no matter how I dress or what I do
- I am trans unconditionally

## Conclusion: How grand, how multiple

> What is transexuality [sic]? An innate feeling? A medical condition (or disorder)? A clinical diagnosis? An identity? A surgery? All of these at once? Or, perhaps, it is one thing here and another thing over there, or a little further along.
>
> (Latham 2017, 177)

Dealing with the rigidity of German health institutions, their cis-normative gatekeeping culture, and the limited range of motion they allow has left me with an institution-induced rage. Transitioning has become an experience that feels at times like 'banging your head against a brick wall' (Ahmed 2012, 26). In this distressing trial-and-error process, I progressively uncovered exactly what kind of transition was possible for me, and on which or whose terms. The violence of this process reminds of this volume's title while also questioning the nature of health 'care', which in my case and others' turned out to be both limited and conditional.

Ironically, this process has revealed the grand multiplicity of trans. The Molian praxiography of trans that I have only begun to lay out here shows that trans not only means different things in different places, but it also means completely contradictory things in those various locations. Trans comes with gaps and discrepancies. It can be very painful to hold and embody all these definitions or implications of trans. At the same time, I experience much awe at how this term works to bring complex variants together, and at how many feelings one person can hold in relation to this one term and its implications.

Trans has potential. It can unify movements: transgender, transnational, transfeminist, translation, and many more (see also Enke 2012; Tudor 2021). It can also be a verb, as Alyosxa Tudor has shown in their article *Dimensions of Transnationalism* (2017). There, 'transing' is defined as 'to go beyond a certain category; to question a category; to deconstruct a category' (Tudor 2017, 21). I have attempted to go beyond the category of trans – to trans being trans – displaying its medicolegal becoming, its effects on me, and my personal development over time. The project is to trans one's social and gendered upbringing and to go beyond what might at times feel like the transnormative path of transition, one where HRT is the ultimate answer, the one-size-fits-all transition package.

When I wander the streets now, I am constantly being misgendered and misread, either as an effeminate gay man, a butch lesbian, or simply as queer (in its original, demeaning sense). How I am being perceived can switch from one moment to the other. Two people in the same room might be at odds about my 'real' gender: for example, 'He is a she' is a quote taken from a recent Zoom call during which my pronouns seemed to have caused confusion. Again, Tudor (2017, 24) has put this beautifully: 'a switching effect is produced', with 'cross-fadings of conventionalised reading habits in an infinite loop'. It can get hard at times not to let the outside gaze get through or into you, and to not let it affect your choices. I often wonder what I should wear and as whom I should try to pass on any given day in order to most effectively protect myself from danger.[10] 'When I walk through the world, the bashers see a fag, the dykes see a butch, and I myself don't have many words' (Clare 2003, 258).

At the end of this investigation of trans as gap, I am ironically left with more gaps. The BGA's transsexuals are not me. The kind of trans that most health providers expect is not me. Maybe this answers the question I posed at the very beginning of this chapter: where am I in all of this? The answer seems to be that I am in multiple locations at once. I am outside, trying to get in – repeatedly coming up against the brick wall of the BGA and its relatives. I am formed within the encounter with, and in opposition to, the BGA: I use it and I resist it.[11] I am in the bullet points that describe my evolution throughout my transition. But I am also not there. Just as 'the gawkers never get it right' (Clare 2003, 258) and 'every reading is a misreading' (Tudor 2017, 36), there will always be this gap, entrenched in the relationship between the signifier and the signified (de Saussure 1974). There might not be the words for me or us just yet; maybe there never will be. But regardless of whether suitable or accurate language ever arrives, we ourselves will always be here, as we always have been: existing, playing, and resisting in the gap.

## Notes

1 This chapter is an extract from my master's dissertation entitled 'Where am I? A personal investigation of non-binary transition in Germany'. The dissertation was submitted in September 2022 at the Centre of Gender Studies, SOAS, University of London. Written in the middle of the pandemic, the thesis wished to criticise certain medical practices while acknowledging the essential workers and scientists who saved the lives of those who were hospitalised and vaccinated.

2 This is argued by (see Latham 2017, 181; Radi 2019; Spade 2006, 316).
3 Melany Cruz and Darcy Luke (2020, 154, emphasis in original) argue that the 'separation of theory and practice' entails 'that the realm of practice is construed as raw material – as data – to be harvested in the research process, whilst theory is seen as detached from geohistorical–political relations', and they find that this 'serves a neo-colonial process of *academic extractivism*'.
4 The technical term 'atherosclerosis' is used by physicians to describe a degenerative change in the vessel walls of arteries. Similar to a house with old pipes, substances accumulate in the pipes over time; as those become more narrow, the flow rate decreases.
5 Excerpt from the German guidelines for trans healthcare, the so-called 'BGA' (GKV Spitzenverband, Medizinischer Dienst der Krankenkassen, and Medizinischer Dienst des Spitzenverbandes Bund der Krankenkassen 2020, 14). All BGA references were translated from German by the author.
6 For recent writing that touches on the harm of standardisation, see Max Liboiron's work *Pollution Is Colonialism* (2021).
7 While this chapter analyses what happens when a trans person does medically transition to alleviate some of their physical gender dysphoria, the latter is not this chapter's focus. See Myriam Sauer's chapter in this volume for a deeper analysis of dysphoria.
8 Taken from my psychotherapeutic report that diagnoses me as a trans man. It follows the BGA's requirements exactly. Translated from German by the author.
9 FtM stands for female to male. MtF stands for male to female. Both terms are mostly outdated and seldomly used by the trans community.
10 Tudor (2017, 29) recognises that even though passing as a concept should generally be questioned, it is at times necessary for protection and survival.
11 For related elaborations on coming up against healthcare systems, medical definitions, and glossaries but concerning chronic pain, see Maria Morata's chapter in this volume.

## References


Ahmed, Sara. 2012. *On Being Included: Racism and Diversity in Institutional Life*. Durham, NC; London: Duke University Press.

Aizura, Aren Z. 2018. *Mobile Subjects - Transnational Imaginaries of Gender Reassignment*. Durham, NC; London: Duke University Press.

Amelung, Till. 2017. *Trans*-Gesundheitsversorgung: Forderungen an die medizinischen Instanzen und an die Politik*. Nachdruck der 1. Auflage. Policy Paper Gesundheit des Bundesverbandes Trans*. Berlin: Bundesvereinigung Trans* e.V.

Anzalduá, Gloria. 1987. *Borderlands: The New Mestiza = La Frontera*. Francisco: Aunt Lutem Books.

Clare, Eli. 2001. "Stolen Bodies, Reclaimed Bodies: Disability and Queerness." *Public Culture* 13(3): 359–366. https://doi.org/10.1215/08992363-13-3-359.

Clare, Eli. 2003. "Gawking, Gaping, Staring." *GLQ: A Journal of Lesbian and Gay Studies* 9(1): 257–261.

Columbia University Institute for Social and Economic Research and Policy. 2019. "Special Initiative on Integrating Biology and Social Science Knowledge (BioSS). Accessed January 11, 2023. https://iserp.columbia.edu/funding/special-initiative-integrating-biology-and-social-scienceknowledge-bioss.

Cruz, Melany, and Darcy Luke. 2020. "Methodology and Academic Extractivism: The Neo-Colonialism of the British University." *Third World Thematics: A TWQ Journal*, 5(1–2): 154–170. https://doi.org/10.1080/23802014.2020.1798275.

Ellis, Carolyn, Tony E. Adams, and Arthur P. Bochner. 2010. "Autoethnography: An Overview." *Forum Qualitative Sozialforschung/Forum: Qualitative Social Research*

12 (November, No. 1) (2011): 1–18. The KWALON Experiment: Discussions on Qualitative Data Analysis Software by Developers and Users. https://doi.org/10.17169/FQS-12.1.1589.

Enke, Anne. (ed.). 2012. *Transfeminist Perspectives in and Beyond Transgender and Gender Studies.* Philadelphia, PA: Temple University Press.

Feinberg, Leslie. 2003. *Stone Butch Blues.* Los Angeles, CA: Alyson Books.

GKV Spitzenverband, Medizinischer Dienst der Krankenkassen, and Medizinischer Dienst des Spitzenverbandes Bund der Krankenkassen. 2020. "Begutachtungsanleitung Geschlechtsangleichende Maßnahmen Bei Transsexualismus (ICD-10, F64.0)."

Jordan-Young, Rebecca M., and Katrina Karkazis. 2019. *Testosterone - An Unauthorized Biography.* Cambridge, MA: Harvard University Press. https://www.kulturkaufhaus.de/de/detail/ISBN-9780674725324/Jordan-Young-Rebecca-M./Testosterone---An-Unauthorized-Biography.

Latham, Jonathan R. 2017. "(Re)Making Sex: A Praxiography of the Gender Clinic." *Feminist Theory* 18(2): 177–204. https://doi.org/10.1177/1464700117700051.

Latham, Jonathan R. 2019. "Axiomatic: Constituting 'Transexuality' and Trans Sexualities in Medicine." *Sexualities* 22(1–2): 13–30. https://doi.org/10.1177/1363460717740258.

Liboiron, Max. 2021. *Pollution Is Colonialism.* Durham, NC: Duke University Press.

Mol, Annemarie. 2002. *The Body Multiple: Ontology in Medical Practice.* Durham, NC: Duke University Press.

Nelson, Maggie. 2016. *The Argonauts.* Minneapolis, MN: Graywolf Press.

Nieder, Timo O., and Bernhard Strauß. 2015. "Transgender Health Care in Germany: Participatory Approaches and the Development of a Guideline." *International Review of Psychiatry* 27(5): 416–426. https://doi.org/10.3109/09540261.2015.1074562.

Nieder, Timo O., and Bernhard Strauß. 2019. "S3-Leitlinie zur Diagnostik, Beratung und Behandlung im Kontext von Geschlechtsinkongruenz, Geschlechtsdysphorie und Trans-Gesundheit." *Zeitschrift für Sexualforschung* 32(02): 70–79. https://doi.org/10.1055/a-0895-8176.

Noble, J. Bobby. 2007. "Refusing to Make Sense: Mapping the In-Coherences of 'Trans.'" *Journal of Lesbian Studies* 11(1–2): 167–175. https://doi.org/10.1300/J155v11n01_13.

Noble, Bobby J. 2009a. "Trans Sex in the City: On the Terrors of the Trans Body." *Women & Environments International Magazine* 78/79: 12–14.

Noble, Bobby J. 2009b. "Trans-Culture in the (White) City: Taking a Pass on a Queer Neighbourhood." *Nomorepotlucks* (blog). https://profiles.laps.yorku.ca/profiles/bnoble/.

Nordmarken, Sonny. 2014. "Becoming Ever More Monstrous." *Qualitative Inquiry* 20(1): 37–50. https://doi.org/10.1177/1077800413508531.

Pearce, Ruth. 2016. *(Im)Possible Patients? Negotiating Discourses of Trans Health in the UK.* PhD, University of Warwick. https://wrap.warwick.ac.uk/id/eprint/88285/.

Preciado, Paul B. 2013. *Testo Junkie: Sex, Drugs, and Biopolitics in the Pharmacopornographic Era.* New York: The Feminist Press at the City University of New York.

Radi, Blas. 2019. "On Trans* Epistemology." *TSQ: Transgender Studies Quarterly* 6(1): 43–63. https://doi.org/10.1215/23289252-7253482.

Rosenberg, Jordy. 2019. *Confessions of the Fox.* London: Atlantic Books.

Saussure, Ferdinand de. 1974. *Course in General Linguistics.* London: Fontana/Collins.

Scialabba, George. 2018. *How to Be Depressed.* Scribd: University of Pennsylvania Press.

Spade, Dean. 2006. "Mutilating Gender." In *The Transgender Studies Reader*, edited by Susan Stryker and Stephan Whittle, 315–332. New York: Routledge.

Stewart, Dafina-Lazarus. 2017. "Trans*versing the DMZ: A Non-Binary Autoethnographic Exploration of Gender and Masculinity." *International Journal of Qualitative Studies in Education* 30(3): 285–304. https://doi.org/10.1080/09518398.2016.1254302.

Stone, Sandy. 2006. "The Empire Strikes Back: A Posttranssexual Manifesto." In *The Transgender Studies Reader*, edited by Susan Stryker and Stephan Whittle, 221–235. New York: Routledge.

Stryker, Susan, and Stephan Whittle. (eds). 2006. *The Transgender Studies Reader*. New York: Routledge.

Tudor, Alyosxa. 2017. "Dimensions of Transnationalism." *Feminist Review* 117(1): 20–40. https://doi.org/10.1057/s41305-017-0092-5.

Tudor, Alyosxa. 2021. "Decolonizing Trans/Gender Studies." *Transgender Studies Quarterly* 2 (8): 238–256.

Wiegman, Robyn. 2020. "Introduction: Autotheory Theory." *Arizona Quarterly: A Journal of American Literature, Culture, and Theory* 76(1): 1–14. https://doi.org/10.1353/arq.2020.0009.

# 12 I am not my MRI

*Maria Morata*

In 2015, pain suddenly entered my life.

Working as a freelance cultural producer in a foreign country, being a single mother and a woman in an ableist and competitive context repeatedly drained my energy and reserves. A thousand times I answered the question 'Have you been stressed lately?' It is one of the first questions you are automatically asked when the industrial health system takes you in and you start your medical odyssey.

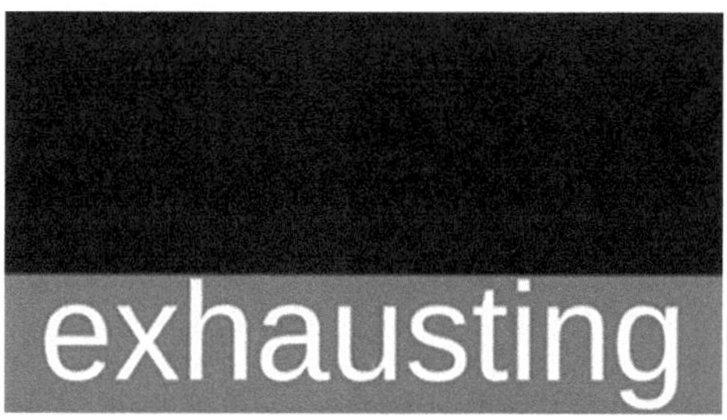


*Figure 12.1* Exhausting, still picture from video. Image credit © Daniele Lucchini

As the pain did not go away within the next three months, the period of time established by the medical-health protocols, it acquired a surname: chronic. It was a condemnation that I lived with for years as insurmountable, which destroyed my emotional and mental structure, and profoundly transformed my being in the world – in all of the worlds to which I had belonged until then. My relationship with pain was influenced by many factors, many agents, many opinions, and many therapies. But no diagnosis. Or, on the contrary, dozens of them, depending on the medical specialty that had assessed me and the frame through which my body was observed. Imaging technologies, governed by a normative, mechanical, and fragmented model of the body inherited from the Western anatomical tradition,[1] gave an account of the morphological and biochemical state of my entrails. Floating and isolated organs, incognisant of their neighbouring tissues and glands, oblivious to shared hormonal storms, were observed and represented by epistemological

DOI: 10.4324/9781032660165-21

spyglasses, looking straight ahead, further, deeper, with more resolution but losing track of the borders, the interactions, the frictions. I can only attest to what the medical anthropologist Francisco Ortega states in his book *El cuerpo incierto* ('The Uncertain Body', 2010) when he observes that this process of fragmentation, inscribed in the culture of the single unique organ, annuls the power of resistance of bodies, disconnecting them from their own phenomenological experience.

*Figure 12.2* Three, still picture from video. Image credit © Daniele Lucchini

The dismantling and depletion of the self occurs subtly through the division of the body into medical specialities, spatially and geographically disseminated in so many waiting rooms of myriad consultants. This continuous back-and-forth deactivated in me not only the perception of my own body but also the truth of my symptoms. They were always under scrutiny and often questioned, or simply ignored as pathology because they were not included in the *vade mecum* totem that rested on the shelves of the consulting rooms and in the minds of many of the doctors I met along the way.

During the first years of this new period of life, I was very far from conceiving of my somatic and mental state as the spiritual change that Virginia Woolf (2012, 3) spoke of in her essay 'On Being Ill' (1930). Very slowly, I am managing to travel with curiosity through 'the undiscovered countries that are disclosed when the lights of health go down'.

Before engaging in my ongoing dialogue with pain, I was dimly aware of the collective, normative, and neoliberal illusion of taking for granted the healthy body that the Mexican philosopher Marco Sanz (2020) claims as one of the theorems of illness. But my illumination was momentary, swiftly extinguished when the temporary discomfort disappeared, fluidity returned to my vital functions, and silence was restored to my organs, a silence that René Leriche (1936) conceived of as health.[2]

The chronicity that settled in my body, the continuous scream and agitation of my nociceptive neurons, made me become familiar with my own fragility and adopt it as a new territory of exploration. My constant encounters with the medical system meant that when I read Jean-Luc Nancy's *L'intrus* ('The Intruder'), not only my thoughts but also my organs resonated with his feeling of 'no longer being dissociable from a network of measurements, of observations, of chemical, institutional and symbolic connections, which cannot be ignored, as can be those of which ordinary life is always woven' (Nancy 2002, 12).

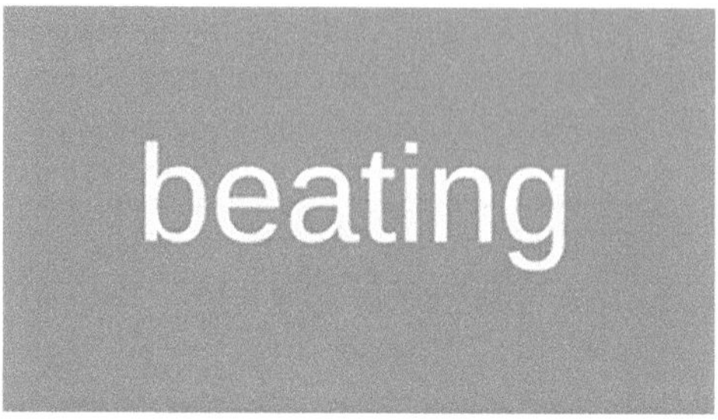


*Figure 12.3* Beating, still picture from video. Image credit © Daniele Lucchini

Chronic pain is not visible. There is no organic, biological, or visual indicator for it beyond the rudimentary Visual Analogue Scale for Pain Intensity (Hayes and Patterson 1921) or the reductionist but scattered McGill Pain Questionnaire (Melzack and Torgerson 1971), which is still in use today. The former is based on a score from 0 to 10: 0 for *no pain at all* and 10 for *worst pain imaginable*. These scores are usually accompanied by coloured smilies, from green to red. The second assesses both the quality and intensity of subjective pain through 78 descriptor words with numerical values, classified into 20 groups.

The results showed no visible traces of organic damage in my body: MRI with no pathogenic signs. It's only in the head. Only in your head.

It's your brain that's producing the pain, or rather it's your brain 'who' is producing the pain. Decades ago, we entered the neurocentric paradigm of science that states that my brain is me. That I am my brain.

Sorry, it's your head.
Sorry, it's your soul, your past, your life.
It is you.
It's your fault.

Nothing but my words could testify that my world was falling apart. But without confirmation from the medical data or legitimation from the technical images that occasionally illuminated the black box of my body, my words were of little value in establishing a diagnosis. And very often they did not even serve to communicate as expected with the nurses, medical students, general practitioners, neurologists, psychologists, psychiatrists, osteopaths, and physiotherapists. My words were not able to articulate my knots, nor could they describe my aching body cramped with fear and anguish. Elaine Scarry already pointed out the fact of the inexpressiveness of pain in her book *The Body in Pain. The Making and Unmaking of the World.* She states, 'Physical pain does not simply resist language but actively destroys it, bringing about an immediate reversion to a state anterior to language, to the sounds and cries human being makes before language is learned' (Scarry 1985, 4). To

Scarry's eloquent prose, I can only add that the exhaustion caused by chronic pain and the accumulated frustration of encounters with the medical system contributed as much to the destruction of my language as the pain itself.

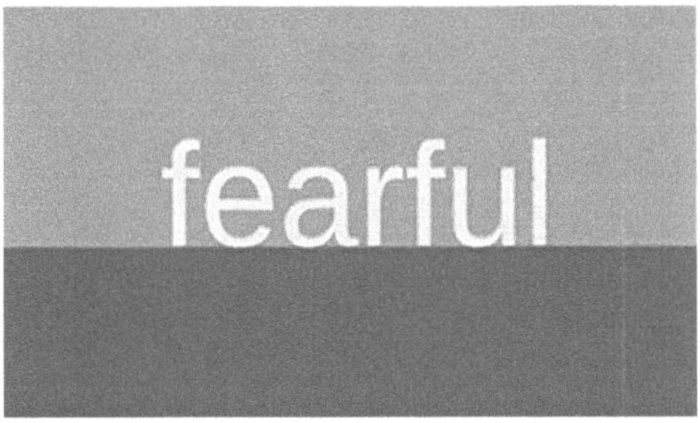


*Figure 12.4* Fearful, still picture from video. Image credit © Daniele Lucchini

I no longer had a voice. I disappeared behind my medical records and my health card. I was just a sick body without a label, spending all my time and energy looking for a name, a treatment, or a solution. I thought I had to be admitted into the realm of Diagnosis. To be a product of this authoritarian naming gesture from the ivory tower of non-intersectional clinical research (Wilson et al. 2019), which ignores the complex overlapping of race, gender, sexuality, education, religion, age, and other identity markers, I thought I was ready to be stamped with the validation of the medical apparati: both ideological and technical.

I longed for those two or three Greek or Latin words of a diagnosis that should give me some proof and legitimation of the existence of my pain – and with it my own existence, because I, all of me, was nothing but pain.

I was quickly classified as a psychosomatic patient. No visible or quantifiable evidence of suffering could be encoded in the figures of my haematogram, in some suspicious shadows of the X-rays, or in the out-of-range coloured areas of my MRI scans. Filled with hope about the possibility of saving my soul and thus saving my body, I entered the military-sanitary regime of psychosomatic clinics. But the well-intentioned mind-body medicine betrayed me, too. I spent weeks walking corridors from one therapy to another, eating suspicious food and feeling in my brain the 24/7 lights-on in the hospital. The promising multimodal approach that was meant to bring my scattered spirit and aching body together in a healing alliance turned out to be a fruitless, confused, and isolated accumulation. Several therapists used old protocols and rusty methods on the ideal patient who starred in their medical learning books, forgetting about my diversity, my deviation, my specific biological and social body. Frustration was served up. In infantilising hours of art therapy, I did, however, learn to weave wicker baskets, to make collective collages of flowers, kittens, and kissing mouths out of old gossip magazines, and to model with clay the animal I identify with. By the way, the animal I identify with is a jellyfish. It is a mixture of my deep desire to be graceful and to liquidly cross the world and the reality of being under constant electrical and chemical nociceptive signals.

Looking for metaphors is both a cultural and rhetorical vice used to approach the incomprehensible, the sublime, and the unspeakable, and a perverse way to

*Figure 12.5* Seventeen, still picture from video. Image credit © Daniele Lucchini

reduce complexities and find social scapegoats, as Susan Sontag denounced in her essay *Illness as Metaphor* (1978). What did my medusa mean then? What social and personal ills did my chronic pain hide?

It was only some time after these Foucauldian experiences with and within the clinic that I was able to immerse myself and float in the words of the philosopher Paul B. Preciado as if they were my own amniotic fluid. Just Beatriz when he started to inspire me with this text, he proposes to think of the body as *Somateca*:

> As a network of organs managed by different biopolitical regimes determined by a set of discursive, epistemological, scientific, pharmacological, economic and visual practices, through immigration and risk management policies, clinical trials, pharmacological techniques, diagnostic practices, media narratives, discursive networks, visual representations and discourses of prevention, control and surveillance.
>
> (Preciado 2013)

My non-disease and my non-diagnosis depend on the technological moment in which I live. Both are contingent on the power-informed visual archaeology which ended up applied to the machines of the clinical system; on the lenses, the frequencies, the rare earth metals that allow chips, memories, and digital systems to live; on the cables; on the thickness of the slices in which my body is scanned, the angles of reflection of light and electrons; on the shock of the magnets that run through me and draw me in a palette of coded electronic colours.

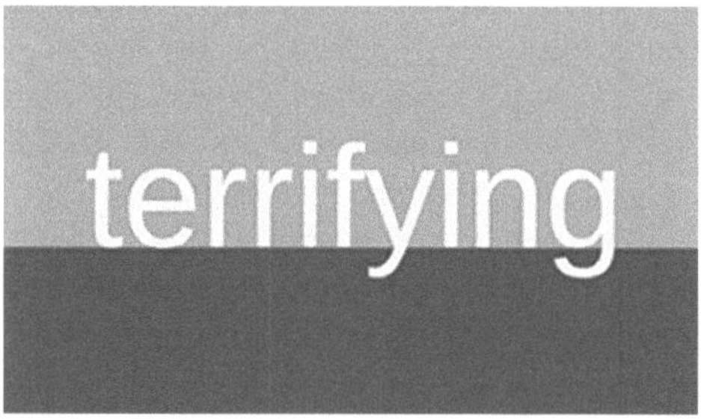


*Figure 12.6* Terrifying, still picture from video. Image credit © Daniele Lucchini

A metallic and mechanical reiki.

An energy emitted at regular programmed intervals, running through me and aligning the molecules and atoms of my organs so that they pose properly in the snapshot of the tomography, of the resonance, of the ultrasound. A magnetic moment of the water contained in my body. The protons of my hydrogen atoms going through an electromagnetic field and becoming tiny magnets that spin, move slightly, and re-emit energy when released. It will be only one of the thousands of still images that will become data, and then fact, then interpretation, and then truth.

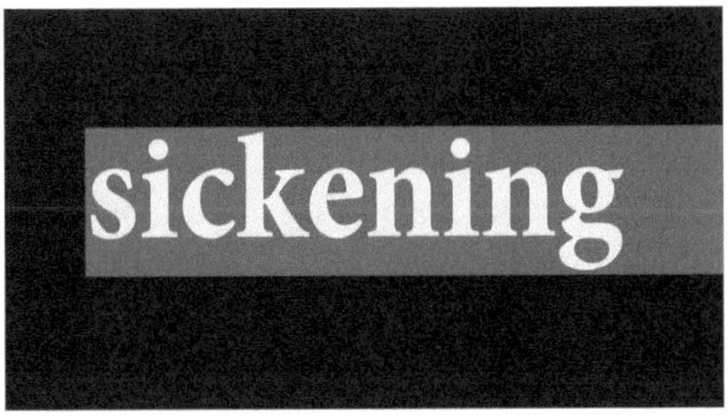


*Figure 12.7* Sickening, still picture from video. Image credit © Daniele Lucchini

Framing, sectioning, fragmenting, slicing the body. Looking for the right field of view. The one which seems to matter. Don't breathe, don't swallow, don't let your heart beat, so the fragile image is readable and becomes a high-quality one. Let the machine create the authoritative knowledge about your body, out of your body.

The echoes of those very small energy displacements translate my tissues, bones, blood vessels, and nerves of my inner me into a technical image. The luminous trace of my body after being magnetised claims to see me without cutting my flesh, but still penetrates my secret, constantly moving humidities. The silent medical image delivered by my body did not fit in the validating diagnostic machinery, which was in charge of revealing the secrets and alterations of my organic life. Body and metals. Technology and flesh. A hierarchical encounter of two black boxes, the one of my body and the one of the imaging machine. An asymmetrical conversation between the unavoidable visual noise of the machine and the pathological noise of my body.

How and when were the normal and desirable values for my body established? Who validated them? In which context, and for whom were they corroborated? Where are the shifts, the displacements, the differences from a me of whom there were no records before? Me, compared to normative and standard anatomies. Are my variations aberrations? False negatives, false positives?

Was my MRI not telling the truth? Was this truth incomplete? What questions have been asked of this image of myself? What did this image say about me? In which language was my MRI addressed? My technical image supplanted me in a dialogue with the health system. What if MRI reading and interpreting are still under the influence of a long photographic scientific culture that attributes to those images the authority of being proof of evidence and truth?

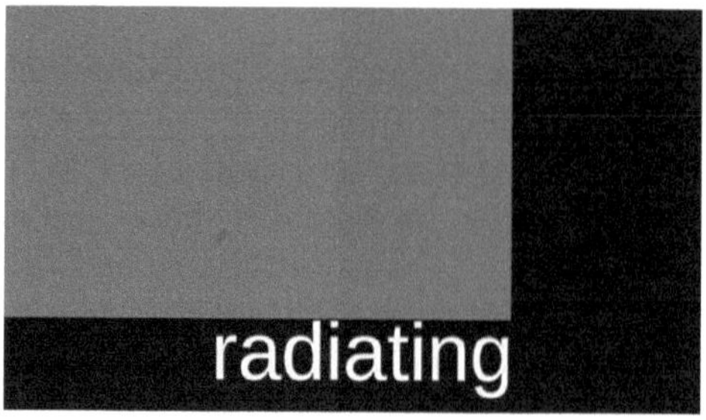


*Figure 12.8* Radiating, still picture from video. Image credit © Daniele Lucchini

MRIs are not unmediated images that provide direct access to my inner body, creating the illusion of image and flesh being interchangeable. They are not neutral, nor are they equivalent to the physical body. A complex cascade of technical operations occurs in the construction of the readable MRI image, which has to be manipulated, corrected, attuned, and calibrated attending to codes of colour, image resolution, and the quality of the machine itself. Body and image are both related, co-constitutive, entangled with many other human and non-human actors in which decisions, agents, values, interpretation, layers of translation, construction, and codification are not revealing the body but creating it.

Seeing does not equal knowing the truth, as medical and scientific methods are not free of bias. Thus, my MRI is not immune to instability or opacity, and neither it is a photograph of the *camera obscura* that is my body. I cannot recognise myself visually in my MRI. Pain has made me attentive to the somatic experience of my body at every moment and this proprioception does not yet know how to dialogue with the MRI image that the machine produces from the aligned atoms of my entrails. The ocularcentrism of science creates a visualisation of my interior that does not correspond to how I feel it. The MRI thereby becomes a fetish image, in which I must believe without understanding, and to which I must subscribe powers, wisdoms, and dogmas from the scientific religion. The clinic is the only one who has access to the tools and technologies that portray me, the only one who knows and controls their codes of interpretation. My tissues and their howls dance to the sound of the medical, technical-scientific paradigm of their time.

## Notes

1 Andreas Vesalius, a Flemish anatomist and physician, published in 1543 *De humani corporis fabrica, libri septem* ('On the structure of the human body in seven books'), a beautifully illustrated volume introducing a new anatomical paradigm based on a culture of dissection. Vesalius let the corpse speak for the living body, opened up the flesh to apply cartography to the human body, and placed the visual at the centre of the scientific knowledge. The path for the pathological anatomy was open, and rapidly claimed as the objective basis for the western clinic method, as Foucault points out and criticises in *The Birth of the Clinic* (1963). Sickness resides now in concrete, visible, and localised lesions inside the body, which explain the symptoms, a truth produced through the objectivity of medical science, an objectivity which I try to disarticulate from my experience.

2 The French surgeon René Leriche (1936) wrote: 'Health is life lived in the silence of the organs' ('La santé c'est la vie dans le silence des organes'). This statement was contested by some members of the scientific community, as pathology can be silent and invisible. Leriche argued that he was speaking from the patient's perspective. I esonated with this empathetic form of speaking as me being an aching body (quoted in Canguilhem 1978, 91).

This text is part of a reading performance realised while projecting and speaking out loud the 78 descriptor words, classified in 20 groups, of the McGill Pain Questionnaire developed by Dr Ronald Melzack and Dr Warren Torgerson in 1971 at McGill University, Montréal, Canada. It was presented at the Conference Violence, Care, Cure: (Self) perceptions within the Medical Encounter, ICI Berlin, 3–4 February 2022.
*Video performance:*
*Concept: Maria Morata*
*Video: Daniele Lucchini*
*Text proofreader: Stassja Mrozinski*
*Speaker descriptor words: Nadja Kolb*

## References


Canguilhem, Georges. 1991. "The Conceptions of René Leriche." In *On the Normal and the Pathological* (1978), 91–102. New York: Zone Books.

Hayes, Mary Holmes Stevens, and Patterson, Donald Gildersleeve. 1921. "Experimental Development of the Graphic Rating Method." *Psychological Bulletin* 18: 98–99.

Leriche, René. 1936. *Encyclopédie Française,* Vol 6. Paris: Société de Gestion de l'Encyclopédie Française.

Melzack, Ronald, and Warren S. Torgerson. 1971. "On the Language of Pain." *Anesthesiology* 34: 50–59.

Nancy, Jean-Luc. 2002. "*L'Intrus,* trans. Susan Hanson." *CR: The New Centennial Review* 2(3): 1–14.

Ortega, Francisco. 2010. *El cuerpo incierto: corporeidad, tecnologías médicas y cultura contemporánea,* Vol. 57. Madrid: Consejo Superior de Investigaciones Científicas, CSIC Press.

Preciado, Paul B. 2013. *Somateca. Producción biopolítica, feminismos, prácticas queer y trans*. Introductory text for the course held by Preciado. Programa de Estudios Avanzados en Prácticas Críticas. Museo Reina Sofia, Madrid. https://www.museoreinasofia.es/sites/default/files/actividades/programas/somateca_dossier_actualizado_1.pdf.

Sanz, Marco. 2020. *La emancipación de los cuerpos. Teoremas críticos sobre la enfermedad.* Madrid: Akal.

Scarry, Elaine. 1985. *The Body in Pain. The Making and Unmaking of the World*. New York: Oxford University Press.

Sontag, Susan. 1978. *Illness as Metaphor*. New York: Farrar, Straus, and Giroux.

Wilson, Yolanda, Amina White, Akilah Jefferson, and Danis Marion. 2019. "Intersectionality in Clinical Medicine: The Need for a Conceptual Framework." *The American Journal of Bioethics* 19(2): 8–19.

Woolf, Virginia. 2012. *On Being Ill* (1930). Ashfield, MA: Paris Press.

# 13 Surprised by the night

## On the traversal of a dysphoric phantasy

*Myriam Sauer*

### A preliminary note

In this chapter, I explore the lived experience of gender dysphoria. My understanding of dysphoria differs from that of conventional psychology. The DSM, for instance, characterises dysphoria as 'the marked incongruence between one's experienced/expressed gender and primary or secondary sex characteristics', being linked to the 'strong desire' for the 'other sex's bodily or psychic characteristics' (APA 2013, 452).

I argue instead that dysphoria is a profound sensual ravaging that accompanies transitioning. It is not something to be overcome or fully left behind. There is no beyond to it, but neither is there a 'before', a place prior to it. Rather, the immanent becoming of trans life is suffused by dysphoria – as growth pain and as a reminder to slow down and return to the calm shores of holding.

I will be switching between prose and theory segments, though these two are not always clearly delimited. It is not so much auto-theory as unsovereign writing; that is to say, it is psychoanalytic writing that eschews the sovereign act of externalising into a clearly delimited subject the travails and tribulations it seeks to understand. Although for purposes of Illustration I will invoke 'Anna', a fictional character, the text itself is dysphoric rather than contained by her. What I am presenting here is not a coherent theory or a systematic exposition. It may be best understood as a map to the trans feminine psychoanalytic understanding of dysphoria. It opens up understanding rather than foreclosing it through systematic exposition.

### Exposure

You traverse a park of modest size, easily accessible from the outside and popular among tourists. You attempt to minimise your considerable physical presence, lest the eyes of cisgender people find and locate you, and address you in a male way. As you see a number of British men approaching, overhearing them referring to each other as 'mates', you start to get apprehensive and try to hide what little of your face is not already covered in hair. Eventually, as they draw closer and do notice you, you cannot help but perceive their curious looks as ridicule. When one of them turns to you, you are now all but certain that the explosion is about to take place. You hear him utter in perfect equanimity, 'excuse

DOI: 10.4324/9781032660165-22

me, do you know where we can find an ATM?', upon which you offer him directions and then leave immediately. The explosion *does take place* – for while the stranger did not gender you incorrectly, you find your entire appearance, most crucially your voice, to be deeply revealing of a lapse before existence itself. A psychodrama, non-transparent to your surroundings, plays out repeatedly in your head. Your mind generates endless replays of your encounter with the British men; in some you are variously humiliated, but in others you are also given an opportunity to actually explain that as a trans woman you find this encounter terrifying. The latter phantasy operates as trauma compensation. Through it, you can stage the resolution of the conflict intrapsychically and establish what was not possible in material reality: the interpersonal resolution and holding of your pain by others.

Later at home, exhausted from your experiences, you decide to go to bed early. As you come to realise that a cough is building up inside of you, you freeze in terror, desperately trying to hold off its production, since you anticipate it to be sonically male. Eventually you do cough repeatedly, sending shockwaves of unease across the body, which loses its coherence and deeper signification, becoming a goo of painful associations and references. Memories of gendered violence experienced as a child evolve into consciousness, and the body flares up, with little fires being created everywhere, which eventually turn into somatic conflagration – a pyromania that eats up the internal psychic structures by corrupting your sense of intimacy. The internalisation of transphobic violence has yielded an internal object world that is destructive and which, if triggered, can tip you into a state of annihilation, where the phantasy of self-destruction marks the final attempt at saving yourself from the self: psychic suicide, which offers at least the promise that the pain will no longer be. Phantasies of self-mutilation intrude into your consciousness: what if you were to reach into your throat and rip out the vocal cords, right here, right now, forever saving yourself from the scourge of living through this pain.

'Please, I cannot', you whimper.

Recognising that the house is on fire and cannot be saved, your attention is seduced by the beckoning call of the abyss. Minutes pass, then hours, and when you wake up, having spent what little sleep you did get in a hazy fog, you are drenched in sweat.

You get out of bed, unsure where to move next. You make your way to the bathroom, where you look into the mirror.

'Avert your eyes', you tell yourself, but then you linger on, staying with the specular image, a reflection of yourself that offers you solace.

'That is really me', you think.

Your eyes examine every pore of your face, trying to find a deceptive impurity, a sign of masculine deformity, yet nothing quite remains in your mind's eye, nothing that would reveal your existence as mistake. You are reminded of the caressing gaze of strangers and of lovers, the carefreeness you gift yourself. You remain transfixed by the beauty of your face, which is only intensified by a brief smile. You step into the shower and let the hot water cleanse your body.

## Explorations

In what follows I will be exploring some of the elements of the prose sketch above, which takes us through a series of events in the life of its protagonist, Anna. What I offer are no more than scattered thoughts generated through reading, personal experiences, and conversations with other trans people. I have two central arguments two make: (1) dysphoria interrupts and modulates the act of knowing; and (2) dysphoria produces a dehiscence of the self. Both of these belong together, and so they need to be elaborated upon in an entangled way.

When speaking of dehiscence, I am borrowing a concept from Jacques Lacan, and when speaking of the interruption of knowing, I have a concept by Wilfred Bion in mind. Dehiscence refers to the opening of a wound. Lacan (1966) uses this concept to express the idea that the psyche can never be properly sutured, and is instead always on the verge of being undone. Bion's understanding of knowing is based upon a distinction between two modes of engaging with the world and its events: by either observing them in an omniscient, manic and paranoid way, or by giving oneself over to the complexity of that world, without immediately insisting on a resolution of that complexity into a positive result. Bion (2014b, 327–328) calls this 'negative capability', a state of mind that is capable of enduring the non-resolution of internal conflict.

Two interrelated questions thus emerge: (1) what does it mean to sustain an act of knowing? and (2) what are the implications of diremption for subject-constitution? Both Bion and Lacan have each in their own way explored these questions, though with little attention being paid to trans issues. I will utilise some of their ideas and bring them to bear on the vignette above, in order to better understand Anna's internal life.

## Imagination

Central to dysphoria is the act of phantasying and engaging in imaginative work. Anna relies heavily on imaginative work both to suture the wound of dysphoria – such as when she encounters herself in the mirror – and to open it. This see–saw of wound-tending is central to the dysphoric condition; it bespeaks a deeper dehiscence of the self. The phantasies that seize Anna are not products of a sovereign mind in the way one may fantasise intentionally about, say, an elephant flying through the room. Phantasy overwhelms and undercuts sovereignty, and as such it draws us closer to an abyssal undoing of being. Phantasy is an intensification of fantasy, because it undoes sovereign control over ourselves. It operates an enabling violence in the sense that it suspends our omnipotent hold on our being while simultaneously being prone to reinscribing a claustric state of mind.

Our phantasies are never fully our own, because phantasies are formations of the unconscious, and our unconscious does not belong to us. Phantasies in that sense lock us in by locking us out: they generate a profound intensity of feeling that comes from outside. The contents, operations, and effects of the unconscious slip away from our conscious grasp, and thereby create a kind of psychic drift that turns our own actions and feelings into something that overwhelms and undermines.

It is in this sense that Freud (1966) notes that 'the ego is not the master in its own house'. We are slipping away from the grasp we have over ourselves, and this fact of slipping away is intensely anxiety-inducing.

The consequence of such anxiety is that we are often in a state of 'minus K', as Bion (2018, 154–155) put it, a state in which we are incapable of wanting to know; thus, we resort to omniscience and the regained omnipotence of phantasy. In her encounter with the British men, Anna faces something she cannot quite understand, something she is unwilling to confront, and this *something* has less to do with the British men as such but rather what they stand for in a larger context: the British men metonymise the patriarchal law.

Once this encounter has taken place, there occurs a shift in her state of mind. Whereas before there was a hesitant interest in learning from experience, the objects she faces quickly become internalised as bad objects, and she starts to engage in a frantic evacuation of them. Her curiosity for learning turns haywire, and her act of knowing turns omniscient: everything she sees and feels is the result of a paranoid-schizoid mind, the contingency of her situation is turned into a definite one, and all the ambivalent signs are turned into foreboding ones. This kind of self-fulfilling prophecy offers a tenuous stability in that it is a familiar space to inhabit, one in which all signs do add up to a meaningful message, one that she is well acquainted with. That message is, 'you are condemned'. This message of condemnation invades her proprioceptive capabilities, and reworks them so that sensuality itself becomes painful.

The loss of knowing leads to the introduction of knowledge. A shift from untrammelled perception to epistemological absoluteness occurs. Knowing requires a special type of sustenance that is as easily gained as it is lost. The real issue of Anna is therefore one of sustenance, of being able to do two things at once: sustaining her act of knowing while being sustained by the other. It means both to endure the frustration of unclear vision and to be embraced by the other as holding and loving.

I believe what is behind these dysphoric feelings is a shattered form of psychosocial attachment; as such, it concerns the other, and its presence in our lives. More specifically, it concerns the *somatisation of this alterity*.

## The Other and the body

Our daily lives are conducted with the assumptions that bodies are to be shaped and reformed in line with the regnant pharmaco-pornographic scheme (Preciado 2013). Paul Preciado invented this concept to refer to a particular constellation of pharmaceutical – hormones, drugs, food – and pornographic objects that have a direct impact on what kind of bodies we find desirable. Bodies are to be optimised in accordance with the images we gather every day through seeing advertisements, through the porn we are watching secretly, or the Other that we are being confronted with in spite of all of our protestations in a Berlin club: beautiful and perfect, drenched in a glistening sweat that magnetises our gazes. I am capitalising 'Other' here to make a larger conceptual point indebted to Lacan. Lacan (1991) distinguished two types of others: the small one, which is a result of our projections, and the big one, which exceeds our understanding and constitutes a form of radical alterity. When I am studying the delicate corporeal contortions of the stranger across the dance floor, *identifying* him (or her, or them; I am not imposing, merely admiring – or am I?) as the object of my desire, then I am turning him into the other, since I allow my identificatory perceptions of him to overdetermine him in his being. In that sense, my encounter with this stranger recalls what Kristeva (1982) would refer to as abjection – my own being is grounded in having cast aside certain traits, corporealities, or genders when I reached a certain critical infantile juncture, and now, as I am being confronted with this Other against all my aspirations, my psyche unwinds.

Lacan urged us to move away from this tendency and bear something in mind when we are observing the Other. He exhorted us to ask ourselves, '*Che vuoi?*' (Italian for 'What do you want?'), an expression Lacan took from a novel by Jacques Cazotte (1871, [1772]). Here, as part of a summoning ritual, the protagonist faces the devil, who appears first as a camel and then as a dog. As the devil approaches the protagonist Alvaro, noticing his trepidation, he amusedly asks him, 'Che vuoi? Che vuoi?'

Alvaro stares at him flabbergasted and musters no more than a few words as response, before eventually collecting himself and telling the devil that he wants to possess him. Fascinated by Alvaro, the devil falls in love with him. He changes shape again, turning into a beautiful woman by the name of Biondetta, who will follow the protagonist – in the beginning as a cross-dressing servant by the name of Biondetto, before eventually settling into her feminine persona. As they grow closer, the protagonist is more and more consumed by Biondetta, who is asking him to truly love her: 'I may only have been a woman for six months', she notes at one point in a decidedly trans feminine fashion, 'but this is who I am, and you must love me'. Biondetta's ulterior motive is to seduce and sleep with Alvaro before their marriage, despite the protagonist steadfastly rejecting her advances in order to project his virginity *and* respect his mother's wish that he only marry a woman she has seen beforehand and accepted as her son's wife.

It is a curious little story, which ends with the devil failing to seduce Alvaro. In a dramatic final scene, they are sitting bedside with Biondetta talking to Alvaro with great urgency, trying to convince him to love her. Alvaro is increasingly persuaded by her, until Biondetta asks him to tell her the following, 'Oh Beelzebub, I love you with all my heart'. Alvaro freezes in terror, upon which a camel peeks through a window, asking them: *Che vuoi?*

Alvaro is mortified by these events – rather understandably, I might add – and hides under his bed. After a while, he returns from his hiding spot and lies in his bed all alone, to be found by a friend hours later, who informs him that Biondetta is gone. They give chase to find her, yet she seems to have vanished from the face of the earth. Alvaro returns to his parents' mansion, where he finds his mother telling him that as long as he listens to his mother, no devil will ever find and consume him.

*The devil in love* was one of the first so-called 'fantasy stories', stories in which it is unclear whether certain events actually took place in the narrative or had been phantasied by the protagonist. They offer a formidable backdrop for the larger question of desire and knowing the other. Can we ever truly understand our phantasies? Would a camel really peek through the window and ask someone in Italian 'What do you want?'

Here is a phantasy of my own: the devil is a trans woman.

The story itself, certainly if read in a Lacanian key, need not be read in this way. After all, the devil merely assumes the *masquerade of femininity*, to seduce the young man who responds by way of *parade* (*parade* in French can also mean 'parry'), rebuffing the Other's beguiling advances, asserting his autonomy from the embrace of trans femininity. I am reproducing this story here because it illustrates how phantasy is its own seduction, and that getting lost in it is its own flight, an escape from the impositions of ideology. Why not allow the Other to enter one's phantasy rather than protecting oneself through Oedipal recourse by calling on the mother. What if there is something awaiting us if maternal possession is abandoned in lieu of a devilish playfulness?

Lacan shies away from allowing himself to be given over to trans femininity's undoing force, insisting instead on the might of the cis-masculine phallus. In some later seminars, to this he adds a number of openly transphobic screeds (Lacan 2007, 2011), where he denounces trans femininity as essentially psychotic. Lacan's transphobia points to a larger problem that one is faced with when doing psychoanalysis as a trans person, a problem that Claude Kempen discusses as well in this volume. The archive is riddled with such violent acts, and yet we are presented with few alternatives. Our way must somehow pass through the archive, animated by the realisation that there are no purities in it. Partially others may step in (Klein, Winnicott, Bion), and partially we are to err all alone, inside and outside of the hegemonic psychoanalytic archive.

So, while Lacan gives us the idea of a radically different Other, he is not the one to show us how to sustain a trans feminine engagement with this radical Other. This is because the Other's devilishness is not merely about unspeakable confrontation, instead alerting us to our insecurities, and opening up a kind of chasm in ourselves that threatens to suck away our attempts at masquerade *and* parade. In this sense – and this is a central claim of this chapter – we are dehiscent at the hands of the Other. Read alongside the Bionian question about sustaining the act of knowing, the essence of dysphoria becomes clearer: *dysphoria interrupts and modulates our attempts at sustaining to know, since we are dehiscent at the hands of the Other.*

However, what is so 'devastating' about this? Its devastating quality stems from the fact that we are not sovereign and that our manifold attempts at resolving this issue of non-sovereignty through hallucinations of potency lack a deeper foundation: all power is illusion. If we are faced with the Other as unbearable confrontation, something that frustrates us so much that we cannot bear to take it in, we proceed to spoil the good object. Envy animates the urge to destroy a good object (Klein 1975, 181). What we cannot bear we turn into an object of our own doing, thereby re-asserting our own potency. We gain omnipotence by reconfiguring through fantasy, for our fantasy belongs entirely to ourselves. Thus enters the small other into our perception, preventing us from facing the transformative capability of the big Other. This intrusion leads to the foreclosure of desire, and its replacement with a mental state inimical to knowing.

Much of this is at work with Anna. She tries to see and understand what is happening to her, but as she is approaching the British men, everything becomes certain: she will fail, she will crash, the explosion will take place – *No.Matter. What.* Dehiscence as a non-foundational experience of subjectivity becomes phobic (what if I cannot suture my inner woundedness?), and so her mind steps in to protect her from sustaining the act of knowing. This is one element of dysphoria.

Dehiscence as a phobic experience is not unique to trans people but rather informs most people's lives, because it touches upon the problem of castration and impotency. To be without potency means to have lost control; it means to become a passive object. To renounce potency is to be at odds with the imperative of taking control over one's body. However, what would it mean to insist on a radically unsovereign body, and to dissolve into the stream of life?

For hegemonic psychoanalysis, which seeks structure through Oedipus, the renunciation of power and of sovereignty would mean chaos. A crucial aspect of Lacanian psychoanalysis is the relationship of the mother and the father, as well as their relationship to castration. Lacan views the mother as overwhelming and potentially dangerous to the child. It is only the father who can prevent the destruction of the child's fledgling sense of symbolic belonging by introducing the name-of-the-father into the child's life, thereby quashing the phantasy of the imaginatively omnipotent phallic mother and securing the symbolic's reliance on metaphor. The father says to the child, 'No, you may not have the mother, and she in fact cannot give you everything anyway' – thereby codifying desire as inherently lacking.

I would like to offer a modified version of this argument. Lacan's transformation of Klein's epistemology of phantasy, in which all mental contents are primarily phantasmatic ones, is profound in that it opens up psychoanalytic thinking to the real and the symbolic as spheres that are distinct from phantasy. However, Lacan – much like Klein – also grafts their formation onto the psychodrama of Oedipal family relations. It seems urgent to me, however, to problematise this Oedipal dependency without altogether throwing out the aspect of holding and attachment. The absence of internalised caretakers and a frail sense of egoic belonging enable transformation, but they can also lead to subjective ruination. Sustained and safe intimacy enables attachment, and intimacy with one's internal objects is established through phantasy. All intimacy is auto-affection – self-touch. To be intimate with oneself is to receive touch from oneself, whether that be through one's fingers, one's own piercing or loving gaze, or one's voice. It is a form of *auto-affection*, in the sense that we affect ourselves and create an internal tension that is emotionally charged. However, can we survive this affective tension?

For Anna, it is the experience of her voice as a seemingly foreign element that perturbs her and intensifies the counterphobia of belonging. It is her specular image and her gaze that offer her solace. Anna experiences her own voice – even her coughing – as masculine, because unconsciously, self-touch, here by the voice, is shot through with transphobic violence, and as such constitutes a form of violence against the self. It is because Anna experienced past intimacy as ungendering, alienating, and foreign to her sensibilities that intimacy both with others and with herself is fractured and painful. Dysphoria may be translated literally here as the unbearable, that which cannot be endured or borne.

In her imagination, she returns to intimacy when contemplating herself in the mirror. The possibility of self-induced wholesome intimacy marks a kind of redemption, a true relief from suffering. It asks her to be capable of sustaining the act of knowing. It means abandoning what André Green (2009) has termed the central phobic position, a state of mind similar to that of the Bionian -K, in which the mind dismisses all new ideas and contents. The phobia is of thinking itself, of actually allowing the unconscious to come to the fore, and dwelling with its contents. If phobia is about panic, about bodies brought into an omniscient state of self-evacuation, then the rare moments of philia gleaned in the introspective moments of mirroring are what keep Anna alive. Her gaze is unperturbed by the unconscious' various formations, because the visual offers her a sense of respite; therein are contained insights, which taken together make up the first elements of healthier nourishment. Psychoanalysis' terms for nourishment are those of introjection and projection, and within Kleinian analysis, what we eat and excrete are objects. Yet, not all objects have a rigorous objective quality; many of them are secrets, *even to us*.

It is perhaps in this sense that dysmorphia – a condition held to be 'repetitive behaviours' of bodily self-examination and obsession (DSM-5: 242–243) – can have a meaning in the context of object-dealing. Dysmorphia then would refer to an unmetabolisable object, which we either hide in a space that is exempt from metabolisation or spit out immediately, so as to prevent its consequences. More generally, dysmorphia is the act of inhabiting one's formlessness which was produced violently, and that is now recast as improperly sovereign.

If dysmorphia is a formlessness of objects, then dysphoria refers to the friction of these processes of metabolisation, and euphoria names those moments, where the phobia of thinking gives way to the pleasure found in engaging the story of life that is never fully finished, an infinite poem sung by the Other. Not all signs are foreboding ones – we are allowed the freedom of love.

## The holding of dysphoric pain

I want to bring our attention to a paper by the psychoanalyst Esther Bick. Bick (2011) extended Klein's understanding of the mind by suggesting that there is a state of 'mental unintegration' that children can fall into when they lack a certain type of care. In this state, nothing coheres into functioning mental principles, and the child is sealed off into what I would call a *crypt of indiscriminate screaming*. It is a non-relational state, one in which the truths of trauma are disallowed from entering our relational understanding and holding.

In this chapter, Bick relates the following vignette, detailing work with a four-year-old girl by the name of Mary. We learn that she was extremely aggressive and would often destroy objects in her surroundings. She came in 'hunched' and 'stiff-jointed', and appeared like 'a sack of potatoes', a phrase that Mary later used herself. Bick's (2011, 136) argument is that the sack of potatoes was a second skin, which 'seemed in constant danger of spilling out its contents', and which existed in lieu of her own muscularity, so that the introduction of a containing object let to an improvement in Mary's situation. I use this argument here to expand on the original sketch of Anna, specifically her frantic attempts to hold together her own mental contents. That Mary would choose the sack of potatoes as a replacement for a somatic grounding in her own being strikes me as reminiscent of Anna's attempts to locate in the other both an absolute phobia and a yearning for being held. It is precisely because she does not experience her own skin (and ears) as capable of auto-affection and intimacy that she seeks to projectively identify certain of her unbearable affects with the phantasy of other cis people being threatening, and yet, as phantasy, they also enable her imaginary fusion with them.

Much can be said about the complicated relationships that cis and trans people, relationships that can be consuming and exploitative in both directions. I want to focus here on one particular example, the interpellation of the cisgendered partner into the role of saviour: trans people enter relationships with cis people (friendships, partnerships, etc.) and recognise in their (often completely phantasised) stability a kind of second skin that can function as a container for one's own unbearable dysphoric suffering. However, to indict such behaviour is to misunderstand the porosity of psychic life as being essentially reliant on interpenetration. This is why the Kleinian concept of 'projective identification' has lost nothing of its urgency, because it speaks to the impossibility of separating self and body.

The 'sack of potatoes' may be understood as a basic metaphor for thoroughly dysphoric bodies, bodies always on the verge of breakdown. Winnicott (1974) once suggested that our fear of breakdown stems from an unmetabolised collapse of the holding environment that happened at a much earlier date. A complicated maternal symbiosis of excessive projective identification and reverie is being set up here (Bion 2014c, 303–304). The most powerful anxiety available to the child is death anxiety. If the mother is incapable or unwilling or simply unavailable to absorb the child's death anxiety, the child will reintroject this anxiety as the 'nameless dread' (Bion 2014a, 159), which has fatal implications for ego-formation. The kind of mental unintegration that Bick describes may now emerge.

The maternal relationship in the trans context is usually interrupted right from the beginning, with a mother (or father, etc.) being unresponsive and even hostile to the gender non-conforming yearnings and anxieties of the trans child. Perhaps it is because cisgender people can resolve death anxiety only by sublimating it into castration anxiety that they do not know how to help their trans kids; if anything, this points to a fundamental ontological impasse in our current understanding of gender's vicissitudes. What I would like to propose is that the kind of frantic anxiety and over-reliance on cis people by trans people stems from this deeper complex of isolation, of not having experienced a reverie of death anxiety. The ways in which many trans people are incapable of finding comfort in their own imaginary is emblematic of an attempt to constantly return to an originary dehiscence and the deep-felt belief that this dehiscence can never be sutured but only repeated. This repetition compulsion stems from the foreclosed holding of the name-of-the-caretaker, which yields psychic disorder whenever one faces a metonymisation of this name-of-the-caretaker, in particular in its violent form as the transphobic paternal name.

I believe then that something very fundamental about dysphoria can be stated thus: the explosion of affect and of searching for the maternal holding environment are aggressive projections of identifications into a horridly empty space, and it is this emptiness that eats Anna up from the inside. What was supposed to be there is a *field of narrative speculation and containment*, in which all emotional life coalesces around the basic fact that the judgment of the law – *you are condemned to fail, so repent by vomiting up the very materials that are meant to lend you form* – is not fate, and that in the loving embrace of the Other the furious waves of dysphoria can indeed find their termination; these are calm shores yet unaccounted for in the mental geography of the dysphoria-addled brain. All trans life is the search for such friendly expanses, and it is predicated entirely on allowing oneself to be surprised by the night's freeing winds.

## Conclusion

Dysphoria is not a purely exogenous affliction or contamination but a unique form of building and establishing corporeality, where creation and destruction enter a symbiotic relationship of decreation. Dysphoria is a profound sensual ravaging that enlivens Anna as much as it hurts and deadens her. I would call the simultaneity of these phenomena the violence of emotion, following Bion (2014c, 278). This violence of emotion is tied to a kind of mental unintegration, a mentality beyond an organising principle that renders sensible the disaggregated particles of experience.

Ultimately, I am suggesting that dysphoria, far from a phenomenon that befalls the mind, is the catachrestic name for an entire sign-production system that affects object-usage and transformation. The violence of emotion felt by the dysphoric subject speaks both to a sense of growth pain and, more significantly, to a unique form of de/creation that accompanies the process of transitioning. The relationship of metaphor and metonymy alerts us to the desire for the intersection of signifying chains, finding in the literality of experience its transcendental intensification. Yet, the trans subject falls back, over and over again, into a type of nonsensical torpor wherein their self is revealed as dehiscent. This state can tip into a state of annihilation, but it can also be transformed in the holding environment, which returns the trans subject to the realisation that the Other is not out to consume and devastate her. Instead, her unique relationship to language and corporeality draws her into the meshwork of gender as a playful co-emergence of all phenomena as metonymy, which in its metaphorisation occasions the blossoming of transitioning.

The trans subject therefore does not pass through dysphoria but moves *by way of dysphoria*, and if it is understood as a system, it becomes clear that while there is no abolition of dysphoria, there is a transformative process wherein the dysphoric and the euphoric reach a point of indeterminateness, which enables the trans subject to learn how to 'bear' both oneself and another.

There are limits to my approach based on clinical concepts. Because the clinic is not the world, the yearnings for a different world will eventually collide with the clinic as political program *itself*. Much clinical work on dysphoria constitutes a kind of anger-management therapy, where there occurs a constant misreading of dysphoria as an individualised system rather than a somatised state of being that indicts the world as such. The dehiscence experienced by the trans subject is the dehiscence that is occasioned by her own radically unassimilable being. It is precisely because trans being opens the seams of conceptual taxonomy in the medical and psychological fields that it can only experience the name-of-the-father as violence. The dehiscence felt by the trans subject is not one that is primarily hers, but the individualised metabolisation of a systemic disorder masquerading as functional paternal law.

Looking back at Anna's associations and the largely unfounded assumptions that guide them, we may say that she is – to paraphrase Adam Phillips (2006) – speaking nonsense, and she does not know when to stop. This incessant speaking of the mind marks an abdication of mental defence, which enables a unique type of creativity, namely, that of dwelling in the oceanic undoing of her psyche. Therein she finds the truth of her trans feminine existence. This truth is as much about the joy of being unrestrained by association as it is about being capable of forgetting one's self.

## Coda

These final reflections bring us back again to the nights and days spent at the clubs – Berlin's true psychoanalytic institutes, where perversion or anal regression are not mere phrases but sought-after realities – beautiful people ensconced in fog, their bodies swerving around, and your eyes following them, curious as much as intimidated. Eventually you find the man you had your eyes on all night, and you see him moving towards the dark room area, turning around to you, winking at you; he is waiting. Can you trust this man? A contemplative moment seizes you – stay here or take the plunge and be transported elsewhere? To a place not quite here, not quite there, somewhere in the interstices, where the weight of gendered signification withers away, making way for a freely associated falling – into his arms or into yours, no matter – as long as something is preserved by the darkness of the room you would find yourselves in, that is, your right to secrecy and not being fully revealed in spite of transphobia's relentless march towards clinical vivisection.

The body returns in those moments – not as rigidity, not as affective ankylosis, but rather as a magma of expression, as dissolution into a pulsating mass. And for the first time in oh so many years, you forget yourself. It is as though you wanted to say to the man over there: 'I have only been a woman for a few years but now you must love me all the more', make up for the lost time, quench the thirst of an entire life of renunciation and loss.

As you are weighing your chances, more mist emerges, with a house line trailing off in the distance: *I want you, I need you, I got to have your love.*

You see his delicate smile, and then dash aside the question that was lingering in the back of your mind of whether or not to trust him. You follow him, for who are you to judge?

The other, after all, is always a polymorphous devil.

And though you know that you should not really embark on this journey that emerges so clearly from your innermost being and draws you towards the Other – it is a queer invitation, one that feels altogether different from the ones that have ravaged you so far – you feel elated and you feel free, and as the devil lays out more and more traces for you to follow, you at last permit yourself to vanish into her embrace, for 'what we love in ourselves is ourselves loving' (Burnside 2006).

## References


American Psychiatric Association (APA). 2013. *Diagnostic and Statistician Manual of Mental Disorders: DSM-5*. Washington, DC: American Psychiatric Association.

Bick, Esther. 2011. "The Experience of the Skin in Early Object Relations." In *The Tavistock Model. Papers on Child Development and Psychoanalytic Training*, edited by Meg Harris Williams, 133–138. London: Karnac Books.

Bion, Wilfred Ruprecht. 2014a. "A Theory of Thinking." In *The Complete Works of W.R. Bion. Volume VI/Second Thoughts*, edited by Chris Mawson and Francesca Bion, 153–161. London: Karnac Books.

Bion, Wilfred Ruprecht. 2014b. *Attention and Interpretation: A Scientific Approach to Insight in Psycho-Analysis and Groups*, edited by Chris Mawson. London; New York: Routledge.

Bion, Wilfred Ruprecht. 2014c. "Learning from Experience." In *The Complete Works of W.R. Bion*, Vol. IV, edited by Chris Mawson and Francesca Bion, 247–371. London: Karnac Books.

Bion, Wilfred Ruprecht. 2018. "Transformations: Change from Learning to Growth." In *The Complete Works of W.R. Bion*, Vol. V, edited by Chris Mawson and Francesca Bion, 115–288. London: Karnac Books.

Burnside, John. 2006. *A Lie about My Father.* New York: Macmillan USA.

Cazotte, Jacques. 1871 [1772]. *Le Diable Amoureux [The Devil in Love]*. Paris: Plon.

Freud, Sigmund. 1966. "Eine Schwierigkeit Der Psychoanalyse [a Difficulty in Psychoanalysis]." In *Gesammelte Werke XII. Werke aus den Jahren 1917–1920*, edited by Anna Freud, 3–12. Frankfurt am Main: S. Fischer Verlag.

Green, André. 2009. "The Central Phobic Position: With a Model of the Free-Association Method." In *Resonance of Suffering. Countertransference in Non-Neurotic Structures*, edited by André Green, 41–74. London: Karnac Books.

Klein, Melanie. 1975. "Envy and Gratitude." In *Envy and Gratitude and Other Works 1946–1963*, edited by Roger Money-Kyrle, 176–235. New York: The Free Press.

Kristeva, Julia. 1982. *Powers of Horror: An Essay in Abjection.* Translated by Leon S. Roudiez. New York: Columbia University Press.

Lacan, Jacques. 1966. "Le Stade du miroir comme formateur du je [The Mirror Stage as Formative of the Function of the I]." In *Écrits*, 93–101. Paris: Éditions du Seuil.

Lacan, Jacques. 1991. *The Seminar Book II: The Ego in Freud's Theory and in the Technique of Psychoanalysis 1954–1955,* trans. Sylvana Tomaselli. New York; London: W.W. Norton.

Lacan, Jacques. 2007. *Le Séminaire XVIII: d'un discours qui ne serait pas du semblant* (The Seminar XVIII: Of a Discourse That Would Not Be of a Semblance). Paris: Seuil.

Lacan, Jacques. 2011. *Le Séminaire XIX: ...ou Pire* (The Seminar Xix: …or Worse). Paris: Seuil.

Phillips, Adam. 2006. *Side Effects*. New York: Harper.

Preciado, Paul. 2013. *Testo Junkie: Sex, Drugs, and Biopolitics in the Pharmacopornographic Era*. Translated by Bruce Benderson. New York: The Feminist Press.

Winnicott, Donald Woods. 1974. "Fear of Breakdown." *International Review of Psycho-Analysis,* 1: 103–107.

# 14 Afterword

## Moral value in medicine: Violence, cure, and care

*Sander L. Gilman*

The louder and more insistent the claim that in scientific medicine both efficacy and empathy could live side by side, and indeed defined medical practice, the less both physicians and patients bought into it by the end of the twentieth century. Their experiences were radically different: alienation on the part of the practitioner and the patient's sense of being treated as a disease or a body part, not as a human being. I experienced this in my own career. After spending a year in residence at the Medical School at Cornell University working on a project on the history of psychiatry, the then-dean invited me in 1978 to join the faculty, as it was understood that medical students needed to be 'humanised'. This was in spite of the fact that I ironically informed him that humanists were the least humane people teaching at any university, as they seemed mainly to quibble about parking spaces. I began a 17-year affiliation teaching the medical humanities. I was certainly not alone, not even in New York City, where the medical school was located, and where other humanists were suddenly drafted into schools of medicine to 'humanise' the new physicians.

I was not completely naïve. In 1975, the barbiturate overdose deaths of Drs Stewart L. and Cyril C. Marcus, identical twins who were both faculty members at Cornell Medical School, where they ran the infertility clinic, made the frontpages of newspapers across the country. The immediate response was, how could such addicts not only continue to practise medicine but, more importantly, how could they continue to teach and research at one of the major schools of medicine in the United States? Evidently, something was amiss with their moral orientation. My function in the greater scope of things was to be proof that the medical school was answering the question of how medical students should be taught to be better people and, therefore, better doctors. Over the following decades, as this case became the stuff of popular culture, such as in David Cronenberg's *Dead Ringers* (1988), my teaching seemed to fill a gap. In 1991, noting the collapse of assumptions about scientific medical praxis, the American Medical Association began a $1,750,000 advertising campaign to polish up the image of the doctor, emphasising the sort of good works that once were the specialties of movie and television doctors.

The 'medical humanities' became a reality across the United States due to the perception that scientific medicine was insufficient in giving physicians-in-training a sense of their moral, ethical, cultural, or political obligations, obligations that

DOI: 10.4324/9781032660165-23

were seen as both more important for this cadre than the 'normal' citizen and at the same time inherently lacking within medical pedagogy. I was raised on the image of the heroic physician in fiction and film. By then, Sinclair Lewis' (whose 1925 novel Arrowsmith was awarded the 1926 Pulitzer Prize) and John Ford's (Oscar nominated filming of 1931) cinematic hero Dr Martin *Arrowsmith* (Ronald Coleman) had been replaced by Dr Judah Rosenthal (Martin Landau), an accessory to the murder of his mistress in Woody Allen's (Oscar nominated) *Crimes and Misdemeanors* (1989).

In my subsequent career, I fulfilled this role at several other schools of medicine, all of which assumed, rightly or wrongly, that I would enrich their curricula by humanising their students. I, too, thought that perhaps I could help reorient them a bit to their role as medical students and then as practitioners, even though most of the students at schools of medicine then found that such courses were a simple waste of their time. They still wanted the *science* in scientific medicine to be foregrounded.

And this debate was not limited to the world of scientific medicine. After the bombings at Hiroshima and Nagasaki, the moral claims of the intellectual triumph of early twentieth-century physics, as represented by Albert Einstein and his pacifist writings after WWI, collapsed into moral opprobrium. C. P. Snow was forced then to counter the claim about the moral force of the humanities at the moment when the humanities still seem to be ascendant and yet were grappling with the legacy of the Third Reich. After the 'problem' of Nazi medicine was resolved (it was assumed) with the Doctors' Trial (officially *United States of America v. Karl Brandt, et al.*) in 1946 and the principle of informed consent was established in theory, if not always in practice, medical science seemed again to claim the moral high ground that it had claimed in the pre-WWII period.

Scientific medicine immediately after WWII had also regained high scientific status as the age of antibiotics, representing an efficient, quick, and present cure, enabled all physicians – or at least those in possession of penicillin – to cure, with or without any moral claims. The filmic moment that fixed this is found in Carroll Reed's account of occupied Vienna, *The Third Man* (1949), in which the horrors visited on post-war Vienna by Harry Lime (Orson Welles) is revealed when he sells stolen penicillin, diluting it, so that it kills instead of cures the children who receive it. Medicine, especially the new antibiotics, would be proof of the claim of science to cure the innocent; but politics kills, Lime observes while looking down from the 'Riesenrad', the Ferris wheel in the Viennese Prater. From that vantage point he compares the miniscule people down below to ants, noting the insignificance of those who suffer due to his penicillin scheme, Lime reveals the full extent of his amorality. 'You know what the fellow said', he explains.

> In Italy, for thirty years under the Borgias, they had warfare, terror, murder and bloodshed, but they produced Michelangelo, Leonardo da Vinci and the Renaissance. In Switzerland, they had brotherly love, they had five hundred years of democracy and peace—and what did that produce? The cuckoo clock.

This is the central moral dilemma of the world after the Holocaust, now trying to recalibrate its moral orientation at the beginning of the Cold War. And what better moral dilemma to trigger this than the sale of ineffectual pharmaceuticals to dying children?

In his 'The Two Cultures and the Scientific Revolution' (1959), C. P. Snow countered the perceived dominance of the moral universe, encapsulated in the humanities of his day, including their claim to make better people, as simply a falsehood proven by their failures. In the age of secularisation which created scientific medicine, one read Shakespeare for moral teaching, not the Bible. This did not make a jot of difference in the best educated, most literate political culture in the world, namely, that of Germany. One could read Goethe in the shadow of one of the beech trees he so admired in Buchenwald, the camp named after them near Weimar, but a walking distance from his home, the site of the murder of innocents. This fact, engraved in our understanding of scientific medicine in the twentieth century, was little different than Harry Lime's claims about the insignificance of humanity.

C. P. Snow, however, demanded a recalibration of the universities to balance the role of the humanities with a new and robust role for the sciences, with their expanded moral force reinforced by the debates following the dropping of the atomic bomb and the 'Doomsday' clock of the *Bulletin of Atomic Scientists*. Snow, who recognised the claims of the humanities on moral education, wanted to state that the sciences could be just as much of a moral force. He argued that there was a 'whole body of literature [...] to demonstrate the intellectual, aesthetic and moral values inherent in the pursuit of science', and that there is 'a moral component right in the grain of science itself, and almost all scientists form their own judgments of the moral life' (Snow 1998, 63). Not that Snow was in any way original in the twentieth century. For example, Sir William Osler (1920, 14) had bemoaned the use of poisoned gas during WWI and the demand of 'a group of medical men representing the chief universities and medical bodies of the United Kingdom was innocent enough to suggest that such an unclean weapon—the use of lethal gases, "condemning its victims to death by long-drawn-out torture", and with infinite possibilities for its further development—should be forever abolished'. These were condemned by public sentiment as unworldly. Unmentioned by Osler is that Fritz Haber, who held the Nobel Prize for Chemistry in 1918 for the synthesis of ammonia, was chiefly responsible for the German poison gas program unleashed in 1915; after the end of the war, he feared being arrested as a war criminal (Charles 2005, 187). Unlike the debate about nuclear weapons, a prohibition against the use of poison gas was agreed to in the 1925 Protocol for the Prohibition of the Use of Asphyxiating, Poisonous or Other Gases, and of Bacteriological Methods of Warfare, commonly known as the 1925 Geneva Protocol, that banned the use of chemical and bacteriological (biological) weapons in war. Not that this stopped their use in Syria in 2018. To this we can add today the subsequent ethical debates about genetic modification, environmental science, vaccination, and other public health interventions, among multitudes of scientific questions debated on moral terms within the sciences themselves.

If the authority of the humanities as the arbiter of moral education began to wane in the world of C. P. Snow, its status collapsed in the twenty-first century.

By the beginning of the twenty-first century, moral education had been abandoned completely – at least for American undergraduates. They were claimed to be on a search for skill-based training, especially in undergraduate fields regarded as free of the sloppiness and uselessness of the humanities. These fields were now summarised by an acronym introduced in 2001 by scientific administrators at the U.S. National Science Foundation (NSF): STEM, standing for Science, Technology, Engineering, and Mathematics. And STEM not only meant 'science'; more importantly, for most American undergraduates it was a code for the pathway to the study of medicine, which remained the highest prestige of all post-graduate fields. The humanities, a form of education without the skills to earn the best possible living, were dismissed; humanities departments that had had a high status in the 1960s, as indicated by their expansion and production of doctorates, were strangled through a radical reduction of funding or closed altogether.

The great irony is that exactly at this moment, STEM suddenly discovered in its struggle to incorporate a new morality into scientific medicine that students, especially those in professional schools such as medicine, indeed needed moral training and the only models available were in the declining fields of the humanities. The 'medical humanities' took centre stage at this moment. The reason for this was that those in STEM fields were suddenly seen as fallible rather than as the idealised practitioners that had inhabited the public fantasies of physicians and engineers, *pace* Ayn Rand, in the twentieth century. That fallible human beings inhabited all professions was true from the Greeks on. Medical training, from the Ancients, was always contested and always charged with producing 'good' or 'bad' physicians, depending on the school's ideology. After the Holocaust, after the Doctors' Trial and the highlighted role that physicians had had in exploiting prisoners in the Death Camps and beyond, the fantasy of idealised perfection was drawn into question. But a nostalgia for a lost age of STEM, that is, a world in which idealised physicians or physicists bore humanities moral burden, was re-inscribed – if not with science as its calling card, then at least the individual physician pursuing truth and justice in an imperfect universe. Here, W. Somerset Maugham (MD, St. Thomas' Hospital, 1897), Lewis Thomas (MD, Harvard Medical School, 1937), Abraham Verghese (MD, Madras University School of Medicine, 1980), and generations of physician-authors peddling a nostalgia about the ethical calling of medicine in a world of institutionalised practice and claims of scientific objectivity were – and are – equally culpable. Such a world never existed before or after Abraham Flexner's radical introduction of scientific medicine into medical education in the pre-WWI era.

The more removed and isolated medical praxis became from the patient, the more spokespeople for these self-same institutions, invested with their authority, played the empathy card. Certainly, individuals in the health care system, drawn into it because of empathy, may attempt to preserve their empathic relationship with the ill and the disabled, but the thrust of the institutions remains scientistic, not empathetic. What motivates individuals may well be empathetic altruism; what motivates a field to shout in the marketplace that it is altruistic and empathetic is clearly neither. For proof, listen to the automatic answering machine at the clinic or the hospital or physician's office: 'Your call is very important to us. Please listen carefully to the following menu as our options have changed'. No matter how humanising education may become, the ideal world of health care only corrupted by the Harry Limes of our world is revealed to have been just as empty, just as vacuous, as that of post-WWII Vienna.

At that moment, paralleling the slow but steady erosion of the moral authority of the humanities, the medical humanities in schools of medicine, staffed by humanists as well as physicians, began to claim that the introduction of the humanities into professional education makes for better people, or at least better doctors. I will use 'Narrative Medicine: A Model for Empathy, Reflection, Profession, and Trust' (2001), an essay by Rita Charon (MD, Harvard University School of Medicine, 1978; PhD, English, Columbia University, 1999) published in the pre-eminent American medical journal *JAMA*, as a touchstone for the claims of the medical humanities in the age of their ascendency. Charon has been honoured repeatedly since then as the creator of 'narrative medicine', so this essay introduces a serious discussion of how scientific medicine had to be transformed in light of the ethical claims of the humanities. Note that it appeared the year that STEM was created as a pedagogical category. Indeed, given that I began work in the field in the 1970s (and taught Rita Charon in a NEH summer seminar on the medical humanities in 1990), I will include myself on the list of those who shaped the field, using arguments that we in the humanities could improve the training of the physician, a belief which then led to funding by such major institutions as the Macy Foundation. In short, Charon's claim is that literature can teach empathy and that empathy is what was lacking in the training of physicians in 2001 to make them

> Better understand the experiences of sick people, the journeys of individual physicians, and the duties incurred by physicians toward individual patients and by the profession of medicine toward its wider culture. [...] Medical educators may find that applicants already gifted with narrative skills are better able to develop into effective physicians than are students deficient in them. [...] Through the narrative processes of reflection and self-examination, both physicians and patients can achieve more accurate understandings of all the sequelae of illness, equipping them to better weather its tides.
>
> (Charon 2001, 1898)

This is exactly what Marjorie Garber (2001, 53–96) labelled decades ago as 'discipline envy', thinking that a field perceived as far from one's own is better able to handle questions than the one in which you were trained. Here, it is assumed that physicians would be best served by methodologies beyond the scope of health care, as only these radically different approaches could assure a true commitment to communicating 'empathy'. Let me bring in the noted literary critic Stanley Fish's (2008) essay in *The New York Times*, perhaps unconsciously responding to the Charon of 2001:

> If it were true, the most generous, patient, good-hearted and honest people on earth would be the members of literature and philosophy departments, who

> spend every waking hour with great books and great thoughts, and as someone who's been there (for 45 years) I can tell you it just isn't so. Teachers and students of literature and philosophy don't learn how to be good and wise; they learn how to analyse literary effects and to distinguish between different accounts of the foundations of knowledge.

As medicine became aware of its inherent deficiencies, it sought remedies beyond itself, and especially *not* in the world of medicine.

Yet, as the physician-educator David Naylor wrote,

> Doctor-patient communication can indeed be facilitated by individual-level decision analysis or formal decision aids. At a simpler level, evidence can be generated and synthesised into forms that are readily accessible to support decision-making by patients and doctors alike. But as the advocates of "narrative-based medicine" argue, these tools cannot replace an empathetic clinician who seeks to understand illness as the patient experiences it, rather than as a disease defined by pathophysiological models, epidemiological evidence, and professional preconceptions. It is ironic, moreover, that the best lessons in "fast and frugal rules of thumb" may well come from understanding the cognitive processes of those master clinicians who consistently make superb decisions without obvious recourse to the canon of evidence-based medicine.
>
> (Naylor 2001, 523)

So, evidence-based medicine can be ameliorated by the idealised 'master clinician', such as Sir William Osler, who linked real science to empathy.

'Empathy' is, of course, a conflicted and contradictory concept. Certainly, within the modern history of medicine, Sir William Osler's view of the new science, the new physician, and the complexity of their distance from the patient still summarises the situation in the twenty-first century. Can we truly 'understand' the internal lives of others, especially those 'put in our care' through our status and investiture, or do we simply project our own sense of self? Jodi Halpern, who is otherwise quite receptive of Charon's message at that moment, becomes rather hesitant when she confronts 'empathy' as the desired outcome of the medical humanities:

> Once empathy is seen as depending on emotional responses, however, a critical problem arises. Emotions are generally outside people's immediate control. How can physicians reliably empathise with patients towards whom they naturally feel little or even negative emotions? Sometimes emotional resonance comes easily. However, busy, overworked physicians may find such responses absent.
>
> (Halpern 2003, 672)

That this is inherent in every system of treatment, the transference and counter-transference, is often unrecognised by both parties. Instead, Charon thinks that the goal should be raising the innate curiosity of the physician, as if that is not equally fraught, given the ambiguous potential of such empathy and curiosity, even detached concern. Taking the Devil's part, we could argue that satisfying curiosity without moral direction is precisely what was condemned at the Doctor's Trial of accused Nazi perpetrators in 1947, in order to put limitations on medical experimentation. Borrowing methodologies from the humanities assumed that these provided some moral limitations for medical education, and they would thus modify the alienation felt by patients and society alike through the abstract claims of scientific medicine, whether real or not.

In 1966, my future colleague at Cornell, the late poet Jon Stallworthy, published an extraordinary poem entitled 'A Letter from Berlin', evoking the medical experiences (fictive or not) of his father, the New Zealand-born Nuffield Professor of Obstetrics and Gynaecology at Oxford University, Sir John Stallworthy (MD, University of Otago, 1939; study in Melbourne, London and Vienna between 1932 and 1938). According to a discussion I had with him in the 1970s, he took an experience narrated by his father after his time as a student of surgery in Vienna in the 1930s, before the Anschluss, and moved its site to Berlin under the Nazis. In the poem, a surgeon performs an operation of great technical brilliance devoid of, or divorced from, any humane purpose, before an admiring coterie of students

> Von Neumann operates at ten
> and would do so if the sky fell in. They lock
> his theatre doors on the stroke of the clock—
> … I knew just as the doors were closing. Last,
> as expected, on Von Showmann's list
> the new vaginal hysterectomy
> that brought me to Berlin.
>                                         Delicately
> he went to work …

The writer of the letter is dazzled by the technique

>             Never had I seen such masterly
> technique. 'And so little bleeding!' I said
> half to myself, half to my neighbour.

But his neighbour was not dazzled, he had seen it all before

>                                         'Dead',
> came his whisper. 'Don't be a fool'
> I said, for still below us in the pool
> of light the marvellous unhurried hands
> were stitching, tying the double strands
> of catgut, stitching, tying. It was like
> a concert, watching those hands unlock
> the music from the score.

Then came the realisation after the surgeon had finished and left:

> I have to apologize. She was dead,
> but how did you know?' Back came his voice
> like a bullet—'saw it last month, twice.

Stallworthy, the poet, reading his father's letter from Hitler's Berlin, saw technical skill as a betrayal of the ideals of medicine and prefiguring much worse:

> Returning your letter to an envelope
> yellower by years than when you sealed it up,
> darkly the omens emerge. A ritual wound
> yellow at the lip yawns in my hand;
> a turbulent crater; a trench, filled
> not with snow only, east of Buchenwald.
> (Stallworthy 1966, 96–98)

Given that literature is a cultural manifestation of the narrative process and that the narrative process should enable us to transcend our own cultural (read: moral) limitations, we seemed to have been in a bind even in 2001. Narratives can teach us, as Stallworthy imagines, about the hidden meanings in an age without empathy, but that age, as we have examined throughout this book, may well seem to lie in the Nazi past, not in our *now*.

What is lacking in the world described by Stallworthy is an acknowledgment of pain, of the simple fact that the death of the patient removes pain as a medical 'problem'. Technique (science) triumphs over healing. I have written much about pain over my career: as an experience, as a historical category, as a key to understanding the shifts and focus of scientific medicine 'following the science' (Gilman 2011, 2014). And pain – as symptom or as the result of therapy – was and is a touchstone of the role of the modern physician to ameliorate suffering as well as to 'do no harm'. At the core of this is the repeated demand that the modern physician alter their objectivisation of the patient (seemingly inherent to scientific medicine) to empathise with their lot.

Sara Ahmed ties these notions of empathy to 'seeing' the patient, an act which, as I have shown since my *Seeing the Insane* (1982), was an intrinsic part of the new medicalisation of medicine but also the creation of the very notion of the patient:

> When we talk of the experience of pain we assume it is 'my pain' because I cannot feel the other's pain. I may experience my pain as too present and the other's as too absent. And yet, others are in pain; I read her body as a sign of pain. I see you grimace, or your face, white and drawn. I watch sadly as your body curls up, curls away. I want to reach you, to touch you. [...] I want to have her pain so she can be released from it, so she doesn't have to feel it. This is love as empathy: I love you and imagine not only that I can feel how you feel, but that I could feel your pain for you. But I want

> that feeling only insofar as I don't already have it; the desire maintains the difference between the one who would 'become' in pain, and another who already 'is' in pain or 'has' it. In this way empathy sustains the very difference that it may seek to overcome: empathy remains a 'wish feeling', in which subjects 'feel' something other than what another feels in the very moment of imagining they could feel what another feels. The impossibility of feeling the pain of others does not mean that the pain is simply theirs, or that their pain has nothing to do with me. I want to suggest here, cautiously, and tentatively, that an ethics of responding to pain involves being open to being affected by that which one cannot know or feel. Such an ethics is, in this sense, bound up with the sociality or the 'contingent attachment' of pain itself.
>
> (Ahmed 2014, 30)

She quite correctly concludes that such a model of empathy

> Is not about feeling the other's pain. Pain is evoked as that which even our most intimate others cannot feel. The impossibility of 'fellow feeling' is itself the confirmation of injury. The call of such pain, as a pain that cannot be shared through empathy, is a call not just for an attentive hearing, but for a different kind of inhabitance. It is a call for action, and a demand for collective politics, as a politics based not on the possibility that we might be reconciled, but on learning to live with the impossibility of reconciliation, or learning that we live with and beside each other, and yet we are not as one.
>
> (Ahmed 2014, 39)

Thus, we return to a debate, triggered by Rudolf Virchow already in 1848, that such categories are those of the 'body politic' in Hobbes' sense, not the world of medical science at all

> Science for its own sake usually means nothing more than science for the sake of the people who happen to be pursuing it. Knowledge which is unable to support action is not genuine – and how unsure is activity without understanding… If medicine is to fulfill her great task, then she must enter the political and social life… The physicians are the natural attorneys of the poor, and the social problems should largely be solved by them.
>
> (Virchow 1848, 2)

The problem is that Virchow and scientific medicine in the age of revolution saw only the upside, and little attention was wasted on what would happen if such views were used to further other models of scientific medicine, such as eugenics and mass murder under the guise of euthanasia, which the Nazis labelled 'T-4'.

In an age where narratives of power could be revealed, the idea that we could focus bio-power for positive change seemed a seductive move, especially when we had behind us the claims of the moral superiority of the humanities in achieving this end. To quote Charon again

> As reflective practitioners, physicians have turned to a study of the humanities, especially literature, to grow in their personal understanding of illness. Literature seminars and reading groups have become commonplace in medical schools and hospitals, both for physicians to read well-written stories about illness and to deepen their skills as readers, interpreters, and conjurers of the worlds of others. Having learned that acts of reflective narrating illuminate aspects of the patient's story—and of their own—that are unavailable without the telling, physicians are writing about their patients in special columns in professional journals and in books and essays published in the lay press. Increasingly, physicians allow patients to read what they have written about them, adding a therapeutic dimension to a practice born of the need for reflection.
>
> (Charon 2001, 1899)

Biopower versus biopolitics? Though there is some debate regarding the specifics of *biopower* and *biopolitics*, the anthropologist Paul Rabinow and the social theorist Nikolas Rose provide a compelling formulation we find useful for our own analysis. For them, biopower

> Entails one or more truth discourses about the 'vital' character of living human beings; an array of authorities considered competent to speak that truth; strategies for intervention upon collective existence in the name of life and health; and modes of subjectification, in which individuals work on themselves in the name of individual or collective life or health.
>
> (Rabinow and Rose 2006, 195)

As a truth discourse, biopower then emerges out of a particular cultural conjuncture where authority over life increasingly becomes concentrated in the hands of modern science, including the psychological sciences. Meanwhile, biopolitics refers to the political struggle over the various problems with human life and death:

> All the specific strategies and contestations over problematizations of collective human vitality, morbidity, and mortality; over the forms of knowledge, regimes of authority and practices of intervention that is desirable, legitimate, and efficacious.
>
> (Rabinow and Rose 2006, 197)

Rabinow and Rose draw an important distinction between *biopower* and *biopolitics*, which is useful for demonstrating how the challenge towards scientific racism presented by some social and behavioural scientists in the pre- and inter-war years involved a fundamental clash over knowledge and authority. This clash resulted in the rejection of one version of biopower, or truth discourse, about the needs for moral education in medicine. However, the rejection of this truth discourse occurred alongside the emergence of a new truth discourse on the role of science in the public sphere. (For all the alternate ways in which *biopower* and *biopolitics* are discussed by Giorgio Agamben in his *Homo Sacer: Sovereign Power and Bare Life* (1995), as well as by Michael Hardt and Antonio Negri in their *Empire* (2001), this critique of the biosciences remains central. Medicine, since the horrors of Josef Mengele's 'medical experimentation' in the death camps, such as Auschwitz, is always the touchstone for bio-power. Note that Josef Mengele had both a Dr Phil in Anthropology from the University of Munich (1935) and a MD from the University of Frankfurt, *cum laude*, in 1938.) The conflict between a collapsing truth regime and an emergent one reflects the relational qualities of *biopower* and *biopolitics*: the emergence of *biopower*, in any given iteration, is always a product of *biopolitics*; and the constitution of *biopolitics* is the consequence of *biopower*. Morality seeks to modulate this. Which moral map is employed is trivial, as all such maps are part of biopolitics. And that is where we find ourselves today: the collapse of the humanities and their survival in STEM as an artefact of truth-seeking coloured by our moral camouflage.

The Alexander Hamilton Professor of American Studies at Columbia University, Andrew Delbanco, in *College*: *What It Was, Is, and Should Be* (2012) sees education as truth-seeking, a priority of the humanities. Science's 'principle of progress' does not translate well into other areas of human life: 'Science tells us nothing about how to shape a life or how to face death [...] It not only fails to answer such questions; it cannot ask them' (Delbanco 2012, 101). He knows that some scientists have predicted that in time 'neuroscience will define and ensure happiness and [...] biochemistry will distinguish truth from falsity among what today are mere opinions about sex and gender', but he doubts 'it will happen'; even if it does, 'none of us will be around [...] and it's not clear that we would want to be' (Delbanco 2012, 99). The straw man here is a science devoid of moral accountability, which flies in the face of all the public debates within science, from the physics of the 1930s to the genetics of the 1990s. But such a utilitarian notion of science is needed if the humanities are to be a counter moral force even within medical education. Of course, the reverse also quickly turns out to be true. Lisa Mendelman (2021, 606) has argued that contemporary literary analysis quickly falls into the language of healing and mental health: 'reparative' and 'recuperative' reading practices are imagined as antidotes to 'suspicious' and 'symptomatic' dissections by critics whose psychospiritual bearing is called into question. Who cures whom remains the question?

The answer is to recognise what my teacher at the Free University of Berlin, the late Eberhard Lämmert, argued in teaching literature, that the humanities and medicine are on one level 'thought experiments'. How do the confrontations of a (too) zealous Norwegian spa doctor, Thomas Stockman from Ibsen's *Enemy of the People* (1882), in the age of Pasteur and Koch provide very different explanations about the relationship between health, society, and politics than the one narrated by another physician, Bernard Rieux from Albert Camus' *The Plague* (1947), in light of the horrors of WWII and the waning of colonialism? What in each case is the 'public's health'? How would we see the implications for us and for our world of post-COVID loss of trust in both or neither? Not as models but as thought experiments for the author, the reader of his times and for us. What if…

In other words, the humanities serve as a sort of contra-factual universe, the 'as if' world postulated at the beginning of the twentieth century by the post-Kantian philosopher Hans Vaihinger in his *The Philosophy of 'As If': A System of the Theoretical, Practical and Religious Fictions of Mankind* (1925). Vaihinger imagines a world populated by counter-possible reasoning, a world in which education (like life) is dealing constantly with counterfactual conditionals. We know that literature is not life, a pitfall that some dealing with medical narratives of all stripes, from novels to case material, often forget. But texts are poor teachers of moral lessons, unless you accept all possible readings as 'moral', even those you find abhorrent. Vaihinger's (1925, 17, 22) view is to avoid seeing our fictions as a copy of reality, but rather as an instrument for finding our way more easily in this world. It is not a copy of our world but a means of orienting ourselves within it, a coping mechanism depending on an infinite variety of variables. Following Vaihinger's lead, they can be a valuable – indeed, a necessary – manner of testing our own blind spots and presuppositions, but perhaps also reenforcing them.

Human beings in general use and test fictions to function in a world of what Anthony Appiah calls dealing with multiple mutually incompatible models. We test each model based on our own location in time and space. It is not an underlying truth, moral or otherwise, but rather 'knowing which lines of inference one should and which one should not follow' (Appiah 2017, 13). Our purpose in using models is not ultimately to obtain the truth about the world, but to navigate it; there is no reason to avoid such inconsistency, moral or otherwise (Appiah 2017, 14–17). I see, along with Vaihinger, that all systems of knowledge, from the 'hard' sciences to the softest humanities, are our own attempts to match our learned sense of the world to the world we experience. This is especially true in medical education. Well before Georges Canguilhem and Michel Foucault, Vaihinger (1925, 23) observed the creation of the 'celebrated statistical fiction […] of a normal, average man. This fiction is not of value for statistics alone, for in medicine we meet the average man in whom all abnormal deviations have disappeared'. And yet the truth is that reality is one of defining difference within all of our fictions against this arbitrary and ever-shifting 'normality'. Friedrich Nietzsche, in the *Twilight of the Gods* (1889), warned us against accepting the commonplace that the *consensus sapientium* establishes the truth in medical terms:

> In every age the wisest have passed the identical judgment on life: it is worthless. […] Everywhere and always their mouths have uttered the same sound – a sound full of doubt, full of melancholy, full of weariness with life, full of opposition to life. Even Socrates said as he died: 'To live – that means to be a long time sick: I owe a cock to the saviour Asclepius.' even Socrates had had enough of it. – What does that prove? What does it point to? – Formerly one would have said (– oh, and did say, and loudly enough, and our pessimists most of all!): 'Here at any rate there must be something

> true! The consensus sapientium is proof of truth.' – Shall we still speak thus today? are we allowed to do so? 'Here at any rate, there must be something sick' – this is our retort: one ought to take a closer look at them, these wisest of every age! Were they all of them perhaps no longer steady on their legs? belated? tottery? decadents? Does wisdom perhaps appear on earth as a raven which is inspired by the smell of carrion?
>
> (Nietzsche 1990, 39)

Vaihinger (1925, 352) roots his argument in Nietzsche's view about being 'beyond good and evil but also beyond truth and falsehood'. Vaihinger then explains not only that trap of dichotomies but also how we use it, and he gives us the tools to autopsy it.

Vaihinger's notion of these fictions as thought experiments is an answer to Wilhelm Dilthey's need in the same moment and the same academic setting to radically separate the humanities from the natural sciences and the new social sciences by making an argument that their critical methodologies simply resulted from their relationship to specific objects of study. The natural sciences uncovered real-existing causal explanations while the humanities (and social sciences) provided explanations for social and historical situations. The latter are fungible, the former fixed. Vaihinger notes that while much attention seems to be paid to what he calls the 'artifice' of the natural sciences as well as the humanities, there does seem to be a radical difference made between the two categories. Exactitude seems to be demanded in the natural sciences, while in the humanities 'exactitude is definitely excluded' (Vaihinger 1925, 10). But look, he says, at fields such as mathematics and even theology, where so-called explanatory presuppositions seem not to work at all. Indeed, beginning his own studies in philosophy, he spent a great deal of time studying pure mathematics. Once you are forced to include all spheres of human activity, from meeting someone for lunch to explaining the universe, universal explanatory models seem unable to explain very much, and yet they are legitimate as well as necessary. This may well be the key message of this very book. Models in medicine are thought experiments, ever juggled and rethought and perhaps even abandoned, as new questions, variables, data, and models become more compelling, that is, truer in the moment for the ultimate clinical goal, the amelioration of suffering, somatic and psychological. Even 'bad' therapies cure; even 'good' therapies kill.

For Vaihinger, reading the fictions of the aesthetic is a perfect manner of framing the medical humanities and then medicine itself:

> The poet shows us imaginary figures, pictures, and individuals, especially in the drama [...] Yet the poetic fiction (in the case of the drama it is a double one, since the actors represent imaginary individuals and deliver imaginary speeches) is of the highest aesthetic importance. How easily the fiction can transform itself into an hypothesis can be seen by the fact that the audience and the reader are not able to maintain the psychical tension of the *as if* indefinitely.
>
> (Vaihinger 1925, 88)

For me, the humanities can add another dimension to the study and practice of medicine, and vice versa. No stronger sense of moral virtue is implied unless we embed this moral goal in one or the other ways of imagining and shaping the world.

In New York City, the German-Jewish exile philosopher Hannah Arendt in her essay 'The Crisis in Education' (1954, 176) condemned the classical moralising tradition that saw education as having a political function:

> It is in fact comparatively easy to do the right thing in matters of education without even pausing to consider what one is really doing, so completely is the specific ethos of the educational principle in accord with the basic ethical and moral convictions of society at large. To educate, in the words of Polybius, was simply "to let you see that you are altogether worthy of your ancestors…".

This Arendt dismisses as merely a form of indoctrination for 'fellowship and authority were in this case indeed but the two sides of the same matter, and the teacher's authority was firmly grounded in the encompassing authority of the past as such'. Real education after the Holocaust is moral in so far as we see ourselves as at

> The point at which we decide whether we love the world enough to assume responsibility for it and by the same token save it from that ruin which, except for renewal, except for the coming of the new and young, would be inevitable.
>
> (Arendt 1954, 194)

This view, which came to dominate such debates in the light of post-modern theory and its supposed claim of the flexibility of values, upheld the seeking after such values in a global, moral sense. Today we can be reshaped by education as an experience in the world but not just in terms of inherited, closed moral systems that refuse to acknowledge the value of difference.

We must remember, as Hannah Arendt gestured at the beginning of her essay, that the Nazis 'with concentration and extermination camps' also saw their undertaking as a moral certainty, and we must always be able to question the system of morality we are advocating, whether in the humanities or the sciences. What, then, if we look to the disciplines not as having intrinsic moral value but instead as 'useful fictions', extending our claim that the humanities are thought experiments to STEM as well, as Vaihinger primarily did in his study? Everyone asks, what would happen *if*? No wonder Albert Einstein was delighted to attend a conference on the philosophical implications of his Theory of Relativity hosted by Vaihinger in 1920, much to the distress of more conservative academic physicists. We can then compare and contrast these claims rather than seeing the one as a necessary corrective to the other. The paradox of the medical humanities is that it then serves exactly the same function in medical education as the sciences, no more and no less. We need to understand that 'because such constructions are devoid of reality they are to be regarded as devoid of utility. This is as incorrect as the inverse inference – from their utility to their validity' (Vaihinger 1925, 22). It is a case of not being 'better than' but 'as good or bad as' but useful in all cases.

My friend Sarah Colvin, the Schröder Professor of German at the University of Cambridge, in reading these observations commented:

> I also agree about the thought experiment, though I think that literature (for example) needs to be taught not as "a" thought experiment but as a model or stimulus for ongoing thought experimentation as a kind of perpetual motion. So not just a "what if?" but a "what if what if were always followed by another what if?" A model of how to be adversarial in a way that is inclusive because it is not about the achievement of a monolithic "winning" point of view.

I would add here the teaching and practice of medicine in all realms, from translational medicine to public health. This is the ambiguity that is present in the undertaking, not the drawing of boundaries between 'doctor' and 'quack', but the acknowledgement that such boundaries, while needing at every moment to be drawn, are fleeting. This is the core of the argument about the parallelism of *all* the disciplines, *pace* Vaihinger. There is a chance that very ability may succeed but also that it may well lead you into dead ends and bad places; you must be always tuned to that potential. And this is as true in *all* interpretative disciplines, including medicine.

## References

Ahmed, Sara. 2014. *The Cultural Politics of Emotion*. Edinburgh: Edinburgh University Press.

Appiah, Kwame Anthony. 2017. *As If: Idealization and Ideals*. Cambridge. MA: Harvard University Press.

Arendt, Hannah. 1954. "The Crisis in Education" reprinted in her *Between Past and Future*, 173–196. New York: Viking Press. 1968. https://www.studocu.com/no/document/universitetet-i-oslo/pedagogisk-psykologi/arendt-crisis-in-education-1954/10603781.

Charles, Daniel. 2005. *Master Mind: The Rise and Fall of Fritz Haber, the Nobel Laureate Who Launched the Age of Chemical Warfare*. New York: Harper Collins.

Charon, Rita. 2001. "A Model for Empathy, Reflection, Profession, and Trust." *JAMA* 286(15): 1897–1902. https://doi.org/10.1001/jama.286.15.1897.

Delbanco, Andrew. 2012. *College: What It Was, Is, and Should Be*. Princeton, NJ: Princeton University Press.

Fish, Stanley. 2008. "Will the Humanities Save Us?" *The New York Times*, 6 January. https://opinionator.blogs.nytimes.com/2008/01/06/will-the-humanities-save-us/

Garber, Marjorie. 2001. *Academic Instincts*. Princeton, NJ: Princeton University Press.

Gilman, Sander. 2011. "Seeing Bodies in Pain: From Hippocrates to Freud." *International Journal of Psychoanalysis* 92(3): 661–674.

Gilman, Sander. 2014. "Seeing Bodies in Pain." In *Health Humanities Reader*, edited by Therese Jones, Delese Wear and Lester D. Friedman, 171–186. New Brunswick, NJ: Rutgers University Press.

Halpern, Jodi. 2003. "What Is Clinical Empathy?" *Journal of General Internal Medicine* 18(8): 670–674. https://doi.org/10.1046/j.1525-1497.2003.21017.x.

Mendelman, Lisa. 2021. "Diagnosing Desire: Mental Health and Modern American Literature, 1890–1955." *American Literary History* 30: 601–619.

Naylor, C. David. 2001. "Clinical Decisions: From Art to Science and Back Again." *The Lancet,* 363: 523.

Nietzsche, Friedrich. 1990. *Twilight of the Gods and the Anti-Christ*, trans. R. J. Hollingdale. New York: Penguin.

Osler, William. 1920. *The Old Humanities and the New Science*. Boston, MA and New York: Houghton Mifflin.

Rabinow, Paul, and Nikolas Rose. 2006. "Biopower Today." *BioSocieties,* 1: 195–217.

Snow, C. P. 1998. *The Two Cultures*. Cambridge: Cambridge University Press.

Stallworthy, Jon. 1966. "A Letter from Berlin." *The Transatlantic Review,* 23: 96–98.

Vaihinger, Hans. 1925. *The Philosophy of "As If": A System of the Theoretical, Practical and Religious Fictions of Mankind*, trans. Charles Kay Ogden. New York: Harcourt, Brace & Co.; reprinted, Petoskey, MI: Random Shack, 2015.

Virchow, Rudolf. 1848. *Die Medizinische Reform. Eine Wochenschrift*. Berlin, 10 July 1848.

# Index

Note: Page numbers followed by "n" denote endnotes.


ableism 34
abortion 33, 121, 127
abstraction, abstract 42, 185, 187, 188
Agamben, Giorgio 3, 47, 55–58, 71n13, 72, 182, 183, 188, 240
agency 4, 13, 74–76, 88, 168, 182, 183
Ahmed, Sara 205, 237, 238
Allan, Michael 141
Almodóvar, Pedro 5, 175–188
alterity 135, 181, 221, 222
ambiguity 34, 55, 69–70, 160, 169, 244
ambivalence 1, 27, 87, 88, 90–92, 95, 135, 175, 176, 180, 188
anatomy, anatomical 5, 30, 40, 179, 180, 184–188, 210, 215, 216n1
animation 182, 184, 185, 187, 188, 191
antipsychiatry, anti-psychiatry 9, 10, 97, 114, 115, 120–122, 125
Appiah, Anthony 139, 241
archive(s) 37, 39, 42, 124, 223
Arendt, Hannah 241
Aristotle 51
art, arts 27, 34, 35, 43, 44, 75, 76, 88, 94, 95, 98, 107, 160, 179–182, 184, 185, 188; and artistic 43, 113, 114; and artist 125, 191; *see also* therapy
artefact(s) 6, 11, 30, 34, 35, 38, 40
artistic research 29, 34, 43, 81, 82, 95
authority 64, 94, 101, 191, 215, 232–234, 239, 243

Bannon, Steve 55
Barthes, Roland 136, 185, 186
Basaglia, Franco 110, 114, 115, 118
de Beauvoir, Simone 163–165, 173
*Begutachtungsanleitung* (BGA) 198, 200–206
Berlant, Lauren 3
bias 1, 11, 19, 21–23, 216
Bick, Esther 225
biography 85, 159
bio-history 62, 67
biology 47, 57, 62, 67, 183
Bion, Wilfred 100, 105, 182, 225–227
biopolitics, biopolitical 3, 4, 12, 31, 33, 47–50, 52, 53, 57, 61, 62, 64, 67, 114, 124–126, 128, 182, 183
biopower 61, 70, 239, 240
birth 17, 19, 20; and birth control 27–32, 37; and birth rites collection 27, 38, 39, 40, 41, 43
body 4, 5, 8, 20, 34, 36, 37, 42, 62–64, 66, 70, 117, 118, 120–122, 125, 126, 138, 145, 152, 154, 157, 167, 175, 178, 180–188, 201, 203, 204, 210–217, 219, 224, 226, 228, 230
Bonz, Jochen 88
Branding 28, 31, 32, 34
Britain 27–30, 42, 109
Brugère, Fabienne 6
Buber, Martin 164
Bühler, Karl 154, 162

Camaraderie 98, 99, 105, 106, 108
Camus, Albert 173, 240
Canguilhem, Georges 8, 68, 241
care 1–10, 12–13, 17, 19–22, 27, 29, 34, 35, 37–39, 43, 61–63, 65–69, 71, 74–76, 115, 152, 153, 155–161, 175–178, 181, 182, 188, 192; and care ethics 5–7, 34–35; and Compulsory care 74, 75
Casa Pound 55
Casado da Rocha, Antonio 156, 162
Catholicism 38, 175
de Certeau, Michel 136
Césaire, Aimé 141

Chamberlin, Judi 75
Charon, Rita 4, 18, 19, 21, 151, 162, 235, 239
China, Chinese 10, 48–54, 57
Clare, Eli 198, 206
class 27, 43, 47, 85, 91, 119–121, 125, 126
clinic 29–31, 33, 36, 37, 39, 105, 113, 114, 118, 126, 127, 134, 140, 142, 178, 180, 181, 214–216, 227; and critique of the clinic 104
Cold War 232
collaborative research 11, 101, 190–192
collage 34, 36, 37
collusion 100–109
colonialism 31, 36, 137, 138, 140, 144, 146
colour blind, colour blindness 12, 17, 21, 22, 142
Colvin, Sarah 244
community,-ies 3, 8–10, 47, 98, 107–109, 114, 115, 118, 127, 134, 154, 159, 163, 164, 166, 167–169, 170–173, 177, 181, 182, 190, 204
consulting room 7, 99, 101
Contagion 1, 37, 56
contemporary art 27, 35, 75, 95, 190
Conti, Nanna (1881–1951) 81, 94, 95
contraception 29–35, 42
Cooper, David 97, 106, 114, 128
counterculture 113, 115, 125
COVID-19, coronavirus 2–5, 10, 20, 21, 37, 38, 47, 48, 55, 56, 67, 90
curation, curating 27, 35
cure 1–8, 10, 12–13, 34, 61, 67, 75, 82, 97, 98, 106, 133, 155, 161, 167, 173, 176, 178, 184, 188, 231
curiosity 186, 211, 221, 235, 236

DasGupta, Sayantani 9, 11, 160
Dechaume, Jean 133
decreation 166, 167
dehiscence 228
Delbanco, Andrew 242
dependency 159, 160, 176
diagnosis 3, 8, 63, 74, 103, 134, 142, 159, 160, 186, 187, 200–204, 210, 212–214
difference 21, 23n1, 82, 108, 119, 122, 126, 153
disease 1, 4, 5, 7–8, 10, 33, 36, 47, 49, 54, 56, 62–66, 68, 140, 152–156, 178, 199, 201, 205, 214, 230, 235
documentary film 1, 95, 113, 118, 124
Dominijanni, Ida 119, 122, 127, 128
Duden, Barbara 5, 8
Dugin, Aleksandr 55
Durkheim, Émile 168
dysmorphia 225
dysphoria 7, 9, 10, 201, 207, 218–227

efficacy 30, 31
Einstein, Albert 231, 243
emotions, emotional 5, 81–83, 95, 104, 192
empathy 1, 11, 19, 178, 230, 233, 235–237
epidemic(s) 49, 56, 57, 65–67
epistemic 3, 114, 132–134, 140, 141, 143; and epistemic injustice 3, 133, 143–146 *see also* injustice; and epistemic violence 74, 75 *see also* violence
Esterson, Aaron 100–105, 110
ethics 3, 66, 68, 135, 139, 156, 163, 167, 168, 170, 172, 173, 180–183, 192; *see also* care ethics
ethnography 127, 128, 132; and autoethnography, autoethnographic method 9
ethnopsychoanalysis 82, 88, 96
eugenics, Eugenics Research Association 27, 31–36, 38, 40, 42, 43
exception, state of, exceptional 51, 55–57
existential analysis 98, 101–102, 109–110
experience(s) 1, 3, 5, 7–9, 12, 13, 27, 39, 42, 43, 74, 75, 82, 83, 88–90, 92, 94, 95, 99–104, 107–108, 114–116, 119, 121, 125, 127, 134–141, 151–153, 155, 156, 158, 160, 163, 165, 167, 169, 171, 175, 176, 179, 183–188, 190–192

famine 49–51
Fanon, Frantz 3, 13, 132–142, 144–146
feminism, feminist 27, 28, 31, 32, 34, 113, 118, 126, 127, 138, 139, 180; and eugenic feminism 38, 42, 43
Fleury, Cynthia 6–8
form 52, 151, 152, 161, 177, 179–187
Foucault, Michel 3–5, 7, 61–73, 114, 134, 142, 146, 153, 154, 216, 241
Freud, Sigmund 98, 136
Fricker, Miranda 133, 143, 144
Fusaro, Diego 54, 55

Galibert-Laîné, Chloé 1–3, 5, 10
Gaze 4, 5, 7, 12, 114, 153, 154, 159, 180, 182, 183, 185, 187, 219
gender 17, 27, 43, 119, 180; and gender medicine 3, 197–206
Genet, Jean 171, 172
Gentile, Giovanni 54, 58
gesture 88, 118, 119, 122, 151, 157, 178, 182, 183, 188

Gilligan, Carol 6
Gilman, Sander L. 4, 7, 10, 11, 13, 47, 237
Ginzburg, Carlo 154, 162
Goffman, Erving 114, 134, 143
Good, Byron 155, 162
Gordon, Lewis 139, 143, 146
Gramsci, Antonio 54, 58n7
Grifi, Alberto 113–128
Guattari, Félix 110, 118, 124, 125, 128

Hardt, Michael and Antonio Negri 241
Hawkins, Anne Hunsaker 8
healing 8, 98, 108, 157, 159, 161, 168, 177, 179, 180, 184, 213, 237, 240
health 4, 8, 10, 12, 19, 20, 27–31, 33, 42, 43, 49, 62–66, 68, 134, 138, 143, 158, 159, 161, 162, 164, 183, 184, 187, 190–192, 210, 211, 213, 240; and political economy of health 64, 65; and public health 27, 47, 65, 66, 232, 244; *see also* mental health
healthcare, health care 4, 5, 9, 10, 12, 13, 19–22, 27–29, 33, 43, 62, 64, 70, 162, 197, 200–203, 233, 234; and reproductive healthcare 28, 29, 42
heritage 74–76
history 7, 8, 10, 35, 38, 40, 43, 62, 63, 65, 75, 81, 82, 86–88, 90, 91, 94, 97, 114, 118, 128n10, 135, 136, 153, 154, 156, 158, 164, 166–170, 172, 173, 181–183, 185, 188, 230, 235
holocaust 134
Hormone Replacement Therapy (HRT) 197, 200, 204, 206
hospital 7, 17, 21, 64, 66, 98, 100, 103–105, 107–108, 114, 115, 125, 142, 175–178, 180–182, 213
humanities 29, 34, 43, 132, 153, 231–234, 239–243
Hume, Victoria 190, 191
hygiene 35, 36, 43, 48–52, 54, 57, 65, 67, 68
*Hyle see* matter
*Hypokeimenon see* substrate

Ibsen, Henrik 240
ideology 31, 32, 34, 36, 38, 114
Igwe, Onyeka 37
Illich, Ivan 157, 158, 162
illness 1, 2, 7–10, 13, 62, 66, 68, 96n2, 103–104, 114, 115, 125, 133, 134, 145, 151–162, 184, 186, 211, 214
imagination 6, 13, 95, 97, 188
imaging technology 5, 210
implicated subject 82
injustice(s) 3, 19, 40, 133, 143–146, 165; *see also* epistemic injustice
installation 85
interdependence 6, 9, 152
interpretation workshop (*Deutungswerkstatt*) 81–85, 88–92, 94, 95
Intersectionality, intersectional 27, 43
Iser, Wolfgang 137, 143

Jervis, Giovanni 115, 125, 127, 128
Johnson, Charles 17, 19, 21, 22
Johnson, Kira 17, 19, 21, 22

Klein, Melanie 99, 176, 178, 223; *see also* paranoid-schizoid, Phantasy
knowledge 12, 30, 32, 37, 40, 43, 61, 63, 64, 67–82, 83, 88, 90, 95, 101, 103–104, 121, 133, 136, 137, 139, 141, 157, 160, 177, 178, 180, 183–185, 215, 216n1
Kraepelin, Emil 132

Lacan, Jacques 119, 128, 222–223
Laing, R. D. 9, 97–112, 114, 126, 127
Lämmert, Eberhard 240
Leriche, René 211, 217
Lévi-Strauss, Claude 50, 51, 54
life 3, 5, 6, 19–21, 35, 38, 61–63, 66–69, 82, 87, 90, 97, 101, 103, 107–109, 116, 119, 125, 135, 137, 139, 141, 152, 161–164, 168, 169, 172, 173, 175, 176, 177, 182–184, 186–188, 198, 199, 202, 210–212, 215, 218, 220, 224–228, 239, 240, 241
Lodrö, Khenpo Tsulrim 52–54
loss 8, 9, 13, 88, 127, 151, 152, 156, 163, 164, 166–170, 173, 179

madness 97, 100–102, 108, 110, 113–115, 118, 122, 124–126, 142, 191
Maran, René 137, 138, 140, 142
Marcel, Gabriel 155, 162
*Married Love* (1918) 29; *see also* Stopes, Marie (Dr.)
Marxism 114
maternal mortality 22, 27; and Black maternal mortality 17, 19–21, 27
maternity 29, 33, 175, 177
matter 29, 34, 35, 37, 38, 39, 43, 51–52
McGill Pain Questionnaire 212, 217
medical 1, 3, 5, 7, 9, 10, 12, 13, 17–22, 30, 34, 61–66, 70, 113, 114, 122, 124, 126, 132, 133, 135, 139, 140, 153–155, 157, 159–160, 175–188, 210–213, 216; and medical apparati 213; and medical

encounter 1, 3–5, 8–9, 11–13, 144–146, 163, 166, 167, 169, 173, 175, 182, 188, 190; and medical education 98, 233, 236, 243; and medical praxis 198–199, 230, 233; and medical school 230; *see also* medical humanities
medical humanities 7, 11, 34, 127n1, 153, 230, 233–235, 242, 243; and critical medical humanities 11, 29, 113, 190–192; and visual medical humanities 11, 34
medicalisation 62, 64, 237
Melzack, Ronald 212, 217
memory,-ies 75, 76, 82, 88, 103, 137, 153, 168, 170, 172, 184; and family memory 85, 88, 89, 90, and inter-generational memory 93
mental 5, 134, 176, 202, 210–211, 224–228; and mental distress 74, 109, 190–192; and mental health 7, 105, 109, 115, 127n6, 240; and mental illness 98, 99, 105–106, 108, 114, 115, 125, 133–135, 142n2
mentalism 74, 76
mice 48–53
midwife 81
migraines 4
misgendering 206
MMBRACE-UK 27
modernity 28, 32, 163, 165, 183
Mol, Annemarie 7–9, 199, 205
MOMMA's bill 22
moral 6, 8, 42, 114, 152, 171, 181, 230, 231, 232, 236, 237, 239, 240–241, 243; and moral dilemma 232; and moral education 11, 232, 233, 240
motherhood 30, 32, 33, 175
MRI (Magnetic Resonance Imaging) 210, 212–213, 215–216
museum(s) 27, 35–39, 42, 43, 75, 190, 191

Nadig, Maya 82, 88, 96
Nancy, Jean-Luc 55–57, 177, 187, 211–212
narrative 1, 3, 8, 12, 13, 18, 21, 22, 32, 52, 75, 76, 94, 117, 137, 151–162, 177, 184, 185, 199, 214, 222, 227, 237, 238, 241; and illness narrative 8; and narrative autonomy 9, 152–162; and narrative medicine 4, 11, 17–22, 153–155, 235
National Socialism 81–83, 85–88, 90, 92, 94
Naylor, David 236
neorealism, post-neorealism 116, 118, 127
Nietzsche, Friedrich 241
Nissen, Camilla (née Conti, 1902–1993) 81, 84–89, 94
Noble, Bobby 198
non-binary 9, 198–206
Nordmarken, Sonny 198
nosopolitics 66
Novalis 4
nurse 118, 120, 125, 175, 177, 178

object relations 97, 99, 105, 176
objectification 13, 141, 144, 146
objectivity 1, 136, 138–140, 144, 146, 153, 216
ocularcentrism 216
organ 5, 133, 140, 175, 177, 180, 187, 188, 210–211, 214–215, 217n2
orientalism 49, 50, 54
Ortega, Fracisco 211, 217
Osler, Sir William 232, 235
other 1, 4, 118, 119, 133, 135, 139, 141, 154, 160, 221–225, 227, 228

pain 3–5, 9, 10, 13, 18, 115, 140, 144, 145, 151, 152, 155–161, 164, 167, 175, 176, 183, 184, 186–188, 204, 210–214, 216–217, 219, 227, 237; and chronic pain 184, 186, 187, 212–214; and pain relief 183, 184
Paranoid-Schizoid 176, 223
Pareigis, Christina 164
patient(s) 1, 4, 5, 7–10, 18, 21, 33, 74–76, 97–102, 104–105, 107, 109–110, 113, 114, 118, 125–127, 135, 140, 142, 140–146, 152–160, 175, 176, 177, 178, 179, 181, 182, 184, 213, 217; and psychosomatic patient 213
perception 7, 12, 19, 100, 108–109, 188; and (self)perception 1, 8, 98, 100, 102
performance 83–85, 93–95, 122, 127, 151, 156, 170, 171
perpetrator studies 95, 96
phantasy 100, 102, 223–224
population 31, 33, 43, 63, 65, 66, 70
power 3–6, 47, 53, 55, 61, 64, 66, 67, 69, 75, 76, 85, 100, 108, 114, 116, 118, 120, 124–127, 133, 140, 144, 159, 161, 168–170, 172, 176, 181, 211, 214, 216
practice 3, 5, 6, 9, 11–13, 17–20, 22, 23, 27, 28, 36, 43, 54, 66, 68, 69, 92, 94, 95, 97–99, 104–106, 108–109, 113, 114,

119, 127, 154, 155, 157, 159, 160; and practice-led research 27
praxiography 198–199, 204–205
Preciado, Paul B. 33, 53, 198, 214, 221
pregnancy, pregnant 19, 21, 22, 27, 34, 117, 178
proprioception 216, 221
prorace cervical cap 27–29, 30, 33–36, 38–44
psychiatric 74, 75, 97, 98, 103, 105–109, 113–115, 119, 122, 123, 125–126, 132, 133, 136, 143; and psychiatric diagnosis 74; and psychiatric survivor 74, 191; and psychiatric violence 74, 113, 114, 119–122, 126
psychiatry 9, 74–76, 97–98, 100, 107, 113–115, 118–120, 124–126, 132–141, 143; and radical psychiatry 113–115, 126–127, 128n12
psychoanalysis, psychoanalytic 96–101, 105, 108, 110, 114, 119, 124, 125, 127, 128, 132, 134, 135, 175, 176, 220
psychosis 98, 101–102, 104, 190
Puig de la Bellacasa, María 6, 29, 34, 35, 43

Rabinow, Paul 239
racism 20, 21, 34, 133, 137, 138, 140, 143, 146
recovery 3, 8, 108, 126, 168
Reed, Carroll 231
*Reichshebammenführerin* 81
remembering 82, 83
reproductive 18, 40, 42, 43, 64, 66, 181; and reproductive choices 31; and reproductive healthcare 28, 42
Reverie 226
Ricoeur, Paul 151, 158, 159, 162
Robcis, Camille 135, 143
Rose, Nikolas 66, 239

Sacks, Oliver 4
Sanz, Marco 211
Sanger, Margaret 31–32
Sartre, Jean-Paul 99, 106, 173
Scarry, Elaine 212–213
Schizophrenia 97, 100–102, 104–107, 109–110, 125
Scholem, Gershom 164
Schwartz, John Alan 53
Science Museum, London 27, 28, 35, 36, 38, 44
self-deception 100, 102, 104
sexual 28, 29, 32, 41–43, 100–101, 136, 143, 178; and sexual difference 9, 113, 118, 119, 122, 126, 127; and sexual reproduction 27, 43, 44
sickness 153, 155–159, 178, 216
silence 151, 154, 156, 157, 160, 161, 165, 187, 211, 217n2
skin 1, 4, 18, 19, 40, 132–139, 141, 142; and *Skin I Live In* 181
Snow, C. P. 231–232
social 1, 3, 4, 7, 9–12, 17–23, 31, 32, 42, 99–106, 108–109, 113–115, 124, 125, 128n16, 132, 134, 135, 137, 138, 144, 153, 158, 161, 213–214; and social intelligibility 100, 104, 106; and social medicine 61, 65–67; and social phenomenology 97–99, 101, 104
Society for Constructive Birth Control and Racial Progress 28–30, 32
somatic experience 216
somatocracy 62
Sontag, Susan 10, 158, 214
Spielberg, Steven 53
Stallworthy, Jon 236–237
STEM: Science, Technology, Engineering and Mathematics 240–241
Stopes, Marie (Dr.) 27–33, 36–38, 42, 43
substrate 48, 49, 51, 52
suffering 3, 6, 8, 126, 133, 134, 137, 138, 140, 143, 151–153, 156–161, 163–170, 172, 173, 176, 184, 187, 191, 213
surgery, plastic surgeon 177–180, 186
symptom 1, 3, 5, 7, 48, 54, 101–102, 104, 106, 107, 134, 140, 144, 145, 146, 153, 154, 156, 159, 190, 211, 216, 237

Taubes, Jacob 164
Taubes, Susan 163–174
Tavistock 97–99, 104
technical image 212, 215
therapeutic community 98, 107–109
therapy 98, 105, 107–109, 115, 132, 202, 204, 213, 228, 237; and art therapy 213; and group therapy 98, 100–101, 105, 108; and individual therapy 100, 102, 106, 110n8; *see also* Hormon Replacement Therapy (HRT)
Third Reich 81, 231
Tibet 52–54, 57n4
Tinnitus 184
Toombs, S. Kay 7, 8
Torgerson, Warren S. 212, 217
Tosquelles, François 144

trans 198–206, 220; and "trans as gap" 9, 198–199, 204–206
transference 82, 235
transphobia 223
transplant 177, 187
Tronto, Joan 6

unconscious 82, 109, 118, 178, 225

Vaihinger, Hans 241–242
Vesalius, Andreas 188, 216n1
video activism 116
violence 1, 3–4, 6, 7, 10–13, 17, 22, 23, 27, 34, 35, 38, 42, 74–76, 106, 119–122, 124–126, 133, 139, 144, 163–178, 180–182, 185–188, 219; and ontological violence 133; *see also* epistemic violence; psychiatric violence
Virchow, Rudolf 67, 238
virus 67, 69
Visual Analogue Scale (VAS) 212
voice-hearing 190–192
vulnerability 4, 6, 156, 162, 175, 177, 180, 188
Vulva 30, 34, 40

Weil, Simone 6, 163–168, 173
Wellcome Collection, London 27, 35, 39, 44
*Wise Parenthood* (1918) 31; *see also* Stopes, Marie (Dr.)
Woolf, Virginia 211
working-class 29, 30, 42, 85

Xun, Zhou 10, 47

Zaia, Luca 48–52, 54, 57

FSC
www.fsc.org
MIX
Papier | Fördert
gute Waldnutzung
FSC® C083411

Kolibri 360 GmbH
Ferdinand-Jühlke-Straße 7
99095 Erfurt, Deutschland
produktsicherheit@kolibri360.de